Food, Nutrition, and the Young Child

• THIRD EDITION

Food, Nutrition, and the Young Child

Jeannette Brakhane Endres
Southern Illinois University, Carbondale

Robert E. Rockwell
Southern Illinois University, Edwardsville

Merrill Publishing Company
Columbus   Toronto   London   Melbourne

Cover Photo: Andy Brunk

Published by Merrill Publishing Company
Columbus, Ohio 43216

This book was set in Melior.

Administrative Editor: David Faherty
Production Editor: Carol Sykes
Art Coordinator: Mark Garrett
Cover Designer: Brian Deep
Photo Editor: Gail Meese

Photo Credits: All photos copyrighted by individuals or companies listed. Robert E. Rockwell, pp. xvi, 26, 43, 48, 54, 65, 75, 86, 92, 100, 131, 136, 138, 170, 171, 178, 183, 191, 242, 260, 270, 281, 294; Cambridge Scientific Industries, p. 63; Robert M. Wagner, pp. 68, 268; U.S. Department of Agriculture, pp. 94, 152, 194, 296, 301; Kevin French, pp. 98, 101, 110, 111, 115, 118, 120, 154, 155, 199, 269; and Merrill, p. 262.

Library of Congress Catalog Card Number: 89-63842
International Standard Book Number: 0-675-21199-9
Printed in the United States of America
1 2 3 4 5 6 7 8 9—94 93 92 91 90

To
Alicia Christina, Teri Lynn, Robert Joel, Amanda Sue,
Kathryn Lee, and Michael Wayne

Preface

Although residents of the United States have perhaps the safest, most adequate, and most nutritious food supply in the world, malnutrition is one of our nation's major health problems. The field of early childhood education focuses on the need to provide total programs that meet the health, intellectual, and social needs of all children.

If young children are to develop to their optimal potential, it is crucial that they be provided with nutritionally sound diets and that they develop the awareness to continue good nutritional habits throughout life.

The purpose of *Food, Nutrition, and the Young Child* is to impart basic concepts about food and nutrition, especially as they apply to the young child. We believe that an effective way of teaching nutrition awareness is to begin with sound nutritional habits and to reinforce these habits as the child grows. For this reason we present techniques that illustrate how the principles of food and nutrition can be integrated into the menu-planning process and the educational curriculum.

This book is intended for students who wish to learn about food and nutrition as they relate to young children and the early childhood curriculum. Students do not need to be in a formal classroom setting for such study; they may be care givers in preschool and day-care settings, nurses, dietitians, or other persons concerned with food, nutrition, and children.

The third edition of *Food, Nutrition, and the Young Child* contains a great deal of new information from the field of nutrition. Our combined coverage of both food and nutrition and early childhood curriculum remains unique.

Chapter 1 presents basic nutrition as it applies to both the child and adult. We address specific factors that influence food choices and identify foods that supply major nutrients to the diet. Following a review of basic nutrition, students are encouraged to make a personal commitment to practice good nutritional habits and are given the opportunity to evaluate their own dietary and exercise patterns. Without physical activity for the child or adult, attention to dietary intake is less meaningful.

A clear and concise presentation of the food and nutritional needs of the infant (birth to 12 months) is given in Chapter 2. A normal feeding and development chart relates nutrition and eating to physical, intellectual, gross motor, fine motor, reflex, oral motor, speech and language, and social-behavioral development. Step-by-step guidelines assist the student in obtaining accurate height and weight measurements and correct interpretations of physical measurements. The chapter also presents information regarding physical fitness activities for infants.

Based on our review of numerous publications on breast-feeding and bottle-feeding and interviews with mothers from various socioeconomic backgrounds, we provide a discussion of the advantages of breast-feeding. When the first edition was written, breast milk was more costly than commercially prepared formulas because of the additional nutritional requirements of the lactating mother; however, there is no longer a significant difference in the cost per day of breast-feeding compared with bottle-feeding.

As children begin their second year of life, they take on unique personalities and characteristics that affect their food needs. Special attention to growth patterns and specific nutrients such as protein, calcium, iron, and fluoride are presented in Chapters 3, 4, and 5. We offer specific guidelines for recommending food intake for each year to assist professionals in the field and students who rely on such guidelines as they evaluate the food intake of the young child.

Because obesity remains a major health care problem, we outline specific steps for its prevention and provide resources for its treatment. Chapter 5, a new chapter, covers the nutritional needs of the school-age child, 6 to 8 years. We present specific recommendations for physical activities that can facilitate energy balance and promote overall fitness. In addition, we discuss influences on the eating patterns of this age group, offer guidelines for choosing nutritious snacks, and address the issue of lowering fat in the child's diet.

Chapter 6 reviews the USDA Child Care Food Program daily food plans for each age group and provides menus that can be used as a reference by students, food service personnel, and care givers. Without the presentation of a well-prepared and well-served meal, little coordination can be achieved between the nutrition and the educational curriculum.

Chapter 7 explores a variety of programmatic approaches used in early childhood programs. One approach is used as a model to successfully teach nutrition concepts to young children. We believe that nutrition can be learned through any programmatic approach with a curriculum that provides enriching experiences and materials and encourages interaction and exploration for the developing child.

Chapter 8 demonstrates how nutrition concepts can be integrated into various curricular areas, enhancing the total early childhood curriculum. Also included in this chapter are new recipes for classroom cooking.

Chapter 9 reflects the importance of working in partnership with parents. Research supports the influence parents have in the lives of young children. We believe that children and their well-being are major concerns for both parents and early childhood educators. This chapter thus presents techniques for successful parent involvement in nutrition education. An expansion of this chapter includes an agenda for a sample nutrition workshop and forms that can be used for communicating nutrition concerns between home and the early childhood program.

Specific Changes in the Third Edition

- Guidelines for exercise and fitness for children from birth through age 8
- An example of a parent meeting that focuses on nutrition awareness
- Forms that can be exchanged between the home and school to communicate nutrition information and concerns
- Food plans that meet the Dietary Guidelines for Americans
- Suggestions for lowering fat in the child's diet
- Guidelines for calculating a lower-fat diet
- Extension of guidelines to include school-age children

ACKNOWLEDGMENTS

A number of people participated in the preparation of the third edition of *Food, Nutrition, and the Young Child*. We acknowledge with sincere gratitude the work of our professional peers who reviewed the manuscript. They represent a diversity of backgrounds, some with orientations quite different from ours. They were thorough, conscientious, and honest, and we appreciate their knowledge and professionalism. We took their suggestions seriously, making the final judgment of what, how, and how much should be written. We are most grateful for their help: Christine Catalini, San Antonio College; Linda C. Claussen, New River Community College; Olivia W. Kendrick, University of Alabama; and Maurine Summers, Aims Community College.

Contents

LEARNING OBJECTIVES

Students will be able to
- **Define nutrition**
- **List factors that influence food and nutrient intake**
- **List the basic nutrients and uses in the body**
- **Identify foods that supply major nutrients**
- **Compare dietary intakes with guides or standards**
- **Evaluate personal dietary and exercise patterns**

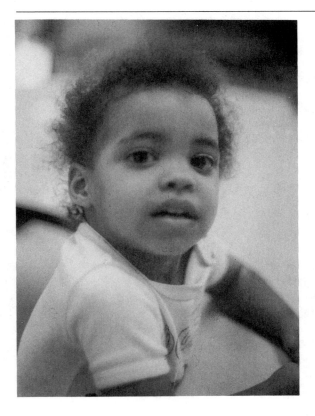

The Nutrients and Food Needs

Before studying the use of foods for children in early childhood settings, a basic knowledge of foods and their nutrient content is necessary. The mass media inform us daily of the latest nutrition controversy, and information on topics such as cholesterol, fat, sugar, fiber, and dietary supplements is often confusing. Parents are concerned not only about their children's dietary intake but their own as well. They turn to the care giver for advice and accurate information. For this reason, factual information about food and nutrition is essential.

This chapter is for you! Using knowledge of basic nutrition principles in your daily food selection will help you have the energy and right combination of nutrients necessary to meet the demands of your profession. In addition, you will be providing a good role model for parents and children.

WHAT IS NUTRITION?

Nutrition is the science of food and how it is used by the body. Nutrition can also be defined as all the processes by which a person—child or adult—takes in food and digests, absorbs, transports, uses, and excretes food substances. Nutrients are substances found in food that must be supplied to the body. When you eat food, your body takes in the nourishment necessary to live, grow, maintain good health, and have energy for work and play. Of course, most people do not eat only for nourishment. Therefore, the study of nutrition must also be concerned with the social, economic, cultural, and psychological implications of food and eating.

Social Factors

Food plays a large part in our social lives. Whether we go to the ballpark, the zoo, the movies, or a party, or stay at home reading a book or watching television, food serves a social role. Rare is the social gathering at which food is not served or sold.

Economic Factors

The cost of living has had an impact on food purchasing. Economic constraints limit the amount and type of food some individuals or families can afford. The wider the variety of foods eaten, the more likely the diet is to contain all the nutrients essential for good health.

Some families with limited economic resources may not be able to purchase a wide variety of foods, and, therefore, it may be more difficult for them to acquire a wide variety of nutrients. Low-income families without adequate transportation may have access only to small grocery stores with limited food selections. Sometimes parents can afford to purchase a wide variety of foods, but time constraints make buying foods from restaurants the economical choice. Families may repeatedly choose to eat only a few selected items from fast-food restaurants, and nutrient intake may be limited if foods are not selected carefully. Thus, variety can be limited either because of the economic inability to purchase nutritious foods or because of the unwise purchase of only a few food items from restaurants.

Cultural Factors

The cultural and ethnic customs of our society influence the food we eat, and ethnic groups in the United States follow various dietary patterns and food preferences. A person's cultural heritage often determines whether a particular food will be eaten, regardless of its nutrient value. However, this country's wide variety of cultures and food habits can make eating interesting and enjoyable as well as a learning experience for children. Following is a brief description of some common types of cultural cooking found in the United States.

Chinese cooking can be identified as Mandarin (north), Shanghai (central), or Cantonese (south). In general, the Chinese use many vegetables and fruits and large quantities of rice. They use few meats and very little milk. Methods of cooking include steaming, boiling, or stir-frying in a small amount of hot fat.

Liberal use of pastas, tomato sauces, and bread characterizes Italian cooking. Many vegetables and fruits, as well as meats and cheese, are used. Milk is seldom consumed except in coffee because it is considered an expensive beverage and is seldom thought of as food.

In the Southern part of the United States a popular dish called chitterlings, intestines dredged with cornmeal or flour and fried crisp, is served. Fish and shellfish are also popular. Many varieties of dried beans are used daily. Cooks season with bacon and salt pork, and hominy grits, hot biscuits, corn bread, and rice are common accompaniments in this region.

Jewish customs, including dietary laws, are observed in varying degrees by Orthodox, Conservative, or Reform denominations. Some families place great value on traditional rituals of the Jewish religion and observe the dietary laws under all conditions. Dietary laws prohibit the use of meat and milk at the same meal, and separate dishes and utensils must be used for preparing and serving meat and dairy products. Orthodox Jews use only the forequarter of animals such as cattle and sheep. Animals and poultry are slaughtered by a ritual butcher (schochet) according to specified regulations. The meat is then koshered. Jewish persons who follow the religious customs do not eat pork products. Likewise, members of the Moslem religion do not eat products prepared from pork.

Vegetarians, for a variety of religious and personal reasons, may restrict meat, milk, and eggs from their diets. Vegetarian diets are discussed in Chapter 4.

Emotional Factors

Emotional factors such as stress or excitement can trigger overeating or a decrease in food consumption. Food can be used as an emotional weapon or crutch. One individual can use rejection or acceptance of specific foods or meals as a method to control the behavior of another.

Students going home from college for vacation who are determined to stay on their diets often find themselves overeating foods prepared by mother. Some nutritional deficiencies cause apathy and depression and are accompanied by a loss of appetite; however, these deficiencies are rare, and variations usually seen in the amount of food consumed from day to day are normal.

Almost every parent believes at some time that his or her child exhibits eating problems. This occurs when the child does not eat vegetables or meat, eats too many sweets, or does not seem to eat enough food. In many cases, eating behavior is a way for children to assert their individuality. A child may have a temper tantrum if the family runs out of a favorite cereal. Another child learns that refusing to eat will usually upset the family and may even result in a reward, a "bribe," for improved behavior. Most of these situations are short-lived and have few consequences. Psychologists often disagree about the cause and cure of eating whims expressed by children, but whatever the cause, psychological aspects of food consumption that originate in early childhood often continue throughout life.

EATING DISORDERS

The eating problems discussed earlier are generally minor and disappear without growth and developmental consequences. Eating disorders that cause obesity or starvation in the United States have a strong emotional component and may have severe consequences that affect the nutritional status of the population [1]. Obesity, a problem believed to be influenced by genetics as well as early childhood feeding patterns, is discussed in detail in later chapters. Emphasis must be on the prevention of obesity, since only 10% to 15% of obese persons are successfully treated in later life.

Self-starvation is practiced by some persons who have a strong fear of becoming overweight. This condition is known as *anorexia nervosa.* Its cause is not known, and in fact it may have multiple causes. It is unclear whether factors related to childhood eating behavior have any effect on later eating disorders. The mass media's campaigns for thinness, specific foods, exercise programs, dietary supplements, and "pill popping" certainly influence some sufferers of anorexia. Some persons, especially women and teenaged girls, take drastic action to control their weight.

Persons diagnosed with anorexia nervosa severely limit food intake to the point where they lose excessive amounts of body weight. They complain of being "too fat" when in fact their body weight is below recommended levels. They believe they "need more exercise" even though they exercise excessively. A constant preoccupation with food may also cause some persons to go on eating binges, gorging on well-liked foods, only to force themselves to vomit or take diuretics and laxatives to bring the weight back down; this condition is called *bulimia.* Extreme thinness provides anorectic and bulimic persons with a sense of control over their lives. Immediate medical, dietetic, and psychiatric measures are needed when anorexia nervosa or bulimia is suspected.

NUTRIENTS IN FOODS

Nutrients are found in foods. Foods may contain a few or many nutrients, and each nutrient has specific uses in the body (see Figure 1-1). Because all foods do not contain the same nutrients or equal amounts of any one nutrient, it is important to understand which foods and quantities of food can provide the combination of nutrients that promotes optimal health.

The body requires six nutrient classes to ensure adequate nutritional status and to maintain good health:

Fat
Carbohydrate
Protein
Vitamins
Minerals
Water

The body must be able to maintain itself through the energy that comes from nutrients. Although some nutrients chiefly provide calories, or energy, others enable the body to grow new cells and tissues. These nutrients are especially important for children and for the repair of injured or old tissue for people of any age. Fat, carbohydrate, and protein provide energy/calories, whereas vitamins, minerals, and water help regulate metabolic processes, including energy

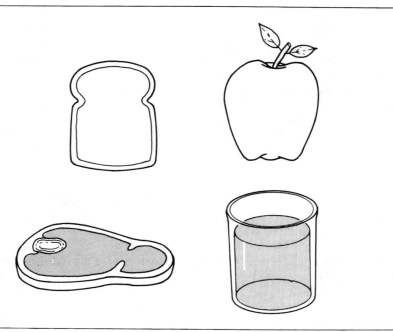

Figure 1–1
Nutrients found in food groups

metabolism, but do not provide energy. Other nutrients function either as part of tissue and biochemical compounds or as regulators of body functions.

Some nutrients are needed in large quantities and others in smaller quantities, but each functions in a specialized manner. The task of providing nutrients to the body in the amounts necessary to ensure adequate nutritional status may seem overwhelming. However, there are shortcuts to selecting the proper nutrients. Using food guides (and standards discussed later in this chapter) will help you select a variety of foods to obtain the nutrients needed for health and life. Because each nutrient is found in a wide variety of foods, the wider the variety of foods eaten, the more likely that the diet will contain all essential nutrients.

Nutrients that provide energy, or heat, are fat, carbohydrate, and protein. *Kilocalories*, or "calories," are a way of measuring the amount of potential energy in a foodstuff. A *calorie* is the basic unit for measuring the energy that will raise the temperature of 1 g of water 1°C. One calorie is a small amount of energy compared with what the human body needs each day; therefore, the term *kilocalorie* (Kcal) is used. A kilocalorie represents a unit that stands for 1000 times as much energy as a calorie represents. When, in everyday conversation, we talk about "calories," we actually mean kilocalories.* With the current trend

---

* The proper shortened form of kilocalorie is *Calorie*, spelled with a capital *C*.

toward adopting the metric system, food energy is also being measured in units called *kilojoules*. One calorie equals 4.18 kilojoules. The values of energy, or the calories, supplied by foods and beverages are approximately 9 kcal/g from fat; 4 kcal/g from carbohydrate; 4 kcal/g from protein; and 7 kcal/g from alcohol.

Appendix I lists the nutrient composition of various foods, as well as their caloric content. Included is the fat, carbohydrate, and protein content along with several vitamins, minerals, and water. A brief look at nutrients in foods follows; however, for a more complete discussion, see additional nutrition textbooks [2,3].

FATS

Most persons associate fat with steaks and chops, cream, butter, or lard. *Lipid* is the name given to a general collection of fats, oils, waxes, and related substances, including cholesterol. Lipids are generally called oils when they are liquid and fats when they are solid.

Fats consist mainly of fatty acids, which can be classified as *saturated* or *unsaturated*. Unsaturated fatty acids are found in the oils of vegetable and cereal products, such as soybeans, rapeseed (canola), corn, cottonseed, and safflower. Rich sources of saturated fatty acids are meats and animal fats, cream, butter, and whole milk. A fat containing a high proportion of unsaturated fatty acids is generally liquid at room temperature, whereas a fat that has a high percentage of saturated fat, such as butter, is solid at room temperature. Vegetable oils are made solid, or saturated, through *hydrogenation,* a process used by manufacturers to add hydrogen to oils. Generally, the more hydrogen added, the harder the fat or margarine. The name given to this product is hydrogenated vegetable fat.

Table 1–1 includes a list of foods that contain varying amounts of saturated fatty acids and unsaturated fatty acids, which are further classified as *monounsaturated* and *polyunsaturated,* depending on their chemical makeup. The Dietary Guidelines for Americans [4] advise people in the United States to consume fats with larger quantities of unsaturated fatty acids and fewer saturated fats and cholesterol.

Function

The body needs many fatty acids, most of which it can synthesize or manufacture. However, at least one essential fatty acid, linoleic acid, must be obtained from foods containing polyunsaturated fatty acids. Without linoleic acid animals experience delayed growth, scaly skin, and hair loss, along with other health problems.

Fat also serves as an energy reserve. When the food you eat contains more potential energy (calories) than you actually use, the food is converted to fat, which is stored, sometimes in excessive amounts, in muscle tissue and around

Table 1-1
Saturated and unsaturated fatty acids and cholesterol from plant and animal sources

Product	Cholesterol (mg)	Saturated Fatty Acids (g)	Unsaturated Fatty Acids* (g)
Cheese and Cheese Products			
1 oz cheddar cheese	30	6.0	0.3
1 C lowfat cottage cheese, 1% fat	10	1.5	trace
2 tbsp (1 oz) cream cheese	31	6.2	0.4
1 oz American cheese	27	5.6	0.3
Eggs			
1 large boiled, hard or soft	274	1.7	0.7
Meat			
3 slices crisp broiled or fried bacon	15	3.3	1.5
3½ oz canned ham	41	1.6	0.4
1 link bratwurst (pork), cooked	51	7.9	2.3
1 beef frank	22	5.4	0.5
Poultry			
3½ oz w/skin, roasted	88	3.8	3.0
½ breast, w/skin, fried	88	2.4	1.9
1 drumstick w/skin, fried	44	1.8	1.6
Dairy Products			
1 C skim milk	4	0.3	trace
1 C whole milk, 3.5% fat	34	4.9	0.2
1 C plain yogurt	14	2.3	0.1
Fruits and Vegetables			
1 medium orange	0	trace	0.1
1 C raw strawberries	0	trace	0.3
⅜ C frozen peas and carrots	0	0.1	0.1
Fats			
1 tbsp butter	36	8.7	0.5
1 tbsp vegetable shortening	0	3.2	3.5

Source: Data from FOOD VALUES OF PORTIONS COMMONLY USED, 14th Edition by Helen Nichols Church and Jean A. T. Pennington. Copyright © 1980, 1985 by Helen Nichols Church B.S. and Jean A. T. Pennington Ph.D. R.N. Reprinted by permission of Harper & Row, Publishers, Inc.

* The amount of unsaturated fatty acids excludes monounsaturated fats.

vital organs. During periods of illness or when energy expenditure exceeds energy intake, the fat reserves are used.

Fats function to provide energy, or heat, for the body. Of all the nutrient classes, fats provide the most concentrated form of energy, supplying 9 kcal/g (29 g = 1 ounce). Fat also supplies a good padding or protection for the liver, heart, and kidneys, the body's vital organs. In addition, fats comprise an essential part of many body tissues such as the brain, bone marrow, and cell membranes. Certain vitamins (A, D, E, and K) are only soluble in fatty substances. Before they can be absorbed from the intestinal tract, these vitamins must be incorporated into a tiny droplet containing fat.

In summary, fat provides (1) an energy reserve, (2) insulation and padding for body organs, (3) a vehicle for the absorption of certain vitamins, (4) essential fatty acids, and (5) a component of certain body tissues.

Sources

Fats are frequently found in our favorite foods for good reason: they enhance flavor and allow us to feel satiated. Fats can be found in both animal and plant foodstuffs, for example, butter and margarine; whole milk; eggs; oils such as corn, soybean, peanut, and cottonseed; and even in the leanest muscle tissue. All fried foods, including popular snack chips, contain fat. Most of the fat eaten in the American diet come from fats and oils, meats, poultry and fish, and dairy products. Other foods that provide energy from fat include mayonnaise, whipped cream, chocolate, nuts, avocados, and coconut.

As previously mentioned, according to the Dietary Guidelines for Americans [4], polyunsaturated fats should be eaten more often than saturated fats. Poultry, fish, and vegetable oils are sources of polyunsaturated fatty acids. The American Heart Association recommends a diet that draws 30% of its calories from fat—less than 10% from saturated fats. In addition, cholesterol should be limited to no more than 100 mg per 1000 kcal, or 300 mg total [5]. The method for determining a diet with 30% of the total calories as fat is explained in Chapter 5.

Cholesterol

Cholesterol belongs to the category of lipids called *sterols*. It does not contribute energy. In some persons cholesterol accumulates in blood vessels and causes a narrowing of the blood vessels leading to the heart, which may result in cardiovascular or heart disease.

Recent evidence suggests that the way cholesterol is carried through the blood, by a substance called *lipoprotein*, may influence the level of risk of heart disease. *Low-density lipoprotein* (LDL) is believed to be a risk factor in the development of heart disease. *High-density lipoprotein* (HDL) is associated with protecting against cardiovascular disease and acts to help "clean up" cholesterol and return it to the liver for excretion. The more HDL one has, the lower the total body cholesterol and, theoretically, the lower the risk of heart disease. HDL level can be maintained or increased by eliminating smoking, maintaining correct weight for height, exercising, and consuming a diet that does not contain too much cholesterol or fat.

Cholesterol is found only in foods of animal origin, especially meats, eggs (yolk), whole milk, some cheeses, and animal fats. Remember that the human body produces cholesterol and thus provides its own supply even if animal products are not eaten in the diet. However, a diet that contains a low level of fat and cholesterol along with unsaturated fatty acids tends to lower the blood's cholesterol level (Table 1–1).

To help lower dietary cholesterol, foods such as chicken with the skin removed should be eaten more often than high-fat meats. Also, low-fat yogurt and reduced-calorie margarine can be substituted for sour cream and butter. Table 1–2 lists foods to substitute when trying to lower dietary cholesterol and fat levels.

Many factors contribute to a high-cholesterol level in the serum: the total amount of cholesterol taken in the diet, the frequency of eating high-cholesterol foods, the type of dietary fat eaten with the cholesterol, age, past dietary intake, and even heredity. Whether everyone, young or old, should lower dietary cholesterol level is still debatable.

Fat Substitutes

Although not approved for marketing in the United States at this time, two fat substitutes have been proposed, Simplesse and Olestra. *Simplesse* is made from egg white or whey protein (milk) by a special method, called microparticulation,

Table 1–2
Food substitutions to lower dietary fat and cholesterol

Eat Less:	Eat More:
Vegetables cooked in butter	Stir-fry vegetables in oil
Bologna	Sliced turkey or chicken, tuna fish, or lean roast beef
Barbecued ribs	Chicken barbecued without the skin
Heavily marbled beef, such as sirloin or New York cuts	Lean beef cuts with all fat removed, such as flank steak, rump steak, or London broil
Lard, meat fat, or shortening made from animal fat	All-vegetable shortenings
Sour cream	Plain low-fat yogurt
Ice cream	Ice milk or frozen yogurt
Butter	Reduced-calorie margarine
American or cheddar cheese	Low-fat cheese, skim ricotta, or skim mozzarella
Whole or 2% milk	Skim or 1% milk
Regular (bottled) salad dressing	Oil plus water, vinegar, and seasoning; reduced-calorie salad dressing
Palm oil, coconut oil	Soybean, corn, sunflower, and safflower oils

in which the proteins are cooked and blended to produce tiny particles. The tongue perceives this protein product as rich and creamy like fat but without the 9 kcal/g that fat provides. The body digests this protein like any other protein substance. *Olestra* is a manufactured sucrose polyester product that tastes like fat. The body doesn't digest, absorb, or recognize it as a foodstuff. Testing continues on both products.

CARBOHYDRATES

Carbohydrates come in different sizes. Simple sugars are called *monosaccharides* because they contain one single unit. *Disaccharides* contain two saccharides or simple sugars. The more complex forms of carbohydrate, or starches, contain more units of sugar and are called *polysaccharides*. Breads and cereals, fruits and vegetables, dairy products, and legumes contain complex carbohydrates. An example of a simple sugar is blood glucose, found in circulating blood. All carbohydrates are converted to glucose in the digestive processes before being absorbed and used as a readily available supply of energy.

Function

Also a source of energy, or heat, carbohydrates provide less energy than fat, yielding only 4 kcal/g. One ounce of fat (2 tbsp oil, margarine, or butter) provides approximately 220 kilocalories, whereas 2 tablespoons of flour or sugar (carbohydrate) provides approximately 100 kilocalories.

Carbohydrates function primarily as a source of readily available energy, since only a relatively small amount can be stored in the liver and muscle tissues. In addition, some carbohydrates act as body regulators or contribute to the structure of certain cells.

Sources

Dextrose and fructose are simple sugars found in many foods. Found naturally in fruits and honey, fructose is obtained commercially from corn. It is the sweetest of all sugars and has been marketed as a table sugar replacement. Crystalline fructose, now available to the consumer, does not appear to raise blood sugar levels in normal individuals, although it does provide energy in amounts similar to table sugar. High-fructose corn syrup, used commercially in soft drinks and baked products as well as in syrup, is not pure fructose but is combined with other saccharides.

The carbohydrate most frequently seen on the table is sugar, or sucrose, a disaccharide, also found naturally in many fruits. However, the carbohydrate found most frequently in foods, especially grains and potatoes and other fruits and vegetables, is starch, a more complex form that takes longer to be broken down by the digestive system when compared with sucrose and the other sugars. Carbohydrates from grains and cereal products are the world's primary source of food, vital to the survival of many persons. The Dietary Guidelines for Americans [4] specifically encourage avoiding sugar and increasing intake of complex carbohydrates and fiber.

Fiber is considered a carbohydrate but it is actually a group of substances, found in plants, that cannot be broken down by human digestive enzymes (for example, cellulose). *Dietary fiber* is the residue of plant food that remains after digestion in the body. *Crude fiber* is the residue of plant food remaining after extraction with dilute alkali in the laboratory—the fiber that remains after chemical digestive procedures. Crude fiber values are used in many food composition tables because the procedure for collecting dietary fiber is complicated, involving collection and analysis of human stool samples over a 24-hour period. Dietary fiber values may be two to three times higher than the crude fiber values. Only recently have analyzed values for specific dietary fiber substances been available.

Insoluble fiber, such as bran, helps move material through the intestinal tract through a process called peristalsis. *Soluble fiber,* such as fruits, vegetables, and oats, provides bulk to the stools and may affect the development of certain diseases. Table 1–3 lists the dietary fiber content of some common foods.

The use of fiber in the diet is advocated to decrease the incidence of atherosclerosis, coronary and aortic disease, appendicitis, disease of the colon, and diabetes [6]. In the United States high-fiber diets have been used successfully to treat persons with colon disease. However, there is no evidence that our consumption of less dietary fiber than people of other countries has led to the development of colon disorders. The claims for a high-fiber diet look promising but are still under investigation. A high-fiber diet causes larger stools and more freqent bowel movements. It is also consistent with current ideas about energy conservation; that is, we should eat more cereal grains directly rather than indirectly from animal products. Foods high in fiber include bran, whole-grain breads and cereals, most fruits and vegetables, nuts, and legumes.

Sugar and Disease

Obesity is the primary nutrition-related health problem today. There is no substantial evidence that table sugar (sucrose) intake causes obesity. Sugar, whether eaten in a sucker or on presweetened cereal, does not cancel the nutritive value of any food or of the total diet. However, consuming sucrose can contribute to tooth decay, so it is important to restrict intake of those sticky carbohydrate foods that feed the bacteria that cause tooth decay.

Nutritionists are often asked whether sugar should be excluded from the diet. The nutrient density of the food in relationship to the total diet must be considered. If a food supplies a high proportion of nutrients in relation to the amount of energy, it is a *nutrient-dense* food; conversely, if it contains a high proportion of energy, or calories, in relation to the amount of nutrients, it is a *calorie-dense* food. For

Table 1-3
Dietary fiber in selected foods

Product	Serving Size	Dietary Fiber (g)
Fruits		
Apple, raw, w/skin	1 fruit	2.8
Blackberries, raw	½ C	4.5
Prunes, canned	⅓ C	5.8
Prunes, dried	3 fruits	3.7
Banana, raw	½ med	1.0
Boysenberries, canned	½ C	5.6
Figs, dried	1 med	3.7
Pear, canned	½ C	3.7
Red raspberries, canned	½ C	9.1
Strawberries, raw	¾ C	2.0
Vegetables		
Artichoke, fresh, cooked	½ globe	7.6
Asparagus, frozen spears	¾ C	4.8
Brussels sprouts, cooked	½ C	3.9
Corn, cooked	½ C	3.9
Corn, creamed, canned	½ C	5.1
Okra, frozen	½ C	3.0
Peas, green, young, canned	½ C	7.9
Pumpkin, canned	¾ C	3.3
Squash, winter, raw (acorn)	¼ squash	4.3
Turnip, green, frozen	½ C	3.7
Legumes		
Beans, butter, cooked	½ C	4.4
Beans, kidney, canned	½ C	7.9
Beans, pinto, cooked	½ C	5.3
Peas, blackeye, cooked	½ C	12.4
Beans, white, cooked	½ C	5.0
Breads/Cereals		
Bread, pumpernickel	1 slice	4.3
Bread, whole wheat	1 slice	1.4
All Bran	⅓ C	8.6
100% Bran	⅓ C	9.1
Wheat germ, plain	¼ C	5.5

Source: Data from Anderson, W.: Plant fiber in foods, Lexington, KY, 1986, The HCF Diabetes Research Foundation, Inc.

example, an orange juice ice pop is more nutrient dense than a sugar-laden soft drink.

A person who requires large amounts of energy because of exercise can consume more foods that are energy rich and calorie dense than a person who is sedentary. The quantity of nutrients needed by an individual remains relatively constant for the same age-sex group. Diets for the elderly and young children, which are relatively low in kilocalories, need to contain nutrient-dense foods unless extra energy is expended through exercise.

PROTEINS

Proteins play an important role in the growth, restoration, and maintenance of body tissues. They contribute 15% of the total body weight. Proteins are made up of about 20 different chemical structures known as *amino acids.* Those manufactured in the body are identified as *nonessential* amino acids, whereas those supplied by proteins in animal or plant foods in the diet are known as *essential* amino acids.

All of the essential amino acids are found in a complete protein. Proteins that contain all the essential amino acids, such as those from animal sources, are known as *complete proteins,* or high-quality proteins. Proteins found in foods from plants lack one or more of the essential amino acids and are therefore called *incomplete proteins.*

Because the body can manufacture many of the amino acids, only seven or eight must come from the daily dietary intake. In the United States the consumption of protein does not appear to be below recommended levels. In fact, persons consume more protein than is needed to meet their daily requirements [7].

Function

Unlike fat and carbohydrate, the primary function of protein is not to supply energy or heat. The principal functions of protein are for growth, maintenance and repair of body tissues, regulation of water balance, help in maintenance of the proper acid base balance within the body, and formation of enzymes, antibodies, and hormones. When sufficient carbohydrates and fats are lacking or when more protein is taken in than the body can use, protein is converted to energy, or heat, supplying 4 kcal/g. When an excessive amount of protein is consumed, it is converted to fat and stored in the fat cells of the body.

Sources

Good sources of complete protein include meats, eggs, and milk. Often foods that provide high-quality protein are also high in fat. However, choosing lean cuts of beef, poultry, and pork, as well as fish, skim milk, and legumes, can provide high-quality protein with only small amounts of fat.

Complementary proteins can be formulated from plant sources to form complete proteins. Two or more foods that contain incomplete proteins and, alone, do not have all the essential amino acids, are combined to form a complete protein containing all the essential amino acids.

A mixture of proteins from unrefined grains, legumes, seeds, nuts, and vegetables eaten over the course of the day will complement one another in their amino acid profiles. It is not necessary that complementation of amino acid profiles be precise and at exactly the same meal. The following food combinations supply complementary proteins:

Baked beans and brown bread
Lentil soup with rice
Hopping John (beans and rice)
Split pea soup with bread
Vegetable pizza with whole wheat crust
Granola with cereal, nuts, and seeds
Tamale pie with beans
Chili with beans and crackers

In the following foods, low-quality protein is supplemented with high-quality protein from milk, meat, and eggs:

Iron-fortified cereal, hot or cold, with milk
Iron-fortified cereal cooked with milk
Cheese sandwich
Toast and eggs
Cheese vegetable casserole
Cheese soufflés
Chili with beans and added meat

Guidelines for Vegetarians. According to the American Dietetic Association [8], vegetarian diets are healthful and nutritionally adequate when appropriately planned. It is important to choose a wide variety of foods from the major food groups and to include a good food source of ascorbic acid (vitamin C) with meals to enhance iron absorption. Children whose nutrient needs are especially high because of growth can meet their requirements following vegetarian diets containing dairy products (see Chapter 4).

Recommendations for selecting vegetarian diets include [9]:

- Keep the intake of calorie-dense foods, such as sweets and fatty foods, to a minimum.
- Choose whole or unrefined grain products instead of refined products whenever possible.
- Use a variety of fruits and vegetables, including a good food source of vitamin C to enhance iron absorption.
- If milk products are consumed, use low-fat varieties.

- Limit intake of eggs to two to three yolks per week to avoid excessive cholesterol intake.
- For vegans, use a properly fortified food source of vitamin B_{12} such as fortified soy milks or breakfast cereals, or take a supplement.
- For infants and children, ensure adequate intakes of iron, vitamin D, and energy.
- Consult a registered dietitian or other qualified nutrition professional.

Well-planned vegetarian diets effectively meet the Dietary Guidelines for Americans.

VITAMINS

Vitamins, like minerals, are not energy producing. Unlike minerals, they are organic and contain carbon compounds; but because they usually are not broken down to carbon dioxide and water (the end products of metabolism), they provide no useful energy. The body cannot manufacture vitamins, yet vitamins are essential for life. They are needed only in small amounts. Their role is to regulate biological reactions required for normal metabolism (chemical changes involved in using nutrients for the functioning of the body) of amino acids, fats, and carbohydrates to produce energy and synthesize tissues, enzymes, hormones, and other vital compounds. Table 1–4 groups the vitamins into those soluble in fat and those soluble in water and provides major functions and sources of vitamins.

Fat-Soluble Vitamins

Fat-soluble vitamins A, D, E, and K are retained by the body. Any conditions that limit fat intake will limit the consumption of fat-soluble vitamins. No one food contains all the vitamins needed, but eating a wide variety of foods from the basic food groups, including fats and oils, will provide an adequate intake. In the past vitamins A and D were not available in necessary quantities in the general food supply and certain foods (for example, fluid milk and other dairy products) had to be fortified.

Vitamin A is required for bone growth, reproduction, stability of cell membranes, healthy linings of skin and mucous membranes, and visual processes. The role of vitamin A in the visual process is best understood and is essential in preventing night blindness. Vitamin A is required in direct proportion to the weight of the individual; Appendix II lists the Recommended Dietary Allowances (RDA) for each age group based on average weights.

The preformed sources of vitamin A include animal products such as butter, liver, and whole milk. Nonfat milk and margarine are often fortified with vitamin A, as are liquid skim, low-fat, and whole milk. Liquid skim and low-fat milk are fortified with the same amount of vitamin A as whole milk, although dry skim milk may not be fortified. Fruits and vegetables contain no preformed vitamin

Table 1-4
Major functions and sources of selected vitamins

Vitamin	Functions	Sources
Fat-soluble Vitamins		
A	Promotes normal growth of bones, epithelial cells,* and tooth enamel; aids in visual adaptation	Liver, kidney, butter, cream, egg yolk, deep yellow and green leafy vegetables, orange fruits and vegetables
D	Regulates absorption and use of calcium and phosphorus; aids in building and maintaining bones and teeth	Direct exposure of the skin to sunlight, fortified milk, margarine, cereals and breads, fish liver oils, small amounts in egg yolk, butter, liver and some fish such as tuna, salmon, herring, sardines
E	Serves as an antioxidant† to reduce the oxidation of vitamin A, unsaturated fatty acids, and vitamin C; helps prevent bursting of red blood cells	Germs of grains; vegetable oils such as corn, soybean, cottonseed, safflower, and coconut; margarine; dark green leafy vegetables; nuts; legumes
K	Required for synthesis of prothrombin needed in normal blood clotting	Main source is synthesized by the intestinal flora; alfalfa, dark green leafy vegetables, liver, egg yolk
Water-soluble Vitamins		
Ascorbic acid (vitamin C)	Promotes formation and maintenance of bone matrix, cartilage, dentin, collagen, and connective tissue; cell wall integrity; acts in metabolic processes of some amino acids; absorption and use of iron; conversion of folic acid into its active form, folinic acid	Citrus fruits and juices, cantaloupe, strawberries, watermelon, tomatoes, cabbage, green leafy vegetables, broccoli, green peppers, cauliflower, turnips, fresh potatoes
Thiamin (vitamin B_1)	Coenzyme‡ required in carbohydrate metabolism for energy production	Whole-grain products, enriched rice, legumes, nuts, liver, pork, green leafy vegetables
Riboflavin (vitamin B_2)	Part of the enzymes§ and coenzymes that accept transfer hydrogen during metabolism; aids in the production of corticosteroids‖ in the adrenal cortex, the formation of red blood cells in bone marrow, glycogenesis¶, breakdown of fatty acids	Milk, cheese, eggs, enriched breads and whole grains, green leafy vegetables, fish, organ meats, lean meats, yeast

Table 1-4
continued

Vitamin	Functions	Sources
Niacin (nicotinic acid)	Constituent of coenzymes‡ involved in the metabolism of carbohydrate, fat, and protein	Yeast, wheat germ, whole grains, soybeans, corn, peanuts, meat, liver, kidney
Pyridoxine (vitamin B_6)	Required for metabolism of amino acids# and use of carbon dioxide, amino, and sulfur groups	Yeast, wheat germ, whole grains, soybeans, corn, peanuts, meat, liver, kidney
Folacin (folic acid)	Required for blood cell formation; coenzyme for use of carbon and hydrogen	Dark green leafy vegetables, mushrooms, organ meats, whole grains, yeast, legumes, orange juice, lemons, bananas, strawberries, cantaloupe, asparagus, lima beans
Vitamin B_{12}	Necessary for normal growth for maintenance of healthy nervous tissue and for normal blood formation; concerned with metabolism that involves single-carbon units; aids in providing energy for the central nervous system; converts folacin into active form	Liver, kidney, meat, fish, poultry, eggs, milk and milk products; primarily found in animal products
Biotin	Required in enzyme systems involving carbon dioxide; releases energy from carbohydrate and fatty acids; metabolizes fatty acids; deaminates protein	Liver, yeast, cauliflower, nuts, chocolate, legumes, egg yolk, milk
Pantothenic acid	Component of coenzyme A for energy metabolism and steroid and cholesterol synthesis	Liver, kidney, yeast, egg yolk, peanuts, whole grains, lean beef, milk, potatoes, tomatoes, broccoli, fish, poultry, legumes; smaller amounts in other fruits and vegetables

*Cells that line the surfaces of cavities and tubes in the body.
†Inhibitor of reactions promoted by oxygen.
‡Small molecule that works with an enzyme to promote the enzyme's activity.
§Large protein molecules that help with the formation of chemical bonds.
‖Fat-related substances that contain sterols. Sterols are compounds composed of carbon, hydrogen, and ozygen atoms arranged in rings with side chains attached.
¶Formation of glycogen, which is the storage form of carbohydrate in animals.
#Amino acids are building blocks of protein.

A but contain specific precursors the body converts to vitamin A. Dark green and yellow vegetables, such as greens, broccoli, and carrots, are especially good sources.

Vitamin D, also called *calciferol,* is important in regulating the metabolism of calcium and phosphorus. It helps in absorption of calcium and phosphorus from the intestine so that proper mineralization of the bones and teeth can proceed. Requirements for vitamin D are not specifically known, but Appendix II provides the RDA for each age group.

Vitamin D can be obtained from food and by the action of the ultraviolet rays in sunlight. Generally, if enough sun is available, deficiencies will not occur. Those persons who cannot get outside in the sun, as well as rapidly growing infants and children, need a food source of vitamin D. Fish-liver oils, egg yolk, liver, cream, fatty fish, and fortified margarines are sources. Growing children who follow strict vegan diets (without milk) risk insufficient vitamin D intake, but careful selection of foods can ensure an adequate supply.

Vitamin E protects vitamins A and C and unsaturated fatty acids from oxidation, a process in which oxygen reacts with and destroys these substances. It is, therefore, called an *antioxidant.*

Vitamin E and polyunsaturated fatty acids are present in the same foods, so increasing the amount eaten of one will increase the other. Vitamin E is found in vegetable and seed oils, shortening, egg yolk, margarine, butter, whole grains, and green leafy vegetables.

Vitamin K is associated with blood clotting. No RDA has been established. Deficiencies are uncommon except in newborn, especially premature, infants, whose intestinal tracts are free of bacteria (a source of the vitamin) and who must rely on maternal stores. The main sources are intestinal bacteria and foods such as dark green vegetables, wheat bran, soybeans, cauliflower, and tomatoes.

Water-Soluble Vitamins

The *B vitamins* are water soluble and are associated together in many foods. Because many of the B vitamins are found in combination with one another as well as with other nutrients such as protein and minerals, a pure deficiency of one B vitamin is rare. There are eight B vitamins: thiamin, riboflavin, niacin, and pantothenic acid are involved primarily in the energy-releasing function of the body, whereas biotin is used for energy storage, pyridoxine for protein metabolism, and folate and B_{12} for blood manufacturing.

The RDA for each B vitamin is listed in Appendix II, and food sources are shown in Table 1–4. In general, the B vitamins associated with releasing energy are needed in larger quantities by persons who have higher energy intakes.

Another water-soluble vitamin, *vitamin C,* or ascorbic acid, is found in many drink mixes and gelatin products in a form chemically identical to the vitamin C found in fruits, vegetables, and rose hips. Although all water-soluble vitamins can be lost from the diet if the cooking juices are not retained, vitamin C is the most unstable. It can be destroyed by copper cookware, heat, and especially alkaline solutions. Vitamin C is oxidized in the air and preserves or protects other substances. In this manner, it prevents fruits from turning brown during food processing.

Scurvy, rarely seen today, is the well-known deficiency disease associated with eliminating vitamin C from the diet. It involves the appearance of pinpoint hemorrhages or bleeding under the skin along with weakness. Vitamin C is, therefore, believed to be needed for proper functioning of connective tissue, the intercellular cement that holds body tissue together and helps support it. In addition, taken with iron-rich foods vitamin C facilitates the absorption of iron. The other exact roles of vitamin C are not completely understood.

Because many products have vitamin C added, most people have little difficulty acquiring the 60 mg RDA. Citrus fruits are the best sources, along with broccoli, cantaloupe, and greens. See Table 1–4 for additional sources.

Fat-soluble vitamins are not destroyed during cooking as are water-soluble vitamins. If possible, vegetables should be steamed to preserve water-soluble vitamins, or the liquid should be used in gravies and soups. Vegetables should be cooked for short periods to retain full nutritional value.

Toxicity

Excessive intakes of water-soluble vitamins are excreted in the urine and present little problem of toxicity. However, dosages that exceed 10 times the Recommended Dietary Allowances may result in the formation of abnormal metabolites of the vitamins or of the interaction of one nutrient with another. Fat-soluble vitamins are more likely to cause toxicity because the excess will be stored in the body and can reach dangerous levels.

MINERALS

A *mineral* is technically defined as an inorganic element containing no carbon that remains as ash when food is burned. Minerals cannot be broken down any further. As many as 40 kinds of minerals may exist, but only 17 are known to be essential to human nutrition (see Table 1–5). Minerals comprise only 4% of total body weight. *Macrominerals* are required in relatively large amounts, whereas *trace elements*, or *microminerals*, are needed in very small amounts. The macrominerals are calcium, phosphorus, potassium, magnesium, sulfur, sodium, and chlorine. Iron, zinc, selenium, molybdenum, iodine, cobalt, copper, manganese, fluorine, and chromium are microminerals.

Mineral function can be classified as either structural or regulatory. *Structural* minerals are part of cell tissues or substances. *Regulatory* minerals help regulate acid-base balance, muscle contractibility, and nerve irritability and also act in coenzyme systems.

An important consideration today is whether the increased consumption of processed and refined foods in which the trace element concentrations have been

Table 1–5
Major functions and sources of selected minerals

Mineral	Functions	Sources
Macrominerals		
Calcium	Strengthens structure of bones and teeth; promotes clotting of blood; promotes water balance; plays a role in the contraction and relaxation of muscle fibers and transmission of nerve impulses; maintains the function of the cell membrane	Milk and milk products, green leafy vegetables, clams, oysters, legumes, almonds, sesame seeds, broccoli, water, dried beans
Phosphorus	Involved in calcification of teeth and bones; acid-base balance; energy metabolism	Liver, meat, eggs, fish, poultry, milk, dairy products, whole grains, legumes, nuts, refined cereals
Magnesium	Catalyst to biological reactions within the cell; aids in the regulation of nerve impulses and muscle contraction	Whole grains, legumes, nuts, green leafy vegetables, meat, molasses, soybeans, cocoa
Sulfur	Component of protein, thiamin, and biotin; involved in oxidation-reduction reactions; activates many enzymes; participates in several detoxification reactions	Meat, eggs, dairy products, nuts, legumes
Sodium	Promotes acid-base balance, water balance, nerve and muscle activity	Table salt, leavenings, monosodium glutamate, soy sauce, condiments, milk, cheese, eggs, sauerkraut, cured ham, fish, water, green leafy vegetables
Potassium	Catalyst in many biological reactions, especially protein synthesis and glycogen formation; promotes water balance, nerve and muscle activity	Bananas, dates, apricots, oranges, cantaloupe, tomatoes, dark green leafy vegetables, liver, meat, milk, fish, bamboo shoots, prunes
Chlorine	Provides hydrochloric acid of gastric juice; acid-base balance; activity of muscles and nerves; water balance	Table salt, egg yolk, meat, cereals, legumes, water

Table 1-5
continued

Mineral	Functions	Sources
Microminerals		
Iron	Carrier of oxygen and carbon dioxide; constituent of hemoglobin in blood and myoglobin in muscles; required element for many enzymes	Organ meats, meat, oysters, leafy green vegetables, legumes, enriched cereals, dried apricots, prunes, peaches, raisins, egg yolk, nuts, whole grains
Iodine	Part of thyroxine, a thyroid hormone that influences growth and rate of metabolism	Iodized table salt, seafood, water, milk, cheese, eggs (if the animal's diet is high in iodine)
Manganese	Essential for normal bone development; activates enzymes; temperature regulation, nerve and muscle activity, and protein synthesis; enhances thiamin storage in the body	Whole grains, legumes, nuts, green leafy vegetables, meat, tea, coffee
Copper	Required for use of iron and enzymes in energy metabolism; necessary in the formation of nerve walls and connective tissue	Liver, shellfish, nuts, legumes, water, mushrooms, whole-grain cereals, gelatin
Zinc	Constituent of hormones and insulin; promotes enzyme activity in metabolism; associated with wound healing; mobilizes vitamin A from liver stores	Seafood, liver, meat, wheat germ, yeast, legumes
Fluorine	Provides resistance to development of dental caries	Water and beverages prepared with water, naturally occurring or fluoridated
Chromium	Required for metabolism of blood glucose, fatty acid synthesis, insulin metabolism	Meat, whole grains, corn oil
Selenium	Antioxidant; substitutes for some of functions of vitamin E	Seafood, meats, grains
Molybdenum	Aids in oxidation reactions	Organ meats, legumes, whole-grain cereals
Cobalt	Aids in maturation of red blood cells (as part of vitamin B_{12} molecule)	Organ meats

reduced or altered will eventually lead to major disease problems. No evidence exists that this has been the case.

Macrominerals

Calcium.   Calcium is found in the body in amounts larger than any other mineral; it is found primarily in the bones and teeth, where it is part of the hard structure. A specific level of calcium is required in tissues and blood. If this level falls, the body takes calcium from bones to restore the tissue and blood levels. Calcium in the tissues and blood acts as a cementing substance, holding cells together, and is used to transmit nerve impulses, to control the movement of substances into and out of cells, and to regulate muscle contractions. Calcium also is used in the blood-clotting mechanism and in the absorption of B_{12}.

For calcium to be available, it must be absorbed. An individual's need for calcium affects how much calcium the body will absorb. Those persons with a greater physiological need—for example, pregnant women and adolescents—will absorb more calcium. Other factors that enhance absorption include lack of stress; taking small amounts throughout the day rather than a large quantity at one time; presence of lactose, which occurs naturally in milk; adequate amounts of vitamin D; and acid conditions in the stomach.

A high-protein diet may cause calcium to be excreted in the urine; thus, individuals taking high-protein diets may require more calcium. Other factors that decrease calcium absorption are lack of physical exercise in persons confined to bed; and presence of phytic and oxalic acids, which bind calcium and are found in common foods. Phytates are present in whole-grain cereals, oxalates in foods such as greens and rhubarb. The harmful effects depend on the quantity consumed. Fortunately, dietary calcium is plentiful, especially in dairy products, compared with the amounts of phytic and oxalic acid found in a well-rounded diet. Excessive fat in the intestine may also reduce calcium absorption, and use of laxatives can cause calcium to move too rapidly through the intestinal tract, thus limiting absorption.

The need for calcium remains throughout life, with the highest intake (1200 mg) required during the adolescent years. The adult RDA is 800 mg, the quantity usually obtained from 16 ounces of milk and a variety of other foods. Adult women need at least 800 mg because more calcium is withdrawn from bone and excreted after menopause. Older adults absorb less calcium than younger adults. In general, children in the United States consume the recommended allowance of calcium. However, women 18 years and older have been shown to consume less than the RDA [7].

A lack of calcium over long periods may result in stunted growth, poorly developed bones and teeth, and rickets. Deficiency diseases resulting from a lack of calcium alone are rare.

Milk and dairy products are the best sources of calcium; broccoli, okra, dried beans, and peas are other sources of the mineral. Chapter 3 includes calcium values in common foods.

Osteoporosis and osteomalacia are two bone abnormalities related to calcium. *Osteoporosis* is a loss in total amount of bone, and *osteomalacia* is the loss of calcium and phosphorus crystals from the bone. Adequate consumption of food high in calcium in childhood and adolescence appears to be needed not only for growth and development, but possibly to assure high bone density and greater latitude for maintenance of skeletal integrity in the face of bone loss in later years [10].

Phosphorus. Like calcium, phosphorus is found in large amounts in bones and teeth. This mineral gives rigidity to bones and teeth and performs more functions than any other mineral element in normal cell metabolism and functioning. Phosphorus is involved in the metabolism of carbohydrate, fat, and protein. It is part of many enzyme systems and plays an important role in the energy metabolism of muscle.

Requirements for phosphorus are the same as those for calcium. Consuming large amounts of antacids may interfere with phosphorus absorption and result in phosphorus depletion. An equal intake of calcium and phosphorus is recommended.

Sources of phosphorus include foods containing calcium and protein. Persons generally need to be more concerned about getting enough calcium than phosphorus. Soft drinks are often overlooked as sources of phosphorus, and frequent intake of these beverages can disrupt the body's calcium-phosphorus balance.

Sodium. The principal element in extracellular fluids, sodium is involved primarily in regulating the acid-base balance in body fluids. Along with potassium, it is important in regulating the body fluid volume. The cells work to keep sodium on the outside of the cell membrane (extracellular) and potassium on the inside (intracellular). If the amount of sodium in the blood changes, the fluid balance of the body is affected.

A safe and adequate intake of sodium ranges from 1100 to 3000 mg daily for adults. There is no RDA for sodium. The kidneys conserve sodium, filtering any excess from the blood into the urine. Too much sodium may lead to an increase in blood volume and extra pressure on the arteries, causing the heart to work harder to pump blood and the blood pressure to rise. Excessive intake of sodium, primarily from table salt (sodium chloride), has been implicated in higher blood pressure. The Dietary Guidelines for Americans [4] recommend a decrease in sodium intake, and it seems appropriate to limit use of salty snacks such as chips, cold cuts, bacon, and pickles.

Sodium is found naturally in greater quantities in animal foods than in plant foods. Cured meats, sausages, canned soups and vegetables, soy sauce, and steak sauces have a high sodium content. Salting of food at the table is unnecessary, except for the athlete who has just lost water and sodium through perspiration. Because over-the-counter drugs may also be a source of sodium, labels should be read carefully.

Potassium. Potassium is an essential mineral that maintains intracellular fluid balance. It is a component of lean body tissue. The need for potassium is increased when there is growth of lean tissue and is lost when muscle breaks down because of starvation, protein deficiency, or injury. Nerve and muscle cells are rich in potassium. Sodium and potassium ions exchange places during nerve transmission and muscle contraction. Therefore, they keep the heart beating regularly. Extreme dieting (liquid-protein diets) may lead to loss of potassium and can cause heart abnormalities.

There is no RDA for potassium, and the daily intake may range from 1900 to 5600 mg. Sources include fruits and vegetables, such as bananas, tomatoes, citrus juices, and potatoes. Although potassium may be prescribed along with certain drugs used for hypertension, it can cause severe reactions if taken in large doses in the form of supplements.

Trace Elements

Iron. Iron is probably one of the most widely known elements. Certain populations in the United States, including children, have an iron intake less than the recommended level [7]. Iron is found in the blood as part of hemoglobin in red blood cells and myoglobin in muscle tissue. Its best-known task is in providing oxygen to the cells of the body. It is also part of enzyme systems.

Iron must be absorbed to be usable. Absorption is enhanced by acids and the presence of vitamin C. When there is a physiological need for iron and when iron is presented in a certain chemical form, it is absorbed more readily. Iron from meats, fish, and poultry, called *heme* iron, is more readily absorbed than the *nonheme* iron of plant origin found in vegetables, legumes, and grains. As with calcium, phytic acid, found in bran, binds iron and forms an insoluble complex that is difficult to absorb. Likewise, fiber may cause food to move through the intestinal tract too quickly, reducing the time needed for complete digestion of foods and iron absorption.

Women need 18 mg per day and men 10 mg. Pregnant women usually receive an iron supplement of 30 to 60 mg (see Appendix II). Iron-deficiency anemia commonly afflicts young children past 6 months of age and adolescents, especially girls. A low iron intake can lead to iron-deficiency anemia and can lower the blood's oxygen-carrying capacity.

Good sources of iron include liver and other organ meats, red meat, whole-grain or enriched and fortified cereals, oysters, clams, dried beans, some fruits, and dark green vegetables. Although the iron from plant sources is poorly absorbed, absorption can be increased by eating a small amount of meat and taking a vitamin C source with the meal.

Iodine. Iodine is necessary for the proper functioning of the thyroid gland; without iodine the thyroid enlarges to capture what little iodine is available in the blood. This enlargement, or goiter, is seen as a swelling in the neck.

The RDA for iodine is 100 to 150 μg per day. The major source of iodine is iodized salt. Seafoods also contain iodine, and iodine is used by some manufacturers as a dough conditioner. Although iodized salt costs a penny or two more than the noniodized form, this small investment goes a long way in preventing goiter, especially when seafood is not eaten frequently.

Zinc.   Present in every tissue, zinc is essential as a component for enzymes involved in vital metabolic pathways. It is necessary for normal growth, prevention of anemia, general repair of all tissues, and wound healing.

The RDA is 15 mg for adults (Appendix II). Zinc deficiency has been noted in children, and it appears that regular intake of zinc through diet, particularly during periods of growth and stress, is necessary. Sources include red meats, milk, liver, poultry, eggs, fish, and seafood, especially shellfish.

WATER

Water is an extremely important nutrient. For a child, the proportion of body surface area to body mass is much larger than for an adult, thus children need proportionately more fluid. The water lost by evaporation from the young child accounts for more than 60% of that needed to maintain the body compared with 45% for the adult. However, it is difficult to determine how much water a child needs, since surface area, activity, and other foods consumed are all contributing factors. Adults lose about 1½ quarts (1.4 L) of fluid per day through urine, feces, and perspiration. At least this much should be replaced from food and beverages each day. A greater quantity of liquids should be taken frequently in warm weather or during strenuous exercise. Anyone who refuses liquids, is vomiting, or has diarrhea can rapidly become dehydrated.

Water is also important for proper elimination. One of the first factors to be considered when a child or adult complains of constipation is the amount of fluids consumed. A recommended practice for anyone is to drink 1 quart (0.95 L) of liquids per day (Figure 1–2).

SUPPLEMENTS

There are few, if any, quick solutions to gaining and maintaining good health. "Popping pills" appears an easy solution to losing weight or making up nutrients missed in dietary intake. However, benefits are largely unproven. Nutrients function together; therefore, an excess intake of one may create a greater need for others. In addition, the use of pills is inappropriate modeling behavior for persons involved with young children. Unless a specific deficiency has been diagnosed in laboratory and clinical tests, the habitual intake of large doses of vitamins and minerals should be discouraged.

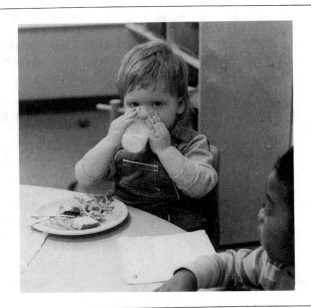

Figure 1–2
Encourage children to drink fluids.

With increased use of vitamin pills to supplement dietary intake, excessive intake of some fat-soluble vitamins has led to overdoses and toxicity. This has occurred primarily in children who consumed vitamins A and D in their diets and were also given supplemental over-the-counter preparations [11].

Both popular and scientific publications have addressed the effects of vitamin C as a treatment for the common cold [12, 13]. Whereas the recommended intake or physiological dosage for vitamin C is 60 mg, which can be met with 6 ounces (180 ml) of orange juice, the pharmacological dosage may be from 100 to 2000 mg. The toxic dose of this same vitamin for the adult is reported to be from 2000 to 4000 mg (2–4 g) [14]; a dosage this size may have harmful effects on the body. Care givers should discourage parents from providing megavitamin (excessive) doses of vitamin C to their children. The Department of Drugs of the American Medical Association substantiates this view, writing that, "until such time as pharmacologic doses of ascorbic acid have been shown to have obvious, important clinical value in the prevention and treatment of the common cold, and to be safe in a large varied population, we cannot advocate its unrestricted use for such purposes" [13].

Vitamin E has also been used in large doses. The health claims that large dietary supplements prevent heart disease and muscular dystrophy and counteract the toxic effects of atmospheric pollutants remain unsubstantiated [15]. Clinical evidence of vitamin E deficiency is almost entirely restricted to premature infants. Today commercially available formulas contain the necessary amount of vitamin E, and parents or care givers need not worry about vitamin E in the formula.

Although large dosages of vitamin B_{12} have been given to many persons, especially the elderly, their effectiveness is still under debate. The red color of the vitamin, along with its almost total lack of known toxicity, makes it an "almost ideal placebo . . . used by megahustlers to make megabucks selling oral tablets containing megaquantities of the vitamin for a wide range of claimed but nonexistent effects" [16].

The list of specific vitamins and their effects on health could continue indefinitely. It is not the purpose of this text to help you remember the role of each vitamin in maintaining proper bodily functions. Rather, the goal is to provide the means by which you can select foods to supply the nutrients needed in your diet and in the diets of those children under your care.

How do you know if you are eating the foods that provide proper nourishment and are participating in exercise that will maintain good health? The following section can help you develop an appropriate diet and exercise program.

GUIDES AND STANDARDS

Several tools may be used to evaluate food and nutrient intake. These include the Modified Basic Food Plan, the Recommended Dietary Allowances (RDA) [17], the United States Recommended Daily Allowances (U.S. RDA), and the Dietary Guidelines for Americans [4].

Modified Basic Food Plan

Nutrients are found in foods, and not every food contains all the nutrients necessary for life. Milk approximates the perfect food, but even it has less fiber, vitamin C, and iron than required. Foods can be grouped according to the specific nutrients they contain. Choosing a variety of foods from these groups will help you select a good diet.

The Basic Four Food Plan, published many years ago by the U.S. Department of Agriculture, is a simple food selection guide [18]. It has been used to plan the foundation for a nutritionally sound diet; however, special consideration must still be given to energy and certain nutrients. The guide has been modified to reflect updated knowledge and information for vegetarians and those who do not consume milk [19].

Table 1–6 gives suggested daily servings of a Modified Basic Food Plan, including meal plans for a variety of special preferences (no meat, no milk, no legumes, and low cost). Foods from the plan are grouped according to their similarity in nutrient content. It is important to choose a variety of foods from the food groups to ensure adequate intake of all nutrients. In comparison with the more traditional Basic Four Food Plan, the modified pattern encourages the more frequent use of whole-grain cereals, green leafy vegetables, and legumes

Table 1-6
Recommended quantity for adults—Modified Basic Food Plan for special preferences and traditional Basic Four

Food Group (quantity/serving)	Modified Pattern (servings/day)	No Meat (servings/day)	No Milk (servings/day)	No Legumes (servings/day)	Low Cost (servings/day)	Traditional pattern (servings/day)
Milk						
8 oz milk or yogurt						
1 oz cheese	2	4	0	1½	1½	2
1½ C cottage cheese						
Meat and alternates						
Animal sources						
3 oz meat, poultry, fish	2	0	4	4	1	2+
2 eggs						
Legumes	2	2	2	0	2	
Nuts	0	1	0	0	0	
2 tbsp peanut butter						
¾ C lentils or beans						
1 oz nuts						
Fruits and vegetables						4 (total)
¾ C vitamin C-rich	1	3	3	2½	0	1
¾ C dark green	1	1½	3	2	1½	*
¾ C other	2	3	0	0	0	
Whole-grain cereal						
1 slice bread	4	6	3	4	9	4†
1 oz cereal						
Vegetable oils						
1 tsp	3	0	0	0	3	As needed

Sources: Modified from King, J. C., Cohenour, S. H., Corruccini, C. G., et al.: Evaluation and modification of the basic four food guide. J. Nutr. Educ. 10:27–29, 1978; and Page, L., and Phiphard, E.: Essentials of an adequate diet, facts for nutrition programs, USDA, Home Econ. Res. Rep. No. 3, Washington, DC, 1957, U.S. Government Printing Office.

*Vitamin A source every other day.

†May be enriched or whole grain.

and provides a pattern that more easily allows for inclusion of foods high in vitamins E and B$_6$, magnesium, and zinc. Discussions in this text of the basic food groups are based on the Modified Basic Food Plan of Table 1-6.

Vitamin E, vitamin B$_6$, magnesium, zinc and folacin, should be included in the diet in greater quantities. Table 1-7 shows good food sources of these nutrients.

Only whole-grain breads and cereals are included in the Modified Basic Food Plan. Many bread and cereal products have been "enriched" in order to replace nutrients found in the bran portion of whole-grain cereals that were removed during the milling process. Table 1-8 shows that enriched rice and bread have substantial quantities of iron and certain vitamins. However, fiber and other vitamins and minerals are more abundant in whole-grain products than in enriched products.

Recommended Dietary Allowances (RDA)

To ensure that the best possible diet has been planned for groups of individuals or for the menus served in preschool or day-care facilities, dietitians often rely not only on the basic food guides but also on the RDA [17]. To do this they compare the nutrients on the menu or the client's food record with the RDA. Although basic food guides answer the question, "Am I getting enough of the right foods?", the RDA best answers the question, "Are the diets or menus providing groups of children with the nutrients needed to meet their needs?"

The 1980 RDA table is found in Appendix II. It lists levels of nutrients considered essential to meet the known nutritional needs of practically all healthy persons. The RDA is based on the judgment of the Food and Nutrition Board and on available scientific knowledge. The allowances are recommendations, not average requirements, and most individuals require less of a nutrient than the RDA values.

Table 1-7
Good sources of vitamin E, vitamin B$_6$, magnesium, zinc, and folacin

Vitamin E (>2.0 IU/serving*)	Vitamin B$_6$ (>0.2 mg/serving)	Magnesium (>20 mg/serving)	Zinc (>1.0 mg/serving)	Folacin (>25 µg/serving)
Nuts	Meat, poultry,	Milk	Milk	Liver
Vegetable oils	fish	Meat, fish	Meat, poultry	Beans
Wheat germ	Legumes	Nuts	Seafood	Leafy greens
Leafy greens	Wheat germ	Legumes	Legumes	Asparagus
		Leafy greens	Whole-grain	Broccoli
		Wheat germ	cereals	
		Wheat cereal	Wheat germ	

Source: Modified from King, J. C., Cohenour, S. H., Corruccini, C. G., et al.: Evaluation and modification of the basic four food guide, J. Nutr. Educ., 10:27–29, 1978.

*A serving equals 3 oz meat, poultry, fish; 2 eggs; ¾ C cooked beans or legumes; 1 oz nuts; ¾ C cooked vegetables or 1 C raw; 1 C milk; 1 tbsp wheat germ; 1 oz dry cereal; ¾ C cooked cereal or pasta; 1 slice bread; 1 tbsp vegetable oil.

Table 1-8
Nutrient composition of whole wheat bread, enriched white bread, brown rice, and enriched rice

Nutrients	Whole Wheat Bread (100 g)	Enriched White Bread (100 g)	Cooked Brown Rice (100 g)	Cooked Enriched Rice (100 g)
Food energy (kcal)	243.0	270.0	119.0	109.0
Protein (g)	10.5	8.7	2.5	2.0
Fat (g)	3.0	3.2	0.6	0.1
Carbohydrate (g)	47.7	50.5	25.5	24.2
Dietary fiber (g)	5.5	2.6	2.1	0.5
Thiamin (mg)	0.3	0.4	0.1	0.1
Riboflavin (mg)	0.1	0.2	0.02	0.01
Niacin (mg)	2.8	3.3	1.4	1.0
Folacin (μg)	62.0	35.0	20.0	16.0
Vitamin B_6 (mg)	0.2	0.04	0.6	0.04
Vitamin E (IU)	2.2	0.2	0.1	0.3
Calcium (mg)	99.0	84.0	12.0	10.0
Phosphorus (mg)	228.0	97.0	73.0	28.0
Iron (mg)	3.0	2.8	0.5	0.9
Magnesium (mg)	195.0	25.0	29.0	8.0
Zinc (mg)	1.8	0.6	0.6	0.4
Potassium (mg)	273.0	105.0	70.0	28.0

Source: Modified from Nutrient data base, Ohio State University Hospitals, Columbus, OH.

The RDA does not provide a definite answer about whether the nutrient needs of an individual are met by a certain dietary intake. For example, if you eat a diet with 45 g of protein daily, the only way to know whether your protein intake is greater or less than your protein requirement is to measure in a laboratory the nitrogen-containing protein waste products lost in urine and feces. Such laboratory tests are rarely necessary. However, the risk of a deficiency increases when intake of a particular nutrient falls below the RDA. Over a period of time or across population groups (for example, children in day-care centers) statements can be made about the extent to which a given group meets the RDA. Using the RDA to evaluate a diet does not allow the dietitian to say a diet is deficient in nutrients but only that the diet did not meet the RDA for the period in question.

Computerized programs have been developed to calculate automatically nutrient intake recorded through dietary recalls or records. One such program, the Nutrient Dietary Data Analysis System [20], has been used for nutrient analysis in this text and for diets and menus nationally [21, 22]. Well-designed and maintained dietary data analysis systems can help the care giver or parent evaluate individual dietary intakes. Not only can an analysis give an estimation of the energy/calories in the diet, but it can also determine how closely the diet meets the Modified Basic Food Plan.

United States Recommended Daily Allowances (U.S. RDA)

The RDA and U.S. RDA are often confused. Whereas the RDA gives a standard against which to evaluate a group of individual diets for nutrient content, the U.S. RDA helps individuals learn about the nutritive value of specific foods from packages or labels.

The U.S. RDA (Table 1–9) was based on the RDA standard for 1968. The values were derived from the 1968 RDA, rather than from the 1980 RDA (Appendix II), to give a single set of values in the U.S. RDA table. This single set of values applies to everyone 4 years of age and older. The U.S. RDA was based on the highest RDA value for each nutrient given in any RDA category according to age and sex. Thus, each value is either equal to or greater than the RDA. Exceptions to this rule are the U.S. RDAs for calcium and phosphorus, which are averages of the RDAs for teenagers (1200 mg) and adults (800 mg).

The U.S. RDA is the legal standard, established by the Food and Drug Administration (FDA), used for nutrition labels on many commercially prepared foods. The U.S. RDA is the most practical and accessible guide for comparing

Table 1–9
U.S. RDA for adults and children over 4 years

Nutrient	Allowance
*Protein	65 g†
*Vitamin A	5000 IU
*Vitamin C	60 mg
*Thiamin	1.5 mg
*Riboflavin	1.7 mg
*Niacin	20 mg
*Calcium	1000 mg
*Iron	18 mg
Vitamin D	400 IU
Vitamin E	30 IU
Vitamin B_6	2.0 mg
Folacin	0.4 mg
Vitamin B_{12}	6 μg
Phosphorus	1000 mg
Iodine	150 μg
Magnesium	400 mg
Zinc	15 mg
Copper	2 mg
Biotin	0.3 mg
Pantothenic acid	10 mg

*Listing of these nutrients is required on all labels; inclusion of other nutrients is allowed but not required.

†If protein efficiency ratio of protein is equal to or better than that of casein, U.S. RDA is 45 g.

the nutrient content of a specific food to approximate nutrient needs of an adult. Although this guide is much less complex than the RDA, it can be misleading unless its source and proper use are understood.

Most foods on the market are labeled according to the percent of adult U.S. RDA. Other sets of the U.S. RDA values are used for labeling products consumed primarily by infants, children ages 1 to 4 (Appendix III), and pregnant or lactating women. The adult U.S. RDA cannot be used to evaluate the diets of young children; however, when children consume "adult" foods, comparisons to the adult standard (Table 1–9) are valid.

Although the U.S. RDA table states the recommended amount of each nutrient in grams, milligrams, micrograms, or international units, you need not learn all these values. Food labels state nutrient content only as a percentage of the U.S. RDA value. You must keep in mind, however, that the percentages of the U.S. RDA values given on packages are based on a specific amount of food, which is noted on the label as the serving size. For example, the label in Figure 1–3

Vanilla Pudding

Nutrition Information

Serving size.................................. ½ C.
Servings per package............................. 4

	Mix to make 1 serving	1 serving prepared as pudding
Calories	100	180
Protein	*	4 g
Carbohydrate	25 g	31 g
Fat	*	5 g

Percentage of U.S. Recommended Daily Allowances (U.S. RDA)

	Mix to make 1 serving	1 serving prepared as pudding
Protein	*	10
Vitamin A	*	4
Vitamin C	*	2
Thiamine	*	2
Riboflavin	*	10
Niacin	*	*
Calcium	*	15
Iron	*	*
Phosphorus	20	30

*Contains less than 2% of the U.S. RDA.

Figure 1–3
Food label using U.S. RDA

shows a serving size of ½ cup of vanilla pudding. To acquire the nutrients—10% U.S. RDA for protein and 180 calories—you would have to prepare the pudding with whole milk and consume ½ cup. If you eat more or less than that amount, the percentage of U.S. RDA of nutrients you consume would be proportionately greater or smaller than the values stated on the label.

The U.S. RDA provides valuable information. It can help you (1) become familiar with dietary sources of specific nutrients and learn information concerning the energy value of a food relative to its protein, vitamin, and mineral content; and (2) plan meals that are nutritionally appropriate by comparing the amounts of a nutrient in different types of food or brands of the same product. For example, if you are considering two different foods, either of which might be used on the preschool menu, U.S. RDA values on labels can help you select an iron-rich vegetable (such as lima beans) or one that is a better source of vitamin A (such as carrots), depending on how much of each of these nutrients has already been provided by the other foods chosen for that day.

The U.S. RDA is not practical for accurately totaling your daily nutrient intake, for several reasons:

1. Many food labels do not include nutrition information, and some foods are usually not labeled (for instance, fresh fruits and vegetables, meats, and so on).
2. Information on some nutrients is lacking, since most labels provide U.S. RDA information only for protein and seven other nutrients.
3. U.S. RDA values are rounded rather than exact values.
4. U.S. RDA values are higher than most of the corresponding RDA values, especially for young children.
5. Allowance must be made for nutrient losses in foods during storage and preparation, the variability in daily intake for some nutrients, and the need for trace elements for which recommendations have yet to be developed.

Dietary Guidelines for Americans

Recently the U.S. Department of Agriculture (USDA), along with the U.S. Department of Health and Human Services (HHS), has been involved in, and supportive of, efforts to encourage changes in certain eating habits. Health problems such as obesity, heart disease, and cancer have been linked to overconsumption of foods containing certain nutrients. Many health professionals believe that the public needs guidance in avoiding excessive consumption of foods with nutrients that appear to be implicated in these disease states.

The Dietary Guidelines for Americans provide the following recommendations:

- Eat a variety of foods
- Maintain desirable weight
- Avoid too much fat, particularly saturated fat, and cholesterol
- Eat foods with adequate starch and fiber
- Avoid too much sugar

- Avoid too much sodium
- If you drink alcoholic beverages, do so in moderation [4]

The Dietary Guidelines for Americans are general statements, whereas the Modified Basic Food Plan provides specific amounts of food to help plan a diet for an individual or a group of children.

Eighty percent of all cancers may be related to the environment and to things we eat, drink, and smoke, rather than to factors we cannot control such as our family background. Research suggests that a diet low in fiber and high in fat, with few fresh fruits, vegetables, or whole-grain breads and cereals, increases the risk of certain cancers [23].

Diet, Nutrition and Cancer Prevention: The Good News, published by the National Cancer Institute, incorporates the Dietary Guidelines for Americans in its guidelines to reduce the risk of cancer [23, 24]. The institute offers the following advice:

- Choose foods high in dietary fiber

  Between 25 and 35 grams daily
  Examples: fruits, vegetables, legumes, and whole-grain breads and cereals

- Choose foods low in dietary fat, 30% of total calories
- Eat a variety of vitamin-rich foods

  Cruciferous vegetables, such as brussels sprouts, cabbage, broccoli, cauliflower, rutabagas, turnips
  Fruits and vegetables containing vitamin A and C

- If you drink alcoholic beverages, do so only in moderation
- If you broil, grill, or barbecue, protect foods from smoke, flames, and extremely high temperatures

A dietary plan for a 7-year-old that meets the RDA and conforms to both Dietary Guidelines for Americans and the National Cancer Institute recommendations is shown in Table 1–10.

YOUR PERSONAL DIETARY INTAKE AND EXERCISE PATTERNS

Looking at your own dietary pattern is one of the most important steps in improving your diet. You will need a sheet of paper and pencil to record your current eating habits. Nutritionists use either a diet record or 24-hour dietary recall.

Diet records are usually sent home with individuals who are asked to record everything they eat and drink for 1 or more days. A *24-hour dietary recall* is usually taken by a trained person (following a specific protocol) during an interview session. Both are means of collecting information about dietary intake to determine the nutrient content of one or more diets. Figure 1–4 shows a completed

Table 1–10
Dietary plan that meets dietary guidelines for 7-year-old*

Meals	Servings				
	Milk	Protein	Fruits/Vegetables	Grains	Fats
Breakfast					
Orange juice, ½ C			1		
Whole wheat toast, 2 slices				2	
Cream cheese, 1 tbsp					1
Jam, 1 tbsp					
Milk 2%, 1 C	1				
Lunch					
Chicken sandwich (3 oz chicken,		1			
½ tbsp mayonnaise-type salad dressing,					1
¼ C lettuce,					
2 slices whole wheat bread)				2	
Legumes, cooked, ½ C		1			
Apple, 1 medium			1		
Dinner					
Baked fish, 3 oz		1			
Broccoli, ½ C			1		
Brown rice, ½ C				1	
Mixed green salad			1		
(spinach, onion, cucumber)					
French dressing, 1 tbsp					1
Grapes, 1 C			2		
Milk 2%, 1 C	1				
Snacks					
Bran muffin				1	
Pear, 1 medium			1		
Milk 2%, 1 C	1				
Jam, 1 tbsp					
TOTAL (servings)	3	3	7	6	3

*Energy requirement may range from 1650 to 3300 kilocalories; this diet includes approximately 2000. Additional foods may be needed to meet energy needs.

diet record, which can also be used for listing foods eaten during the past 24 hours (see forms in Appendix IV).

For the purpose of analyzing your own dietary intake, you may combine the two methods. For example, you may keep a record for 2 days preceding or following the 24-hour recall. Just write down all the foods and beverages eaten, when these foods were eaten, how prepared (for example, frying, steaming), and the amount consumed. Whenever dietary habits are studied in order to modify an

Name M. Sawicki

Address

Date: From 1/11/89 To ——

Number of feeding periods   Day 1 5   Day 2 ——   Day 3 ——

Pregnant ( )   Nonpregnant (X)

Ht. 65 in.

Wt. 128 lb.

Age 20

Sex F

Time	Food and preparation method (e.g., fried, baked, creamed)	Amount (e.g., C., tsp., tbsp.)	
7:00 AM	Orange juice	3/4 C.	
	Scrambled egg	2	
	Whole wheat toast	2 slices	
	Milk, 2%	1 C.	
	Margarine	1 tsp.	
12:00 PM	Great northern beans, cooked	1½ C.	
	Cooked cabbage	1 C.	
	Fruit cocktail, canned	3/4 C.	
	Corn bread	1 piece	
3:00 PM	Milk, 2%	1 C.	
6:30 PM	Salmon loaf	3 oz.	
	Creamed pototoes	3/4 C.	
	Broccoli, frozen, cooked	1 C.	
	Enriched bread	1 slice	
	Margarine	2 tsp.	
	Coffee	1 C.	
10:00 PM	Apple, raw	1 large	
	Corn, popped	2 C.	

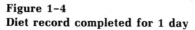

Figure 1–4
Diet record completed for 1 day

undesirable pattern, you may want to include where the food was eaten, with whom the food was eaten, and your mood or feeling when the food was eaten. In addition, how much exercise you get may also be important for controlling weight (Figure 1–5).

Recording the amount of food eaten and your exercise patterns will make you more conscious of what you eat. However, this is true only if the recording or recall is completed in the time interval immediately following food intake. Begin with whatever you consumed most recently or are consuming right now and record the items eaten from this time yesterday. Now take a look at the diet. Is your diet adequate? If you continue to eat this way, will your food intake ensure good health and prevent nutritional deficiencies? How do you know? What standard did you use? You now have the tools used to evaluate your food and nutrient intake.

Check your diet. How many different kinds of food did you consume? Five? Seven? Ten? Fifteen? In general, the wider the variety of foods eaten, the more likely the diet is to be adequate. At least 12 to 15 different items chosen from a wide variety of foods, not fortified foods, are needed to meet the RDA. However, if a diet consists of candy, soft drinks, and other foods with low nutritional value or density, the diet will be inadequate, no matter how varied.

Remember that all persons throughout life have the need for the same nutrients, but the amounts may vary. Nutrient needs can change depending on age, sex, size, activity, and state of health. Of all the guides mentioned, there

Food and Exercise Record					
Amount of Food/ Duration of Exercise*	Description	Time	Where/With Whom (location of eating/exercise)	Mood†	Kcal Consumed/ Expended††
2 C	Popcorn	3:30–4:00	Watching TV	b	+ 200
½ hr	Walked 1½ miles	4:00–4:30	Park/alone	c	– 160
*May calculate activity in minutes at miles per hour. †a = anxious, b = bored, c = content, d = depressed, e = angry, h = happy, t = tired. May be omitted when recording for a child. ††Record calories for foods eaten only if those expended in exercise are not available.					

Figure 1–5
Food and exercise record

are two you can use for determining whether the diet contains all the necessary nutrients. These guides are the Modified Basic Food Plan and the RDA. These are really similar, but the basic food guide as modified is a simple and convenient food selection guide to obtain the RDA for nutrients considered necessary.

How Does Your Diet Compare?

In comparing your diet to the basic food groups, it is easier if you first list the basic food groups and then compare the number of servings of each food consumed with the recommended quantity. Figure 1–4 shows a 24-hour dietary recall for a 20-year-old woman. On examining the diet, you may note that you eat more or less frequently and that your choice of foods differs from the example given. Many combinations of foods can supply the nutrients the body needs to function properly. We compared the diet to the Modified Basic Food Plan (Table 1–11). It appears to have all the constituents so commonly discussed (e.g., vitamin C in juice, protein in beans, eggs, and fish); however, it lacks one serving of whole-grain products.

This diet was also compared with the RDA (Figure 1–6) by using a computer. The results show that intake of vitamin B_6 is less than 65% of the RDA. One additional serving of whole wheat bread or brown rice would have increased the intake of B_6 to more than 66% RDA.

The student can manually complete a form similar to that in Figure 1–4 by taking the foods from the diet and converting them to nutrients found in the food composition table (Appendix I). The major nutrients for each food can be totaled and compared with the RDA (Appendix II) and a percentage calculated.

Computerization provides a much easier method for analyzing the nutrient content of the diet. However, use of the Modified Basic Food Plan does an adequate job of determining if your diet or that of the children in the center meets most nutritional needs.

A person's dietary intake may not be judged adequate or inadequate based on an evaluation of 1-day recall. However, the 24-hour recall can help in making decisions on how to modify your own dietary intake or for screening purposes to determine whether a child needs further evaluation of nutritional status.

Determining Calorie Requirements

When you eat too many foods that contain large amounts of potential energy in relation to the amount of energy you actually use, the excess is stored as fat. One primary indication of excess fat stores in the body is when an individual weighs more than what the charts estimate to be a desirable body weight (DBW) in relation to that person's sex, age, height, and body frame. Desirable body weight can be calculated with the following formulas:

For women: Allow 100 pounds for your first 5 feet of height. For each additional inch over 5 feet, add 5 pounds (for each inch under, subtract 5 pounds).

Table 1-11
Comparison of sample diet with basic food groups

Consumed Quantity of Food in Sample Diet	Servings of Basic Food Groups							
		Protein Foods		Fruits and Vegetables				
	Milk	Meat, Fish, Poultry	Legumes and Nuts	Vitamin C	Dark Green	Other	Cereal Products	Fats and Oils
¾ C orange juice				1				
2 scrambled eggs		1						
2 slices whole wheat toast							2	
8 oz milk (2%)	1							
1 tsp margarine								1
1½ C cooked beans			2					
1 C cooked cabbage						1⅓		
1 piece corn bread							1	
¾ C fruit cock-tail						1		
8 oz milk (2%)	1							
3 oz salmon loaf		1						
¾ C creamed potatoes						1		
1 C broccoli					1⅓			
1 slice enriched bread*†								
2 tsp margarine								2
8 oz coffee								
1 large apple						1		
2 C popcorn†								
TOTAL	2	4		1	1⅓	4⅓	3	3
Basic food guide	2	4		1	1	2	4	3
Difference	0	0		0	(+)	(+)	(−)	0

*Because of the limited amounts of magnesium, zinc, B₆, vitamin E, and folacin, enriched bread has not been equated to one serving of whole-grain cereals.

†Not considered part of the Modified Basic Food Plan.

```
TOTAL          NUTRIENT      %RDA 0%       20%    33%  40%       60% 66%    80%         100%
----------------------------I--------I-----I---I---------I--I------I----------------I
2009.6 KCAL ENERGY           96% XXXXXXXXXXXXXXXXXXXXXXXXXXXXXXXXXXXXXXXXXXXXXXXXX
  93.4 GM   PROTEIN         212% XXXXXXXXXXXXXXXXXXXXXXXXXXXXXXXXXXXXXXXXXXXXXXXXXXX
7472.6 IU   VITAMIN A       187% XXXXXXXXXXXXXXXXXXXXXXXXXXXXXXXXXXXXXXXXXXXXXXXXXXX
 214.8 IU   VITAMIN D        72% XXXXXXXXXXXXXXXXXXXXXXXXXXXXXXXXXXXX
  21.4 IU   VITAMIN E       214% XXXXXXXXXXXXXXXXXXXXXXXXXXXXXXXXXXXXXXXXXXXXXXXXXXX
 302.2 MG   VITAMIN C       504% XXXXXXXXXXXXXXXXXXXXXXXXXXXXXXXXXXXXXXXXXXXXXXXXXXX
 483.4 MCG  FOLACIN         121% XXXXXXXXXXXXXXXXXXXXXXXXXXXXXXXXXXXXXXXXXXXXXXXXXXX
  15.7 MG   NIACIN          112% XXXXXXXXXXXXXXXXXXXXXXXXXXXXXXXXXXXXXXXXXXXXXXXXXXX
   2.3 MG   RIBOFLAVIN      178% XXXXXXXXXXXXXXXXXXXXXXXXXXXXXXXXXXXXXXXXXXXXXXXXXXX
   1.7 MG   THIAMIN         158% XXXXXXXXXXXXXXXXXXXXXXXXXXXXXXXXXXXXXXXXXXXXXXXXXXX
   0.9 MG   VITAMIN B6       45% XXXXXXXXXXXXXXXXXXXXX
   3.4 MCG  VITAMIN B12     112% XXXXXXXXXXXXXXXXXXXXXXXXXXXXXXXXXXXXXXXXXXXXXXXXXXX
1309.5 MG   CALCIUM         164% XXXXXXXXXXXXXXXXXXXXXXXXXXXXXXXXXXXXXXXXXXXXXXXXXXX
1916.7 MG   PHOSPHORUS      240% XXXXXXXXXXXXXXXXXXXXXXXXXXXXXXXXXXXXXXXXXXXXXXXXXXX
  18.8 MG   IRON            105% XXXXXXXXXXXXXXXXXXXXXXXXXXXXXXXXXXXXXXXXXXXXXXXXXXX
 294.7 MG   MAGNESIUM        98% XXXXXXXXXXXXXXXXXXXXXXXXXXXXXXXXXXXXXXXXXXXXXXXXXX
   9.7 MG   ZINC             65% XXXXXXXXXXXXXXXXXXXXXXXXXXXXXX
-----------------------------I--------I-----I---I---------I--I------I-----------I
```

Figure 1–6
Nutrient analysis of woman's diet in Figure 1–4 (*Source:* NDDA Laboratory, Southern Illinois University at Carbondale.)

For example, at 5'5": 100 pounds (for first 5 feet)

                <u>+ 25</u> pounds (for remaining 5 inches)

                125 pounds = DBW

For men: Allow 106 pounds for first 5 feet of height. For each additional inch, add 6 pounds (for each inch under, subtract 6 pounds).

For example, at 6':   106 pounds (for first 5 feet)

                <u>+ 72</u> pounds (for remaining 12 inches)

                178 pounds = DBW

Table 1–12 estimates the calories needed to maintain desirable body weight and avoid gain with age. First determine whether you are very inactive, sedentary, moderately active, or very active. Locate the calories per pound of desirable body weight (column 2) for your activity level, and calculate your total calorie needs. If your DBW is 125 pounds and you are sedentary, you would need approximately 1625 calories (125 × 13 = 1625) to maintain desirable body weight.

Exercise

You have learned to record, calculate, and improve your dietary intake. What about your output of energy? You don't have time to exercise? You can't put forth the time and effort of the jogger you watch each day? Only 90 minutes of brisk exercise per week or 30 minutes of vigorous exercise three times a week is recommended. Of course, exercising daily can more easily become part of a routine.

Exercise does affect the amount of energy you need. What you eat and how much you exercise must be considered together when evaluating your dietary intake. Table 1–13 presents the average calories spent for 30 minutes of exercise by a 150-pound person. Energy burned in a particular activity varies in proportion to one's body weight. A 100-pound person would reduce the calories by one third, whereas a 200-pound person would multiply by 1⅓. An additional benefit of exercise is that it keeps the body's appetite control mechanism functioning properly. A person may miss internal cues for hunger and satiety without

Table 1–12
Estimation of calorie needs (Adults at DBW. Calories appropriate to maintain weight and avoid gain with age.)

Activity Level	Kcal./lb. DBW	Kcal./kg. DBW
Very inactive or obese	10	22
Sedentary	13	28.6
Moderate	15	33
Strenuous	20	44

Source: Modified from Chicago Dietetic Association and Southern Suburban Dietetic Association of Cook and Will Counties: Manual of Clinical Dietetics, Philadelphia, 1981, W. B. Saunders Co.

Table 1–13
Average energy expended by a 150-pound person in one-half hour

Activity	Energy Expended (kcal)
Bicycling 3 miles	120
Bicycling 6 miles	205
Cross-country skiing per ½ hour	350
Jogging 2¾ miles	330
Jogging 3½ miles	460
Jumping rope per ½ hour	375
Running in place per ½ hour	325
Running 5 miles per ½ hour	640
Swimming 25 yards/minute for ½ hour	137
Swimming 50 yards/minute for ½ hour	250
Tennis, singles per ½ hour	200
Walking 1 mile	120
Walking 1½ miles	160
Walking 2¼ miles	220

Source: National Institute of Health: Exercise and your heart, NIH Pub. No. 81–1677, Washington, DC, 1981, U.S. Government Printing Office.

exercise. Weight loss through diet and exercise is likely to be 98% fat, whereas diet alone produces a weight loss of 75% from fat and the remainder from muscle tissue.

You are now ready to record what you eat along with how much you exercise on a form similar to the one presented in Figure 1–5. We have included one of our daily food and exercise records, but 3- to 7-day records can better help you determine changes required in your diet and exercise patterns.

EXERCISE CONCERNS AND CAUTIONS FOR CHILDREN

With the increase in incidence of obesity, care givers are becoming concerned about energy balance as it affects not only energy intake but also energy expenditure. Positive energy balance produces weight gain in excess of needs for growth and development. When this happens the care giver may turn to exercise to increase the young child's energy expenditure, especially when the child is at the 90th percentile height for weight. The child's parents may also be pressuring the care giver to modify the child's dietary intake and exercise patterns.

Cautions regarding preschool exercise programs come from both the early childhood and the health care professions. Elkind feels that exercise programs at too early an age put infants and young children in inappropriate learning situations as well as expose them to risk of physical and/or psychological damage.

Most children can get all the exercise they need by doing what they do naturally as they use their senses and movements to explore their world [25]. (See Figure 1-7).

Further cautions come from the American Academy of Pediatrics [26]. After a 2-year study of preschool exercise programs, the academy concluded that infant exercise programs do nothing to improve a baby's physical fitness. The academy advises general play until age 6. Exercise programs geared to children under age 3 do not enhance the development of the healthy child.

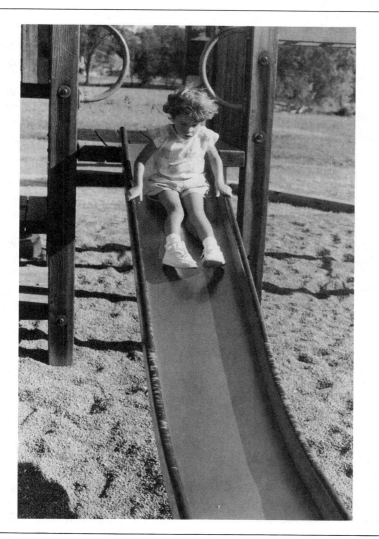

Figure 1-7
Doing what comes naturally is an excellent physical fitness program for children.

Structured exercise programs do not belong in the early childhood curriculum. Care givers should provide a physical environment that provides freedom of movement and exploration. Specific recommendations for physical fitness activity are provided in Chapters 2, 3, 4, and 5.

SUMMARY

- Nutrition is the science of food and how it is used by the body. The study of nutrition involves the social, economic, cultural, and emotional factors that affect the intake of food.
- There are six classes of nutrients with specialized functions in the body.
- Dietary fat, carbohydrate, and protein are major nutrients that have specific functions but also supply heat, or energy, to the body.
- Each of the nutrients is found in a wide variety of foods. Therefore, the wider the variety of foods one eats, the more likely the diet will contain all essential nutrients.
- Supplementing the diet with large amounts of vitamins and minerals is not advisable. Megadoses of specific nutrients should be prescribed only after appropriate clinical and laboratory tests confirm the need.
- Applying the basic principles of nutrition to your personal diet provides experience in learning what factors to evaluate in diets of children in the center and practicing good nutrition principles helps care givers to be good role models for parents and children.
- Several guides may be used to evaluate dietary patterns or intakes. Each guide was developed to be used for a different purpose.
- Following the Modified Basic Food Plan allows the care giver to obtain the Recommended Dietary Allowances.
- Completing a daily record of what has been eaten and the amount and kind of exercise performed are steps in understanding an individual's total dietary intake needs.
- Structured exercise programs are not necessary for children under the age of 6.

DISCUSSION QUESTIONS

1. Describe the nature, functions, and use of the essential nutrients.
2. Which of the nutrients supply energy to the body, and which one supplies energy most efficiently?
3. In addition to the specific nutrients found in foods, which other factors must be considered when the subject of nutrition is studied?
4. Are there consequences of exceeding nutrient requirements?
5. Why should you as a care giver practice the principles of good nutrition?
6. How can you calculate which nutrients you are getting in your diet each day?

7. Which guides and standards can you use to evaluate dietary intake?
8. Is it possible to evaluate both dietary intake and exercise?
9. Discuss structured exercise programs for adults and children under age 6. What differences exist and why?

REFERENCES

1. Satter, E. M.: The feeding relationship, J. Am Diet. Assoc. 86:352–356, 1986.
2. Hegarty, V.: Decisions in nutrition, St. Louis, 1988, Times Mirror/Mosby College Publishing.
3. Hamilton, E. M. N., Whitney, E. N., and Sizer, F. S.: Nutrition: concepts and controversies, ed. 4, St. Paul, 1988, West Publishing Co.
4. U.S. Department of Agriculture and U.S. Department of Health and Human Services: Nutrition and your health: dietary guidelines for Americans, Washington, DC, 1986, U.S. Government Printing Office.
5. American Heart Association, Nutrition Committee: Dietary guidelines for healthy adult Americans, Circulation 74:1465A, 1986.
6. Vahouny, G. V., and Kritchevsky, D.: Dietary fiber in health and disease, New York, 1982, Plenum Press.
7. National Center for Health Statistics, U.S. Department of Health and Human Services, Public Health Service: Dietary intake source data: United States, 1976–80, DHHS Publication No. (PHS)83-1681, Hyattsville, MD, 1983.
8. American Dietetic Association: Position of the American Dietetic Association: vegetarian diets, J. Am. Diet. Assoc. 88(3):351, 1988.
9. American Dietetic Association: Position of the American Dietetic Association: Vegetarian diets—technical support paper, J. Am. Diet. Assoc. 88:352–355, 1988.
10. Sandler, R. B., Slemenda, C. W., Lapporte, R. E., et al.: Postmenopausal bone density and milk consumption in childhood and adolescence, Am. J. Clin. Nutr. 42:270–274, 1985.
11. Hazards of the overuse of vitamin D, Nutr. Rev. 33:61, 1975.
12. Pauling, L. C.: Vitamin C and the common cold, San Francisco, 1970, W. H. Freeman & Co.
13. Dykes, M. H. M., and Meier, P.: Ascorbic acid and the common cold: evaluation of its efficacy and toxicity, J.A.M.A. 231:1073–1079, 1975.
14. Hodges, R. E.: Ascorbic acid. In Nutrition reviews: Present knowledge in nutrition, New York, 1976, The Nutrition Foundation, Inc.
15. Bieri, J. G.: Vitamin E. In Nutrition reviews: Present knowledge in nutrition, New York, 1976, The Nutrition Foundation, Inc.
16. Herbert, V.: Vitamin B_{12}. In Nutrition reviews: Present knowledge in nutrition, New York, 1976, The Nutrition Foundation, Inc.
17. Food and Nutrition Board, National Research Council: Recommended Dietary Allowances, ed. 9, Washington, DC, 1980, National Academy of Science.
18. Page, L., and Phipard E.: Essentials of an adequate diet: facts for nutrition programs, U.S. Department of Agriculture, Home Econ. Res. Rep. No. 3, Washington DC, 1957, U.S. Government Printing Office.
19. King, J. C., Cohenour, S. H., Corruccini, C. G., et al.: Evaluation and modification of the basic four food guide, J. Nutr. Educ. 10:27–29, 1978.
20. Endres, J., and Sawicki, M.: Guide for the use of the Nutrient Dietary Data Analysis System, Carbondale, IL, 1980, Southern Illinois University.
21. Sawicki, M., and Endres, J.: Energy and nutrient calculations using an optical character reader system, J. Am. Diet. Assoc. 82:138, 1983.
22. Endres, J., Dunning, S., Poon, S. W., et al.: Older pregnant women and adolescents: nutrition data after enrollment in WIC, J. Am. Diet. Assoc. 87:1011–1019, 1988.
23. National Cancer Institute: Diet, nutrition and cancer prevention: the good news, U.S. Department of Health and Human Services,

Washington, DC, NIH Publication No. 87-2878, 1986, U.S. Government Printing Office.

24. National Cancer Institute: Diet, nutrition and cancer prevention: a guide to food choices, U.S. Department of Health and Human Services, Washington, DC, NIH Publication No. 85-2711, 1984, U.S. Government Printing Office.

25. Elkind, D.: Miseducation: preschoolers at risk, New York: 1987, Alfred A. Knopf, p. 13.

26. American Academy of Pediatrics: Sports and your child: a position statement of the American Academy of Pediatrics, Chicago, 1987, The Academy.

LEARNING OBJECTIVES

Students will be able to

- **Identify tools used to evaluate nutritional status**
- **State advantages and disadvantages of breast milk for infants**
- **Describe infant formulas**
- **Discuss the introduction of solid foods during the first year**
- **Evaluate an infant's dietary intake and feeding and eating skills**
- **Discuss nutrition-related problems of the infant**
- **State several components included in the policy statement related to nutrition in an infant center**

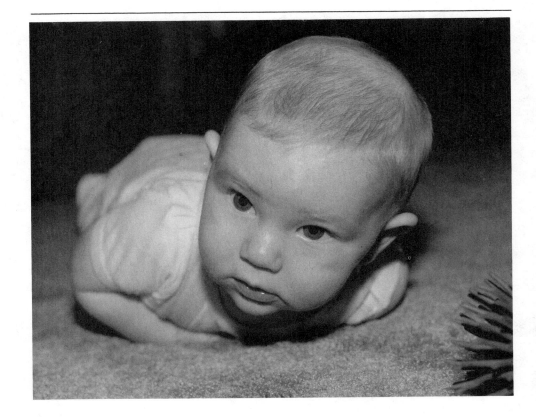

2

The Infant
(Birth to 12 Months)

Some of you reading this for the first time may never have held or cared for an infant. On the other hand, some of you may have several children of your own and feel comfortable with the infants brought to the center for care. In either case recent reports of studies conducted with infants and the recommended practices resulting from studies related to nutritional care should be interesting to both groups. They should also help you provide the best nutritional care for the young child in the center. You are urged to consult the references for an in-depth study of growth, development, nutrition needs, feeding practices, and common problems of the infant and to refer parents to local public health nutritionists or dietitians for additional guidance.

PHYSICAL CHARACTERISTICS RELATED TO FOOD

After the first year the child will never again grow so rapidly. Each month during the first year brings a new set of joys and problems for parents and care givers until finally the infant emerges at 12 months as an individual and "proper person" [1]. During the first year the child is dependent on the care giver for physical, emotional, and social needs, and the cry is the main form of communication.

At birth the normal child is able to suck but cannot lift its head, roll over, or in any other way signal for food. When the infant is at least 8 months old, the experienced care giver can easily distinguish between the distress cry (for example, for food or a dry diaper) and the "I'm-bored-and-frustrated" cry, which often characterizes to the parent the 1-year-old "whiny or demanding child."

By this time the child is finger-feeding and is well into eating with a spoon. Some of the eating behaviors expected of the child during the latter part of the first year of life are chewing and feeding finger foods, holding a bottle, drinking from a cup, holding a spoon, and attempting to feed self if a spoon is dipped into food.

Critical Periods

As a child grows, a care giver will note critical periods characterized by certain oral, adaptive, and gross motor skills. Table 2-1 summarizes normal feeding development during these critical periods for the infant to 12 months. Referring to the developmental milestones in areas related to feeding and nutrition, the care giver can observe the child's behavior in relation to the standard. Further evaluation is necessary to determine any delay. In infancy critical periods have special meanings in relation to food intake. When a baby is born, a sucking reflex provides a method for obtaining nourishment. Not until the 3- to 5-month period does the sucking motion become modified enough for the infant to accept semisolid food from a spoon.

By 7 months the infant has learned to chew. At this time the infant is developmentally ready to accept foods with a texture other than pureed. Table foods chopped, mashed, or cut in small pieces are well accepted. Experience with developmentally delayed children shows that if foods of varied textures are not offered at this time, the infant may refuse food, refuse to chew, or even vomit unfamiliar foods when they are offered. This is rarely the case with a child who is developing well and is allowed to interact with the family. This child will take food while being held by someone who is eating and will explore tastes and textures.

ANTHROPOMETRIC AND LABORATORY MEASURES RELATED TO NUTRITION

Among the measures that the care giver can use in determining the proper intake of food and nourishment are the anthropometric measurements of length and weight. These measurements should be accurately taken on a monthly basis in the center, or parents should arrange to attend local public health or private clinics for such measurements. Although it is advisable and recommended for the center to have a properly constructed measuring board, in some cases the changing table, a tape measure, and an immovable head piece have been used. In all cases it requires two persons to measure an infant. Figure 2-1 (page 54) shows the proper procedure.

Table 2–1
Stages of development for infants*

Stage	Physical	Nutritional	Intellectual
Fetal: Conception to birth	Development of anatomic characteristics followed by growth and elaboration of all systems	Receives nourishment via placenta; maternal weight gain first trimester 1 to 2 kg with 0.4 kg per week gain for remainder of pregnancy	Brain grows to about 25% of adult size
Newborn: Birth to 10 days	Average weight—3.4 kg; average height—50 cm; average HC†—35 cm; has large head, round face and chest, prominent abdomen, and short extermities; loses weight	Seeks source of nourishment by rooting reflex from bottle or breast, consuming colostrum or prepared formula	Brain growth continues; coordination of senses and motor functions begins
Infancy I: 10 days to 2 months	Regains birthweight; sitting height equal to 57% of body length; rapid growth of head and body	Continues to nurse mature breast milk or formula; not developmentally ready for solid food (orally or physiologically, e.g., renal solute load)	Inspection of surroundings begins; differentiation of self from others
Infancy II: 3 to 5 months	Doubles birthweight; increases length; posterior fontanel closes; deciduous teeth begin erupting	Continues to be nourished by breast milk or formula; iron stores begin to be depleted	Attention span increases; hand-eye coordination begins
Infancy III: 6 to 9 months	Subcutaneous fat reaches peak by 9 months; closure of anterior fontanel by 9 months	Oral mechanism ready to accept solid food; cereal introduced first in a very thin consistency; consistency thickened, as tolerated; new foods introduced, as tolerated	Imitation of others begins; understands a few words
Infancy IV: 10 to 12 months	Triples birthweight; average HC† of 47 cm equals chest circumference; 6 to 8 teeth present	Tooth eruption progresses to tolerated transition from pureed to chopped foods; formula or breast milk recommended until end of the first year	First words; concept of object permanence develops; brain weight now about 75% of adult's

*This chart provides the health professional with a standard tool for assessing feeding levels.
†Head circumference.

(continued)

Table 2–1
continued

Stage	Gross Motor	Fine Motor	Reflex
Fetal: Conception to birth		Sucks thumb in utero	
Newborn: Birth to 10 days	Flexed adducted posture	Grasp reflex; palmomental reflex; inserts thumb when hand is brought to mouth	Sucking, rooting, gag, asymmetrical tonic neck reflex (ATNR) present; moro and tonic labyrinthine reflexes emerge
Infancy I: 10 days to 2 months	Flexed-abducted posture emerges; head extension in prone (60° at 3 months); head lag when pulled to sitting; midline positioning of head begins in supine; forearm propping	Grasp reflex continues; hands often open; ulnar side of hand strongest; mouthing of fingers and mutual fingering	Rooting (3 months) and sucking (2 to 5 months) disappear; phasic bite reflex present
Infancy II: 3 to 5 months	Extended-abducted posture emerges; extended arm position in prone; rolls prone to supine and back; head erect in supported sitting (6 months); sits propping on arms	Raking fingers; immediate approach and grasp on site, then eyes and hands combine in joint action; radial fingers begin to dominate	Grasp reflex disappears (4 to 6 months) and moro disappears (5 to 6 months); tonic labyrinthine disappears (6 months); symmetrical topic neck reflex (STNR) emerges at 6 months
Infancy III: 6 to 9 months	Rotational patterns emerge; sits erect with hands free; re-erects self in sitting and comes to sitting independently; pivots on stomach; pulls to standing; crawls on stomach	One hand approach to objects; transfers objects; thumb begins to move toward forefinger	Protective extension forward in upper extremities begins (9 to 10 months); phasic bite develops to munching
Infancy IV: 10 to 12 months	Independent mobility by crawling (9 months), creeping (12 months), or walking (12 to 15 months); pivots on hips in sitting; walks holding onto furniture	Finer adjustment of digits; inferior-pincer grasp; pokes with forefinger; beginning of voluntary release and neat pincer grasp with slight extension of wrist (10 to 11 months)	Protective extension sidewards in upper extremities begins at 7 months; STNR disappears (8 to 12 months); tilting responses in sitting begin at 7 and 8 months

Oral/Motor	Speech and Language	Social/Behavioral
Embryological development of oral structures: lips, tongue, hard palate, soft palate, peripheral muscles		
Rooting reflex; gag reflex; sucking (flexor tone in neonate); suckling, phasic bite reflex; palmomental reflex; smooth coordination of suck, swallow, breathing	Birth cry; cry becomes longer; strong, rhythmical breathing	
Suckling, phasic bite reflex, palmomental reflex continue	Smiles; visually localizes speaker; breath stream lengthens; coos (vowel sounds); uses special cry for hunger	Regards face; eye contact; smiles
Suckling; cup-drinking; spoon-feeding begins; phasic bite reflex develops to munching	Controls breath stream; varies pitch; vocalizes vowel sounds (nonimitative); begins to babble (consonant sounds); responds to name	Laughs aloud; responds to talking
Sucking; cup-drinking continues; more refined spoon-feeding; chewing	Recognizes some familiar names; plays peek-a-boo, pat-a-cake; stops to "no"; gestures to some familiar words or requests (come, byebye, up); babbles imitatively; jargons	Differentiates family members; fearful of strangers
Sucking, cup-drinking, spoon-feeding, and chewing continue	Follows simple verbal requests (put that down); understands simple questions (where?); attends to speech; gestures appropriately; first words (mama, dada, byebye); jargons	Plays peek-a-boo and pat-a-cake

Source: Modified from Harvey-Smith, M., et al.: Feeding management of a child with a handicap: a guide for professionals, Memphis, 1982, University of Tennessee Center for the Health Sciences.

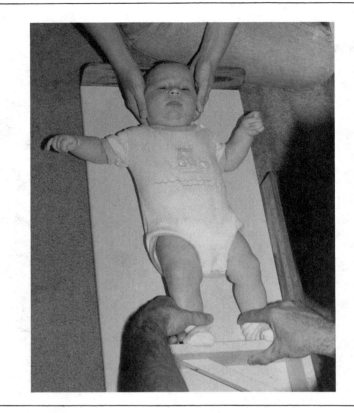

Figure 2-1
Care givers measure length of infant.

Measuring

The infant is measured using "recumbent" length (the child is lying down).* The standards until age 2 years are based on recumbent length, ideally measured on a table with an immovable head piece and movable foot piece. A measuring tape (preferably graduated in millimeters) runs along the table's length. The child is placed face up with the head brought against the head piece and is held there with gentle pressure. The head, shoulders, hips, and feet are oriented in a single line as they would be for a standing measurement. The knees are held flattened against the table, and the toes point upward. The movable board is brought against the bottom of the feet, heel touching board, with gentle pressure. Ideally, each measurement should be repeated at least three times with any necessary adjustments in body orientation. Immediate accurate recording of each of the three measurements is essential. The three measurements may then be averaged

* One measuring device is available from Ward Cabinet Works, 114 Maureen Dr., Hendersonville, TN 37075.

and recorded; in practice taking three measurements may not be possible.

Weight should be measured using a beam-balanced scale with nondetachable weights. As little clothing as possible should be worn; however, the same amount of clothing should be worn each month. For infants, scales weighing to the nearest gram are desirable. The balance of the scale should be checked before each weighing. An infant should be laid on the scale (if body size permits) or seated at the exact center of the scale [2, 3].

Individual charts for infants (for determining normal values) can aid in determining if the child is growing and developing at a satisfactory rate. These charts, shown in Figures 2–2 to 2–7, can be obtained from the National Center for Health Statistics (NCHS) or several drug companies.

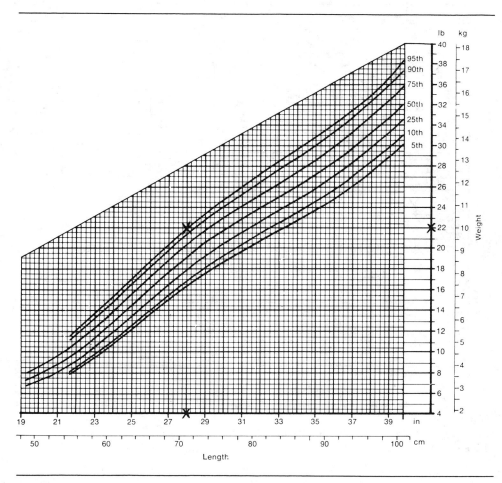

Figure 2–2
Girls' growth chart from birth to 36 months showing weight for length at 95th percentile (*Source:* U.S. Department of Health, Education and Welfare, National Center for Health Statistics, 1979.)

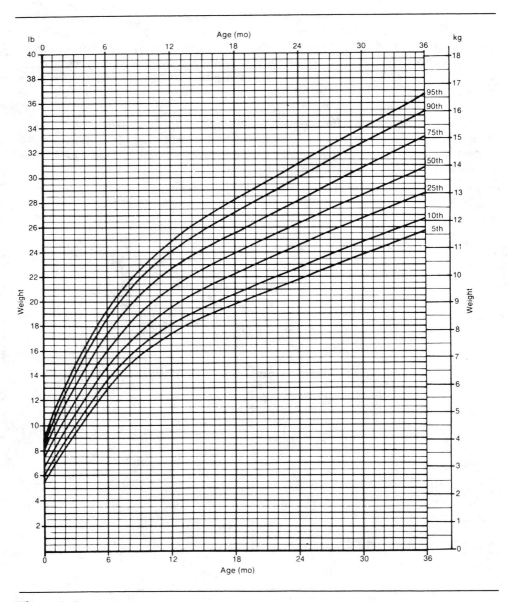

Figure 2–3
Girls' weight-for-age growth chart from birth to 36 months (*Source:* U.S. Department of Health, Education and Welfare, National Center for Health Statistics, 1979.)

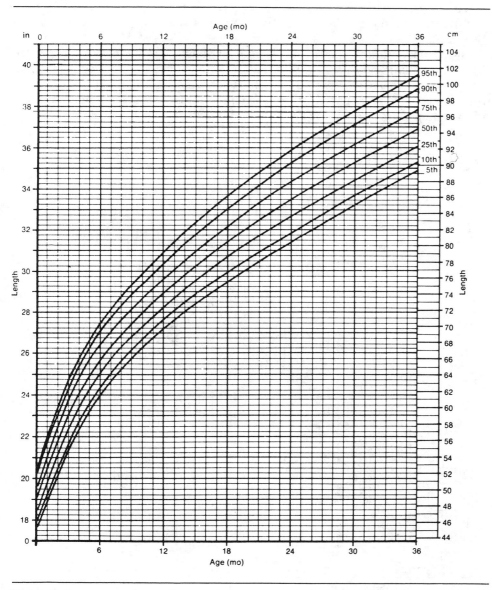

Figure 2–4
Girls' length-for-age growth chart from birth to 36 months (*Source:* U.S. Department of Health, Education and Welfare, National Center for Health Statistics, 1979.)

The charts are intended to record the growth of the individual child; they were constructed by the NCHS in collaboration with the Centers for Disease Control [2, 3]. The charts are based on data from the Fels Research Institute, Yellow Springs, Ohio. These data are appropriate for young girls and boys in the general U.S. population. Their use will direct attention to unusual body size, which may be a result of disease or poor nutrition. Height and weight charts can aid both the care giver and the parent in making minor adjustments in the dietary intake of the child. Girls' weight for length is charted in Figure 2–2, weight for age in

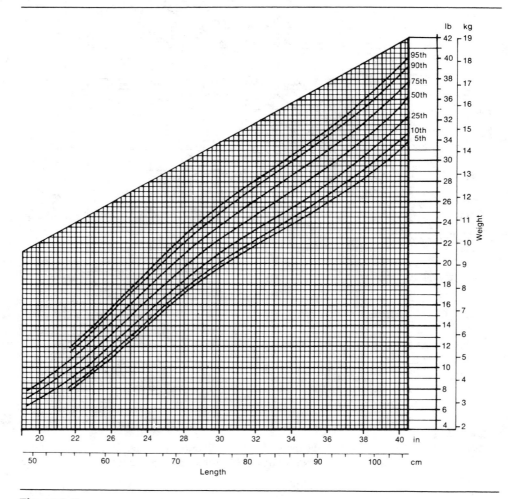

Figure 2–5
Boys' weight-for-length chart from birth to 36 months (*Source:* U.S. Department of Health, Education and Welfare, National Center for Health Statistics, 1979.)

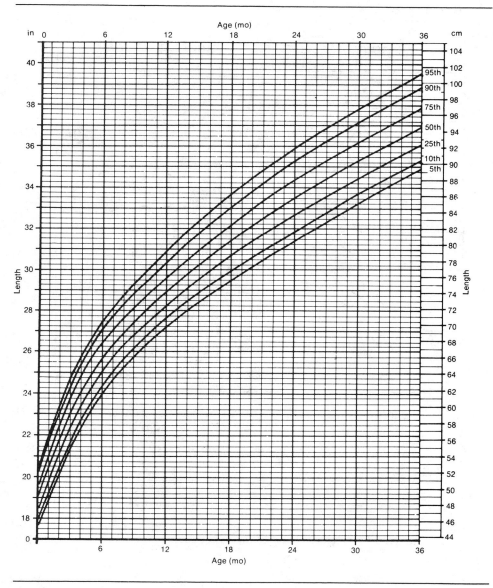

Figure 2-6
Boys' length-for-age growth chart from birth to 36 months (*Source:* Department of Health, Education and Welfare, National Center for Health Statistics, 1979.)

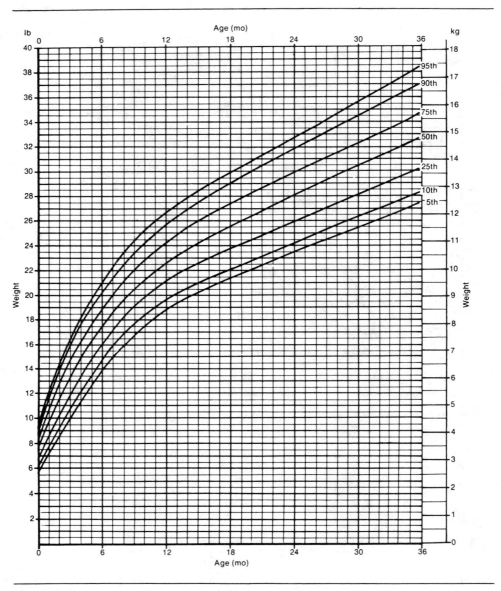

Figure 2-7
Boys' weight-for-age growth chart from birth to 36 months (*Source:* U.S. Department of Health, Education and Welfare, National Center for Health Statistics, 1979.)

Figure 2-3, and length for age in Figure 2-4. Similar charts for boys are found in Figures 2-5, 2-6, and 2-7.

Recording

First, take all measurements and record them. If three measurements are taken, the average should be plotted on the appropriate chart. For example, to plot a girl's length for age, find her age on the horizontal scale (Figure 2-4); then follow a vertical line from that point to the child's length measurement on the vertical scale. Indicate with a mark where the two lines intersect. In charting a boy's length for weight, find his length on the horizontal scale in Figure 2-5 and place a mark where the length crosses the weight on the vertical scale. When the child is measured again, join the new set of marks to the previous set by straight lines.

Interpreting

Many factors influence growth. Therefore, growth data alone must not be used to diagnose nutritional deficiencies, although they do allow you to identify unusual growth patterns in children. Each chart contains a series of curved lines, numbered to show selected percentiles. These refer to the rank of a measurement in a group of 100 children. If a child's weight is taken and a mark is placed on the 95th percentile of weight for age, it means, hypothetically, that only 5 children among 100 of the corresponding age and sex have weights greater than that recorded.

Practice taking lengths and weights, and inspect the set of marks you make. If any are particularly high or low (for example, above the 95th percentile or below the 5th percentile), you may want to check the accuracy and, if correct, refer the child for further evaluation. Compare the most recent set of marks with earlier sets for the same child. If the child's weight for height has jumped from one percentile level to another, you may also want to again check the accuracy of the measurements and discuss any changes with the parents before referring the child for further evaluation. Rapid changes are less likely to be significant when they occur within the range from the 25th to the 75th percentile. Measurements that fall between the 10th and 25th or 75th and 90th percentiles may be normal or abnormal and must be judged against previous and subsequent measurements and genetic and environmental factors that affect the infant.

Table 2-2 provides a quick reference of lengths and weights. If the child weighs more or less than indicated in the table, his or her measurements can be plotted on the length and weight charts to determine the individual child's pattern. The length and weight charts are more appropriate for regular use in the center over a long period.

The normal full-term infant gains more than an ounce a day between the eighth and forty-second day of life. A baby who weighed 8 pounds at birth could weigh between 11 and 12 pounds when brought to the center at 2 months of age. Weight gain can vary depending on many factors, including genetics. Short-statured

Table 2-2
Lengths and weights at 50th percentile for various ages

	Weight (pounds)		Length (inches)	
	Males	Females	Males	Females
Birth	7¼	7	20	19¾
1 month	9½	8¾	21½	21
3 months	13¼	12	24	23½
6 months	17¼	16	26¾	26
9 months	20¼	18¾	28½	27¾
12 months	22½	21	30	29¼

Source: National Center for Health Statistics, Health Resources Administration, DHEW, Hyattsville, MD, 1977. Data from the Fels Research Institute, Yellow Springs, OH.

parents are more likely to have a shorter child. Likewise, the premature infant, a child of multiple births (twins), and a low-birth-weight infant (birth weight of less than 2.5 kg or 5½ pounds) will generally be smaller. Consequently, it is important to note the child's family and medical history when a child enters your care in order to accurately interpret the results of the measurements.

An additional anthropometric measurement taken by health professionals is the skinfold thickness. Figure 2–8 shows the Lange Skinfold Caliper, which can be used to measure the amount of fat under the skin (subcutaneous fat). This measurement has been most widely used (1) in hospitals to determine the subcutaneous fat and nutritional status of a patient having surgery, (2) to monitor obesity in a clinical setting, and (3) in controlled research studies. We are not advocating the wide use of this instrument by every care giver. When a child has height and weight measurements that appear to need further evaluation, the dietitian or pediatrician will be able to provide additional information using the skinfold calipers. The care giver should understand the skinfold measurement as an additional tool to help evaluate the young child's total growth and development.

The use of skinfold thickness in the assessment of nutritional status of children is based on the assumption that increased subcutaneous fat, resulting from either high calorie intake or low energy expenditure, reflects a greater calorie reserve [4]. Measurement of skinfold thickness can provide an indirect estimate of body fat and may be used to screen children who are overweight or underweight. Along with length and weight, skinfold thickness should be taken at regular intervals during routine health checks by trained staff or when the child visits the health center.

Laboratory Measurements

Measurements of hemoglobin and hematocrit are laboratory procedures that provide yet another index of nutritional status. *Hemoglobin* is the iron-containing

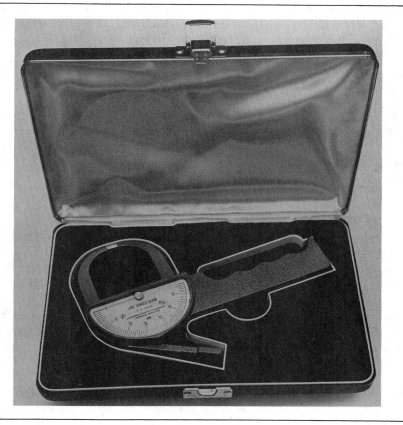

Figure 2–8
Lange Skinfold Caliper (Cambridge Scientific Industries, P.O. Box 265, Cambridge, MD 21613.)

protein in red blood cells and provides the bright red color. *Hematocrit* is a measure of the packed red blood cells after separating the solids from the plasma in the blood. When the red blood cells are few in number or are of poor quality, *anemia* is diagnosed. If the child has iron-deficiency anemia, the red blood cells will be small and light in color (indicating less hemoglobin) and will carry less oxygen than normal red blood cells.

Measurements of hemoglobin or hematrocrit are often taken to determine nutritional risk factors for children in programs such as the Supplemental Food Program for Women, Infants and Children [5]. The first assessments are usually taken after children reach 6 months of age. For the 6- to 12-month-old infant the acceptable hematocrit value is 31%, and the acceptable hemoglobin level is 10 g/100 ml [6].

It should be emphasized that abnormal data from any one measure alone are not indicative of malnutrition but must be coupled with other medical, laboratory, and dietary indexes before the parents or care giver become alarmed.

BREAST-FEEDING OR BOTTLE-FEEDING

The nutritional needs of infants from birth to at least 4 months of age are unique, are well-documented, and can be met with breast milk or iron-fortified infant formulas. The care giver makes few decisions regarding the kind and amount of food to give the young infant. These decisions have already been made by the parents with the pediatrician.

Breast-feeding

The incidence of breast-feeding in hospitals (Figure 2–9) has increased from slightly more than 50% in 1980 [7] to about 58% in 1987 [8]. A revival of interest in breast-feeding began in the early 1970s, and both incidence and length of breast-feeding increased substantially between 1971 and 1982. During this period, the use of whole cow's milk and evaporated milk as well as prepared infant formulas decreased. Since then, the increase in breast-feeding has leveled off to approximately 56%. Continued increases will depend on raising breast-feeding levels in those groups who currently show the lowest incidence of breast-feeding: blacks, mothers younger than 20 years of age, and lower-income families [7].

Advantages of Breast-feeding. Human milk is the most appropriate nutrient supply for human infants and also gives significant immunological protection against infection. Infants who are breast-fed have a lower incidence of infection and require fewer hospitalizations than infants who are fed formula exclusively [9].

Breast-feeding should become the established norm. Nursing for only a few weeks or months is better than not nursing at all. The positive factors usually given by medical professionals [10] should also be stressed by the care giver:

- Nutritional superiority and easy digestibility
- Lower incidence of infection, illness, and allergy in breast-fed infants due to the bacteriologic safety of breast milk and the presence of immunologic components
- Opportunity for optimum mother-infant physical contact and bonding
- Likelihood of a more rapid uterine involution due to oxytocin secretion
- Likelihood for the mother to return to prepregnant weight within 2 to 6 months if maternal fat stores are used to supply part of the caloric needs for breast-feeding

Limitations of Breast-feeding. Although we strongly advocate breast-feeding, a few of the commonly described complaints are [11]:

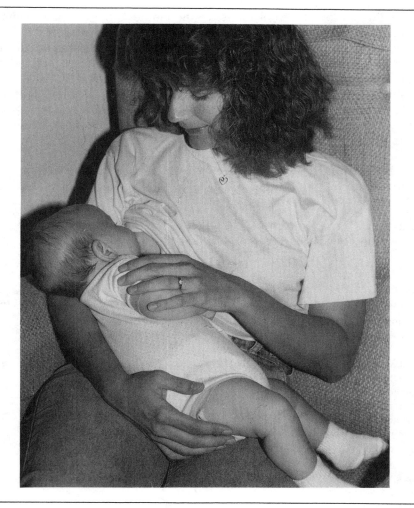

Figure 2–9
Mother breastfeeds infant.

- More frequent feedings during first week
- Milk leakage from the breasts
- Enlarged breasts
- More gradual weight loss
- Less rest for mother during first weeks
- Less opportunity for fathers (or other family members) to participate in feeding the infant
- A softer and more frequent infant stool

Depending on the choice of foods for the mother's diet, breast-feeding may or may not be more costly than bottle-feeding. Table 2–3 compares the daily cost of bottle-feeding to the cost of supplemental food choices for the nursing mother. A mother needs between 500 and 1000 additional calories and additional nutrients to meet the RDA for lactating women. Both diets in Table 2–3 provide sufficient energy, but only diet A provides all necessary nutrients (supplemental foods are in addition to a diet that meets the RDA for a nonpregnant adult woman). When legumes are substituted for meat the cost is similar to bottle-feeding.

Storing Breast Milk. Working women may pump their breasts in order to leave milk with their child at the center. The milk can be collected in containers and,

Table 2–3
Comparison of costs per day of breast-feeding and bottle-feeding

Additional Foods for Lactating Women			
Diet A (630 kcal)* Food and Quantities	Cost/Day	Diet B (500 kcal)† Food and Quantities	Cost/Day
Whole milk, 2 C (total 4 C)	$0.45	Milk, 2% (additional 4 C)	$0.90
Meat, 2 oz	0.45		
Vegetables, dark green or deep yellow, 1 serving	0.32	TOTAL	$0.90
Citrus fruit or other good sources of vitamin C, 1 serving	0.25		
Other fruit or vegetable, 1 serving	0.20		
Whole-grain bread or cereal, 1 serving	0.04		
TOTAL	$1.71		

Commercially Prepared Formulas and Basic Equipment	
Item	Cost/Day
All formulas, double strength, 13 oz can	$1.22
Unbreakable bottles (12 @ $0.89 each)	0.07
Nipples (12 @ 2 for $0.99)	0.04
Liners (12 @ 125 for $3.99)	0.18
TOTAL	$1.51

*Meets RDA for breast-feeding woman.
†Does not meet RDA for breast-feeding woman.

if refrigerated, safely used within 24 hours [10]. Breast milk may be frozen for longer periods; however, freezing and thawing can destroy its cellular structure. If freezing the milk, do so immediately after hand or mechanical expression into a container (such as a disposable bottle liner). Before use, place the frozen milk in the refrigerator for several hours to thaw, or defrost milk in a microwave using only the defrost setting. After thawing, do not refreeze. The thawed milk may need to be mixed to distribute the cream. Check to be sure that milk warmed in the microwave is not too hot.

Center Assistance for Breast-feeding Mothers. The center staff can assist the mother in breast-feeding the youngster by verbally reassuring the mother of their support for her effort. Specifically, the center can:

1. Provide a room or screen a portion of a room for working mothers to feed infants during their breaks.
2. Provide refrigerator space for hand or mechanically expressed milk so the infant can be fed during the day if mother is not available.
3. Provide literature and referrals for the mother; for example, topics might include techniques of maintaining milk supply, resources for using or renting breast pumps, names of other breast-feeding mothers. (See Appendix 2–A for sources of educational materials.)
4. Encourage the mother not to begin using pacifiers or supplemental bottles unless a feeding pattern has been established. Bottle-feeding may cause nipple confusion and decrease milk supply [12].
5. Refer low-income families at nutritional risk to the Special Supplemental Food Program for Women, Infants and Children (for more information, see Appendix 2–B).

Bottle-feeding

The bottle-fed baby should be held closely when feeding, and a close relationship should be established between parent and infant (Figure 2–10). Any signal that the bottle-fed baby is satisfied with the quantity of formula given should cause the care giver or parent to stop feeding even if only 1 ounce (30 ml) of formula remains in the bottle. Forcing the last ounce into baby may set the pattern for overeating for the toddler, preschooler, and adult. This can be associated with "cleaning your plate" or forcing the last bite of mashed potatoes; consequently, patterns leading to obesity may develop.

Formula. If formula is to be used, an iron-fortified commercially prepared formula is the complete food for the infant. Iron-fortified formulas contain vitamins and iron; therefore, no supplements are necessary. If fluoride is not available in the water supply, supplemental fluoride should be given. Most formulas come in ready-to-serve, concentrated, or powdered form. We believe what is probably the most important thing for care givers to remember when bottle-feeding is to

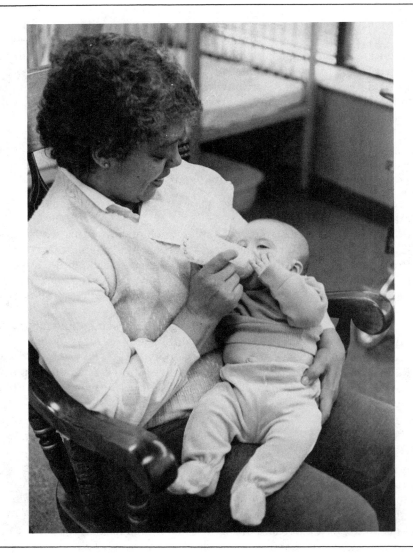

Figure 2-10
Care giver holds infant close while bottle-feeding.

always hold the baby close to the body and focus attention on the child. Feeding should provide not only food but a feeling of security and love. There should be no "propped" bottles in the center!

After 3 months of age relatively few infants consume more than 6 ounces (180 ml) of formula per kilogram of body weight per day (3 ounces or less per

Table 2-4
Recommended dietary allowances for infant

Nutrient	0 to 6 Months*	6 to 12 months†
Food energy (kcal)	kg × 115	kg × 105
	(lb × 52.3)	(lb × 47.7)
Protein (g)	kg × 2.2	kg × 2.0
Vitamin A activity (IU)	1400	2000
Vitamin D (IU)	400	400
Vitamin E activity (IU)	4	5
Ascorbic acid (mg)	35	35
Folacin (μg)	30	45
Niacin (mg)	6	8
Riboflavin (mg)	0.4	0.6
Thiamin (mg)	0.3	0.5
Vitamin B$_6$ (mg)	0.3	0.6
Vitamin B$_{12}$ (μg)	0.5	1.5
Calcium (mg)	360	540
Phosphorus (mg)	240	360
Iodine (μg)	40	50
Iron (mg)	10	15
Magnesium (mg)	50	70
Zinc (mg)	3	5

Source: Based on Food and Nutrition Board, National Academy of Sciences—National Research Council: Recommended Dietary Allowances, revised 1980.

*Weight 6 kg (14 lb), height 60 cm (24 in.).

†Weight 9 kg (20 lb), height 71 cm (28 in.).

pound per day). For an 11-pound (4.95 kg) baby the quantity might be 32 ounces (1 quart; 960 ml) of formula per 24-hour period. Generally, 26 to 32 ounces of formula will satisfy infants during the first 4 months of life. However, if the child is bottle-fed at 6 months of age and doesn't eat solid foods, 32 ounces or more of formula may be necessary to meet the child's energy needs. A 14- to 15-pound (6.3 to 6.75 kg) baby will need more than 700 kcal or 1 quart of formula per day. The child younger than 6 months of age needs approximately 52 kcal per pound of body weight. Table 2-4 provides formulas for calculating daily energy and protein needs and lists recommended allowances of vitamins and minerals.

Formula for most infants supplies 20 kcal per ounce, and 32 ounces of formula supplies 640 kcal (20 kcal per ounce × 32 ounces). By the time the child weighs 15 pounds, without supplemental foods he or she would need 39 ounces (1170 ml) of formula to meet the energy allowance (15 pounds × 52.3 kcal per pound = 784 kcal). The American Academy of Pediatrics recommends that the amount of formula or cow's milk should be limited to less than 1 L (33.8 fl oz) or about 1 quart per day [13]. When calorie needs reach over 640 kcal, supplemental food should be provided to increase the calories to recommended levels.

Table 2-5
Composition of milk and infant formulas

| Name of Product | Energy Contribution | | | Comments (commercial source) |
	Carbohydrate (%)	Protein (%)	Fat (%)	
Human milk	39	6	30 to 55	Breast milk
Whole milk	30	21	49	3.5% fat; pasteurized
2% low-fat milk	38	27	35	2% nonfat milk solids added; 2% fat; pasteurized (not recommended)
Skim milk	57	38	5	0.1% fat; pasteurized (not recommended)
Goat's milk	26	20	54	
Advance	40	15	45	Milk-based formula for older infants with cow's milk and soy protein isolate, corn and soy oils, corn syrup, lactose, vitamins, and minerals (Ross)
Enfamil	41	9	50	Cow's milk and whey, soy and coconut oils, lactose, vitamins, minerals; also available with iron (Mead Johnson)
Isomil	40	12	48	Milk-free formula made with soy protein isolate, coconut and soy oils, corn syrup, sucrose, vitamins, minerals; for milk-sensitive infants; also available without sucrose (Ross)
Lofenalac	50	15	35	Low phenylalanine product for infants and children with phenylketonuria; chemically treated casein hydrolysates to remove phenylalanine and supplements of methionine, tryptophan, and tyrosine; added corn oil, mixed carbohydrates, vitamins, minerals (Mead Johnson)

Table 2–5
continued

Name of Product	Energy Contribution			Comments (commercial source)
	Carbohydrate (%)	Protein (%)	Fat (%)	
Meat base (MBF)	38	16	46	Hypoallergenic formula for infants sensitive to milk; made with meat protein (beef heart), sesame oil, sucrose, vitamins, minerals (Gerber)
Nursoy	40	12	48	Soy protein isolate, oleo, coconut, oleic, safflower, and soy oils, sucrose, vitamins, minerals (Wyeth)
Nutramigen	52	13	34	Milk-free, casein hydrolysate formula with corn oil, sucrose, modified tapioca starch, vitamins, minerals (Mead Johnson)
Pregestimil	53	11	36	Milk-free casein hydrolysate formula with corn and MCT oils, corn syrup solids, modified tapioca starch, vitamins, minerals (Mead Johnson)
Prosobee	40	12	48	Milk-free formula with soy isolate, coconut and soy oils, corn syrup solids, vitamins, minerals (Mead Johnson)
Similac	43	9	48	Cow's milk with corn and soy oils, lactose, vitamins, minerals; available with or without iron (Ross)
Similac PM 60/40	41	9	50	Whey and casein protein, corn and coconut oils, lactose, minerals, vitamins, 60% lactalbumin and 40% casein in protein, vitamins, minerals (Ross)

(continued)

Table 2-5
continued

Name of Product	Energy Contribution			Comments (commercial source)
	Carbohydrate (%)	Protein (%)	Fat (%)	
S-M-A	43	9	48	Cow's milk formula with whey, oleo, coconut, oleic, safflower, and soy oils, lactose, vitamins, minerals; available with or without iron (Wyeth)
iSoyalac	39	12	49	Milk-free formula with soy isolate, soy oil, sucrose, tapioca dextrins, vitamins, minerals (Loma Linda)
Soyalac	39	12	49	Milk-free formula with soybean solids, soy oil, corn syrup, sucrose, vitamins, minerals (Loma Linda)

Sources: Data on human milk from Composition of foods, Agriculture Handbook No. 8-1., U.S. Department of Agriculture, Agricultural Research Service, revised 1976, item 170.01-107; data on whole, 2%, and skim milk from NDDA Laboratory, Southern Illinois, University at Carbondale, 1980; data on formula composition from information provided by formula companies, May 1988.

A wide variety of formulas are available on the market. The composition of these formulas is given in Table 2-5. Some formulas have a specific purpose, and this table can be used by the care giver to compare each formula to human milk and to cow's milk.

Whole Cow's Milk. "Undiluted" whole cow's milk is not an acceptable alternative to human milk as long as milk or formula supplies the major source of calories. Protein content of cow's milk is above the acceptable range, and the carbohydrate content is lower than in commercially prepared formulas or breast milk. The amount of fat is consistently high in cow's milk, whereas the fat content of breast milk increases as nursing continues. Breast milk is lower in fat content when nursing begins and higher at the end of the breast-feeding period. Evaporated milk, modified only by dilution with water, has the same characteristics as whole milk.

The low-income, high-risk infant should be given iron-fortified formula as the most reliable source of calories and iron until 1 year of age. For the diets of other infants we agree with the American Academy of Pediatrics [13], which has stated,

"Although many mothers will continue to breast-feed or formula-feed their babies through the first year of life, there is at present no convincing evidence from well-designed research studies that feeding whole cow's milk after 6 months of age is harmful if adequate supplementary feedings are given." On the basis of knowledge of the types of solid foods commonly given to infants and the composition of these foods, it has been reported that the protein, fat, and carbohydrate content of the diet will probably remain within desirable limits if the transition to whole cow's milk is made after the infant is consuming the equivalent of at least 1½ jars of strained foods (about ¾ cup) daily. If whole cow's milk and strained foods are used, the infant will probably not be receiving adequate iron (see "Supplementation").

Skim and Low-Fat Milks. Skim and low-fat milks are unacceptable alternatives to human milk during infancy. Skim milk provides 38% of calories from protein and 5% from fat, and "2 percent" milk provides 27% of calories from protein and 35% from fat. Thus, both are too high in protein, and skim milk is too low in fat in comparison with prepared formulas or human milk (6% to 16% protein, 30% to 55% fat).

Infants fed skim milk as the main source of calories generally are not able to consume the daily energy allowance and probably have to mobilize stores of body fat to meet energy needs. This is potentially dangerous, since it depletes energy reserves and any illness that interferes more than briefly with food intake may become life threatening.

Preparation of Formulas. It is important in the infant center to remind care givers of the proper method to be used in preparation of all formulas. Sterile water should be used during the first months even if the parent has discontinued such practices at home. If either a powdered or concentrated formula is used, sterile water will be needed. Proper sterilization techniques for bottles are included in Appendix V. Preparation of single feedings may be preferable to preparation of all feedings for a 24-hour period. It is advisable in a center with only a few infants to purchase sterile water and/or disposable bottles of ready-to-feed formula for use during the first 2 to 3 months of life to ensure the child's safety. Often powdered formulas are convenient if the infant is at the center for a short time. It is best for the formula to be used in the 24 hours following preparation (Chapter 6). Breast-fed babies should have a supply of mother's milk in the freezer in case of emergency or to be used when the mother is delayed in returning to the center.

Supplementation

The American Academy of Pediatrics [14] recommends that during the first few months of life, the breast-fed infant receive supplementation of iron, vitamin D, and fluoride, if the child is not taking fluoridated water. Parents and care givers may initially react adversely to the recommendation to supplement diets of breast-fed infants since they believe that human milk is a complete and ideal food for the infant. Fomon [15] has discussed several explanations for the failure of human milk to meet certain nutritional needs of infants under living conditions prevailing in industrialized countries. Supplementation of specific nutrients serves the best interests of both mother and infant.

Breast milk and cow's milk contain little iron, but the iron is very well absorbed from breast milk. At least one study suggested that the iron in breast milk is sufficient to meet the needs of an infant who is *exclusively* breast-fed until tripling birthweight, at about 1 year of age [16]. However, the American Academy of Pediatrics [17] recommends that *all* infants receive iron supplementation by 4 months of age (term infants) or 2 months of age (preterm infants).

Iron-fortified infant formula is recommended for infants as an alternate and predictable source of iron in place of an iron supplement. If the infant is fed a commercial formula without supplemental iron, or is fed a "homemade" formula made from fresh or evaporated milk, supplemental iron should be used.

Once a child has started eating solids, iron-fortified cereal can provide an excellent source of iron. One-half cup of iron-fortified dry cereal will provide over 50% of the recommended amount of iron. Mothers generally feel more comfortable feeding infant cereals than providing medicinal iron.

Gastrointestinal disturbances such as diarrhea or constipation and certain feeding problems have been attributed to formulas containing iron. There is little evidence, however, that this is a significant problem.

Although the RDA for specific nutrients is presented in Table 2-4 the care giver need worry little about the acquisition of specific nutrients by infants who are breast- or bottle-fed with iron-fortified formula. In summary, by 4 months of age children should be receiving:

Breast milk with vitamin D and iron supplements; or
Iron-fortified formula only (supplements already added to formula); or
Formula (non-iron-fortified) with addition of iron-fortified infant cereal; or
Breast milk with iron-fortified infant cereal and vitamin D supplement; and
Fluoride if (1) water is not given infants who are breast-feeding; (2) fluoridated water is not used for dilution of concentrated formula; or (3) ready-to-feed formula is used without additional water from a fluoridated supply.

The use of iron-fortified formula or cereal is recommended during the first 12 to 18 months of life.

SOLID FOODS

Currently there is a debate over the introduction of solid foods before the age of 6 months. Years ago mothers were told that they might introduce cereals at the first or second week or even the second day of life. This theory has now given way to the introduction of solid foods at a later time—4 to even 6 months. Most parents are providing their infants with some solid foods at approximately 4 months of age. It is probably better if this food is limited to iron-fortified infant cereal. If formula or cow's milk is limited to 1 quart (0.96 L) per day, when solid foods are introduced depends more on the weight of the baby than on an arbitrary age of 4 or 6 months.

By the age of 4 months some infants are physiologically capable of accepting foods from a spoon and transferring them from the front of the mouth to the back for swallowing. Some children at this time will be able to sit in a high chair or baby seat and lean forward with mouth open indicating a need or desire to eat. Turning the head, closing the mouth, and pushing food away should be signals to you that the infant is satisfied (Figure 2–11). Thus, the infant now has some control over how much is consumed. The parent or care giver who is responsive to the child's needs should stop feeding when the baby is satisfied and thereby prevent the possibility of overfeeding and obesity.

When introducing solid foods, parents often wonder what dietary restrictions, now advocated for good health, they should apply to their children's diets.

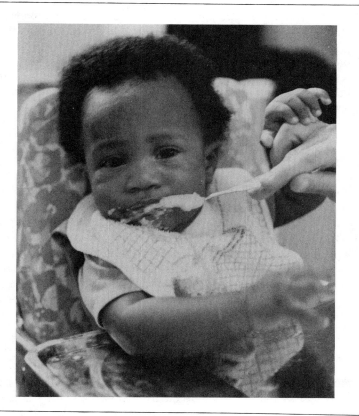

Figure 2–11
Baby signals care giver to stop feeding.

However, much of the nutrition information for adults is not appropriate for infants. These following guidelines developed by Gerber are consistent with the positions of the American Academy of Pediatrics, Committee on Nutrition, and the American Dietetic Association. A good overview of points to remember when feeding infants, the guidelines can be used by care givers and parents to safeguard infants from overly restrictive diets.

- Build to a variety of foods.
- Listen to your baby's appetite to avoid over-feeding or under-feeding.
- Don't restrict fat and cholesterol too much.
- Don't overdo high-fiber foods.
- Sugar is okay, but in moderation.
- Sodium is okay, but in moderation.
- Babies need more iron, pound for pound than adults.*

Infant Feeders

For a child with normal development, cereals and other pureed foods should never be put through a bottle with a large opening or into an infant feeder. In essence, this is force feeding. Unfortunately this type of feeding is usually provided by overanxious parents of young infants whose needs would be met by formula or breast milk alone. The extra energy provided by foods may lead to excessive weight gain. Parents who are using bottles with large holes in the nipple or infant feeders should be discouraged from such practice.

How Much Food?

Table 2–6 provides a guide to the amount of foods for infants, with the energy contribution of each item. In this case small amounts of cereal were added when formula intake reached 32 ounces (960 ml).

Table 2–7 illustrates the nutrient needs and food intake of one 5-month-old infant. The total energy in the diet (733 kcal) slightly exceeds the recommended level (732 kcal) for this child's body weight. Formula provides most of the calories and protein, which in this case is several grams higher than recommended. Note that single-grained infant cereal (rice) is used. High-protein cereal is unnecessary when infants are taking formula. Usually high-protein cereals are more costly to purchase and add unnecessary protein to the child's diet.

First Finger Foods

At 6 to 7 months the infant will also enjoy finger foods and will be eager to self-feed. Acceptable finger foods include hard toast (whole wheat), grapefruit and

---

* Dietary guidelines for infants were developed by Gerber Products Company and based on American Academy of Pediatrics, Committee on Nutrition, 1989.

Table 2-6
Guide to amounts of foods for infants

Age (months)	Weight	Foods*	Energy (kcal)
Up to 1	Up to 9 lb (9 lb × 52 kcal/lb = 468 kcal)	23 fl oz formula	460
2 to 3	Up to 12 lb (12 lb × 52 kcal/lb = 624 kcal)	32 fl oz iron-fortified formula	640
4 to 5	Up to 14 lb (14 lb × 52 kcal/lb = 728 kcal)	32 fl oz iron-fortified formula 8 tbsp dry baby cereal	640 83 ___ 723
6 to 7	Up to 16 lb (16 lb × 48 kcal/lb = 768 kcal)	32 fl oz iron-fortified formula 6 tbsp dry baby cereal 4 fl oz baby fruit juice 5 tbsp baby vegetables	640 62 56 15 ___ 773
8 to 9	Up to 18½ lb (18½ lb × 48 kcal/lb = 888 kcal)	32 fl oz iron-fortified formula 6 tbsp dry baby cereal 4 fl oz baby fruit juice 7 tbsp baby vegetables 6 tbsp baby fruit 3 tbsp baby meat, cooked legumes, or tofu	640 62 56 23 61 47 ___ 889
10 to 11	Up to 20 lb (20 lb × 48 kcal/lb = 960 kcal)	32 fl oz iron-fortified formula 8 tbsp dry baby cereal 4 fl oz fruit juice 8 tbsp vegetables 8 tbsp fruit 1 oz meat or equivalent meat alternate	640 83 56 24 76 75 ___ 954
12	Up to 22½ lb (22½ lb × 48 kcal/lb = 1080 kcal)	32 fl oz formula 8 tbsp dry baby cereal 6 fl oz fruit juice 10 tbsp vegetables 8 tbsp fruit 2 oz meat or equivalent	640 83 84 30 76 150 ___ 1063

*Because variation in individual recipes creates difficulties in calculating calorie content of homemade foods, commercial foods were used. "Table foods" should begin around 6 months of age. This guide may be used in screening dietary intakes of infants to help identify those with very excessive intakes. Activity levels can make a big difference in requirements, and a healthy infant may eat more or less. The infant who consumes more milk may need less of other foods. Use the table as a guide, not a rule!

Table 2-7
Nutritional needs and diet for 5-month-old infant (weight 6.4 kg (14 lb); height 26 in.)

Nutritional Needs

Requirements

Calories	732 kcal (kg × 115 kcal or lb × 52.3 kcal)
Protein	14 g (kg × 2.2 g)
Iron	10 mg

Food intake provides

Infant Food	Amount	Energy	Protein	Iron
Cereal*	9 tbsp dry	93 kcal	2.0 g	11.5 mg
Formula†	32 oz	640 kcal	14.7 g	12.0 mg
TOTAL		733 kcal	16.7	23.5 mg

Food Pattern for 5-Month-Old Infant

Time	Food	Amount
7:00 AM	Formula	8 oz
7:30 AM	Cereal with formula	5 tbsp + 3 oz formula
11:30 AM	Formula	6 oz
3:00 PM	Formula	2 oz
6:00 PM	Cereal with formula	4 tbsp dry + 2 oz formula
	Formula	6 oz
10:00 PM	Formula	5 oz

Source: Calculations from NDDA Laboratory, Southern Illinois University at Carbondale.
*Nutrient values for rice.
†Infant formula provides 20 kcal/oz standard dilution.

orange sections, other cooked fruits and vegetables, corn bread, whole wheat crackers, and bite-size pieces of soft cheese. Experiment, and do not overcook vegetables and fruit. The food should remain as a vegetable or fruit "stick" and not "melt" in the child's mouth. Young children when hungry will try a variety of cooked foods such as carrots, green beans, and cooked dried beans; even strong-flavored vegetables—turnips, broccoli, cabbage, and cauliflower—are enjoyed by young children. Often children will eat these foods warm or cold. Before the meal, when the infant is particularly hungry, try placing a stick of cooked vegetable, warm or cold, on the child's tray instead of crackers or bread. You may be surprised to find that the child readily accepts these foods.

Fresh blackberries and strawberries, as well as more common fruits such as oranges, grapefruits, peaches, pears, and apricots, are all acceptable and provide the child with a variety of tastes. The most important point is that variety introduced now will set the pattern for food habits throughout life.

THE CUP

The child can approximate lips to the rim of a cup by 5 months and can begin drinking from the cup by 6 months. No more than 2 to 3 tablespoons should be put in the cup when the baby is learning to drink. Two tablespoons are much easier to clean up from the floor than 4 ounces. A refill is also more rewarding for the child and the care giver or parent.

EATING WITH UTENSILS

At about 8 to 10 months of age, baby will be interested in using a spoon for feeding. Use a spoon with a flat, wide bowl for easier scooping; a dish with sides also makes scooping easier. Remember to be prepared for spills and messes that accompany the first attempts at self-feeding. It is best to place a vinyl or plastic cloth underneath the high chair or to spread papers on the floor. At 6 to 8 months, when baby is learning to experiment with foods, give the child every opportunity to learn about foods and how to eat them. These exciting learning experiences are expressions of independence and should certainly be encouraged and enjoyed. Try to understand and even see some humor in the sweet potatoes on the nose, chin, and hair. Adopting the child's perspective rather than an adult's helps make the experience tolerable and even enjoyable.

EVALUATING THE DIET

Until this point you have had an opportunity to examine some of the measures related to nutritional status as well as to examine the food needs of the very young child. The following exercise will assist you in evaluating an infant's diet. Table 2–8 is an example of a child's diet. After studying the diet, exercise and the height and weight information given in the text, write comments about the diet.

Table 2–8
Dietary intake for 9-month-old child

Food	Amount	Food	Amount
Breakfast		*3:00 PM*	
Infant cereal	3 tbsp	Whole milk	½ C
Applesauce	¼ C	Oatmeal cookie	1
10:00 AM		*5:30 PM*	
Whole milk from a bottle	1 C	Strained peas	1 jar
12:00 noon		Junior* vegetables and ham	1 jar
		Whole milk	½ C
Strained vegetables and chicken	1 jar	Oatmeal cookie	1
Mashed potatoes and gravy	½ C	*8:00 PM (bedtime)*	
Whole milk from a bottle	1 C	Ice cream	½ C

*Commercially prepared baby foods can be purchased either as "strained," which are pureed, or "junior," which are finely chopped and require a little chewing.

The diet is that of a girl, 9 months of age, weighing 8 pounds (3.6 kg) at birth, who weighs 22 pounds (9.9 kg) and measures 28 inches (70 cm) for length. When plotted on the girls' [weight-for-length] chart (Figure 2-2), her measurements fall on the 95th percentile. The length for age is on the 50th percentile, and weight for age is on the 95th percentile. With the available data from the past 9 months, one may become concerned about the child's weight gain.

Look first at the nutritional content of the diet (you may wish to refer to Appendix I). The child is consuming 3 cups of milk with the addition of a small amount of ice cream. As noted in Chapter 1, this supplies the calcium and protein for the diet. However, the milk is whole milk fortified with vitamins A and D but not with iron or vitamin C, which the child requires at this age. A further look at the diet indicates that the child is consuming no food sources high in vitamin C, although potatoes and strained mixed foods will contribute some vitamin C to the diet. Citrus fruits or fortified fruit juices contain the largest amounts of vitamin C, and they are absent.

The infant cereal probably supplies iron for the day. The diet is excessive in energy, providing 55 kcal per pound of body weight. As noted in Table 2-6, the recommended amount is 105 kcal per kilogram or 48 per pound. Figure 2-12 is the computer printout from this diet analysis. Note that four nutrients were consumed in amounts less than 66% of the RDA. This is a result of discontinuation of formula and absence of whole-grain cereals, vegetable oils, fruits, and vegetables.

Probably more distressing than the nutritional content of this diet is the kind of food being offered to the child. The care giver should note that the child is receiving cookies and mixtures of strained foods such as vegetables and ham or vegetables and chicken. These foods are not enhancing the child's learning experiences but provide excessive energy when compared with the nutritional value. This diet contains no meats other than those found in combination foods. This is not of concern, since the amount of protein received is 47 g. Milk alone supplies 24 g of the 20 g recommended (using the formula given in Table 2-4: 10 kg × 2.0 g protein).

An additional factor to be considered is the few foods, including fruits and vegetables, that require chewing. Although it is obvious that the child has the ability to chew (she chews the oatmeal cookie), the opportunity is not provided with mashed potatoes, applesauce, and junior and strained foods. For a child 9 months of age, it would be wise for the parent or care giver to plan the meal so that most, if not all, of the solid foods are table foods—whole-grain cereals, cooked vegetables and fruits, and soft meats (possibly ground).

ROLES OF CENTER AND FAMILY

An infant's first experience with the parent and care giver revolves around feeding. Family experiences are a result of cultural and religious influences as well as the physical environment. Many practices cannot and should not be

```
TOTAL           NUTRIENT  RDA(%) 0%        20%   33% 40%       60% 66%    80%       100%
---------------------------I---------I-----I---I---------I--I------I---------I
1214.6 KCAL ENERGY      116 XXXXXXXXXXXXXXXXXXXXXXXXXXXXXXXXXXXXXXXXXXXXXXXXXX
  43.6 g    PROTEIN     218 XXXXXXXXXXXXXXXXXXXXXXXXXXXXXXXXXXXXXXXXXXXXXXXXXX
5732.9 IU   VITAMIN A   287 XXXXXXXXXXXXXXXXXXXXXXXXXXXXXXXXXXXXXXXXXXXXXXXXXX
 300.1 IU   VITAMIN D    75 XXXXXXXXXXXXXXXXXXXXXXXXXXXXXXXXXXXXX
   1.4 IU   VITAMIN E    28 XXXXXXXXXXXXXX
  20.6 mg   VITAMIN C    59 XXXXXXXXXXXXXXXXXXXXXXXXXXXXX
  64.0 µg   FOLACIN     142 XXXXXXXXXXXXXXXXXXXXXXXXXXXXXXXXXXXXXXXXXXXXXXXXXX
   4.8 mg   NIACIN       60 XXXXXXXXXXXXXXXXXXXXXXXXXXXXXX
   1.8 mg   RIBOFLAVIN  295 XXXXXXXXXXXXXXXXXXXXXXXXXXXXXXXXXXXXXXXXXXXXXXXXXX
   0.7 mg   THIAMIN     139 XXXXXXXXXXXXXXXXXXXXXXXXXXXXXXXXXXXXXXXXXXXXXXXXXX
   0.5 mg   VITAMIN B6   86 XXXXXXXXXXXXXXXXXXXXXXXXXXXXXXXXXXXXXXXXXXX
   3.2 µg   VITAMIN B12 216 XXXXXXXXXXXXXXXXXXXXXXXXXXXXXXXXXXXXXXXXXXXXXXXXXX
1134.8 mg   CALCIUM     210 XXXXXXXXXXXXXXXXXXXXXXXXXXXXXXXXXXXXXXXXXXXXXXXXXX
1010.9 mg   PHOSPHORUS  281 XXXXXXXXXXXXXXXXXXXXXXXXXXXXXXXXXXXXXXXXXXXXXXXXXX
   7.6 mg   IRON         50 XXXXXXXXXXXXXXXXXXXXXXXXX
 107.8 mg   MAGNESIUM   154 XXXXXXXXXXXXXXXXXXXXXXXXXXXXXXXXXXXXXXXXXXXXXXXXXX
   5.9 mg   ZINC        118 XXXXXXXXXXXXXXXXXXXXXXXXXXXXXXXXXXXXXXXXXXXXXXXXXX
---------------------------I---------I-----I---I---------I--I------I---------I
```

Figure 2–12
Nutrient analysis of infant's diet in Table 2–8 (*Source:* NDDA Laboratory, Southern Illinois University at Carbondale, 1984.)

changed; however, it is the role of the infant center to provide the parent with sound information that encourages the parent to provide the child with nourishing food. Likewise, it is important for the center, through practices of the staff and written menus, to foster good nutrition principles.

The provision of nourishment has been an important aspect of the mother's role in family life. With changing roles in life-style, the mother does not always plan and prepare the family menus. Other family members or persons outside the home often provide daily meals. With this in mind, the need for nutrition education for the father and mother seems apparent (Chapter 9). Knowledge of basic nutrition, nutritional needs of the life cycle, menu planning, and food preparation is essential for all persons caring for the children in the family unit.

NUTRITIONAL-RELATED PROBLEMS

The care giver may be confronted with questions regarding iron-deficiency anemia, lactose intolerance, food allergies, and obesity. Perhaps even more common are concerns about constipation, diarrhea, and spitting up or vomiting.

Iron-Deficiency Anemia

The diagnosis of iron-deficiency anemia is left to the physician or health clinic. However, the care giver can help prevent the onset of iron-deficiency anemia by being informed of the foods that contain iron and helping parents see the importance of using sources of iron for prevention of this problem. The RDA for iron for the young infant, birth to 6 months of age, is 10 mg; for the 6- to 12-month-old child it increases to 15 mg (Table 2–4). The full-term baby's iron stores are depleted by 6 months of age, and this occurs earlier for preterm infants. Iron-deficiency anemia often becomes apparent after the first 6 months of life and through the preschool years.

Care givers can remind parents that the American Academy of Pediatrics recommends that all infants receive iron supplementation [12]. As discussed earlier, if iron-fortified infant formula is used, iron is already in the formula and is a constant, predictable supply. If the baby is breast-fed, is fed a commercial formula without supplemental iron, or is fed a "homemade" formula made from fresh or evaporated milk, iron-fortified infant cereal or supplemental iron should be used [17].

Lactose Intolerance

Lactose is the natural sugar in milk that is digested with the help of an enzyme called *lactase*. Full-term infants nearly always tolerate lactose well, even if they are from populations where there is a high prevalence of lactose intolerance among adults. When lactose intolerance occurs in infancy, it is usually temporary, a secondary symptom of illnesses that affect the intestinal mucosa (lining), producing diarrhea. When lactose intolerance is suspected, it should be confirmed by a physician before being treated by feeding a lactose-free formula. Unlike the infant, older children may have less of the enzyme lactase and may develop an intolerance to lactose [18].

Food Allergies

The gastrointestinal tract is permeable to macromolecules (larger molecules) during early infancy, at least to 7 months of age. If some proteins are not completely broken down to amino acids, the protein may be absorbed intact and a food allergy produced. If solid foods are introduced after 6 to 7 months of age, allergies present little problem. It is recommended that the use of commonly allergenic foods (eggs, cow's milk, soy protein) be delayed until after 6 months [12].

Only one new food should be introduced into the infant's diet at a time, and the food should be continued for several days. Single foods are preferable to mixtures of foods in the early months (for example, peas would be a more appropriate choice than mixed vegetables). If allergic symptoms appear when this procedure is followed, it is easy to identify the food. If allergic symptoms appear after mixed vegetables are eaten, it is impossible to tell which vegetable caused the reaction. Children with a family history of allergies are more susceptible to allergies and in infancy should be fed single-grain cereals and individual vegetables and fruits. If no symptoms occur, mixed foods may be offered. Mothers of potentially allergic infants should be encouraged to breast-feed, since infants are rarely allergic to breast milk. Common food allergy symptoms include hives, rashes, vomiting, excessive gas, and diarrhea. In addition, a wide variety of other symptoms including respiratory problems may result from an allergy. Cookbooks and other materials are available to assist parents in preparing allergen-free meals [19].

Obesity

Evidence of obesity is increasing in the United States. Because obesity is associated with numerous medical problems and is difficult to cure, attention must be focused on prevention. Many factors can contribute to an excessive intake of food. Several suggestions can be made to assist in preventing obesity:

1. A family history for obesity should be obtained for each infant, since a child born to obese parents is at risk for obesity.
2. Accurate measurements of length and weight should be taken routinely during visits for health care and plotted on growth charts. Rapid weight gain, especially without a proportionate increase in length, should alert the professional and care giver to the need for follow-up.
3. The infant's food intake should be assessed for energy value periodically; when possible, the parents' good dietary practices should be reinforced.

4. Parents should be made to understand what constitutes sound eating and feeding habits and the need to develop them during infancy, since a pattern of overfeeding in infancy may persist into adult life.
5. Mothers should be encouraged to breast-feed for at least 6 months. Nevertheless, if every cry is interpreted as hunger, breast-feeding can produce an overweight baby. A mother who bottle-feeds should not pressure the baby to empty the bottle during feedings.
6. Care givers and parents should not use food as a reward or pacifier for any form of distress. Both breast-fed and bottle-fed babies have used the nipple as a pacifier.
7. Solid foods should not be added to the infant's diet before 4 to 6 months of age. Mothers should have some idea of the caloric density of common foods to assist in making sound food choices.
8. Regular physical activity should be encouraged beginning in infancy.

Should an infant become overweight or obese, parents should be advised to obtain consultation from a professional dietitian or other health professional. The treatment goal generally is the slowing of the rate of weight gain in proportion to linear growth, not an actual loss in weight. Dietary restrictions that are too severe may reduce fat-free tissue, inhibit growth, and deplete energy reserves needed for periods of stress.

Gastrointestinal Tract Disturbances

Parents often come to care givers complaining that the child is constipated or has diarrhea. The definition, incidence, and treatment of constipation are all subjects of dispute. It is generally agreed that a hard, dry stool passed with straining characterizes *constipation*, not the frequency of the stool. Some babies may have a stool only three or four times a week. A daily stool is unnecessary. Constipation rarely occurs in breast-fed infants who receive adequate milk or in non-breast-fed infants who receive an adequate diet [20].

Stools of breast-fed infants usually appear loose and are frequent; however, it is not uncommon for a totally breast-fed infant to have no stools for 1 or 2 days. When solid foods are introduced, stools change in appearance and frequency.

When solid foods have been introduced, mild constipation may be alleviated by increasing use of whole-grain cereals, fruits, or vegetables. Check the child's current diet, including fluid intake, and modify it with food and additional fluids. With the decreased consumption of milk, other fluids may not be sufficient to meet the child's needs. If repeated episodes of constipation occur, an evaluation of the infant's diet by a health professional should be made and appropriate counseling given.

Diarrhea is the passage of frequent, unformed, or watery stools. The term usually implies a change from the infant's usual stool pattern. Acute diarrhea is frequently brief in duration—1 to 4 days—and represents a problem primarily with water and electrolyte (especially sodium and potassium) balance. If the infant is not severely dehydrated, an attempt should be made to feed the infant while treating diarrhea. However, foods that have been recently added to the diet should be avoided. If the infant is dehydrated, the pediatrician will prescribe replacement therapy for water and electrolytes. An infant is likely to become very irritable if given inadequate calories for long periods [21].

When mild diarrhea lasts for more than 3 days, attention should be focused on providing adequate calories and nutrients and on maintaining water balance. The mother should consult a physician. Diarrhea accompanied by a temperature over 101°F, diarrhea accompanied by vomiting that lasts more than 24 hours, or severe diarrhea with stools more than 10 times per day with a large volume of water lost requires immediate medical attention [22].

Spitting up, or *regurgitation*, is the return of small amounts of food during or immediately after eating. *Vomiting* is more complete emptying of the stomach, especially when it occurs sometime after feeding. Spitting up should not concern the care giver or parent. A limited amount of regurgitation is a normal occurrence in the first 6 months of life. It can be kept to a minimum by burping the baby during and after each feeding, handling the baby gently, allowing the baby to nap on the side or abdomen after feeding, and making certain that the head is not lower than the body during naps. Spitting up usually diminishes by 8 months.

Vomiting is common in infancy and is associated with a great number of problems that vary widely in severity. A physician should always be consulted.

Bottle Mouth Caries

The use of a bottle as a pacifier may contribute to development of *bottle mouth*, or *nursing bottle caries*, a condition that can destroy the baby teeth. The nursing bottle syndrome occurs when the child's teeth are exposed to carbohydrates for long periods, such as when the child falls asleep with the bottle in the mouth. Sweetened drinks, fruit juices, formula, and breast milk can all cause caries. The baby should be held while taking the bottle. Some pediatricians advise wiping the teeth after each feeding; however, this may be impractical for the baby's care giver. If mother and baby sleep together, nursing on demand through the night may also lead to caries because the breast milk may pool in the mouth and remain in contact with the teeth for an extended period of time. Preferably, juices should be unsweetened and not offered until the infant is able to drink from a cup.

EXERCISE AND PHYSICAL FITNESS FOR INFANTS

The National Association for the Education of Young Children suggests the following physical fitness activities for infant center care givers:

Physical fitness for infants—If you have time, you can play physical fitness games with babies for a minute or two once or twice a day. Move the arms gently in a rhythmic pattern. Make the legs "ride a bike." Firmly holding the baby under the arms, boost the infant slightly above your face so the child can laughingly look down at you. Hold the baby under the arms in a standing position on the lap and dance the child briefly up and down. Encourage sluggish babies, but don't force them. For example, motivate the sedentary crawler by holding an attractive toy inches in front of the child and see if the child will creep to get it. Don't tease, though, if the baby appears to be frustrated. It seems pompous to call this "curriculum". These are the things most mothers have done for centuries. But it is part of what people trained as infant workers are shown how to do because all these activities in gentle moderation are good for babies. [23]

The following movement skills were observed during a visit to an infant-at-risk program [24]:

- Tumbling
- Care giver exercising extremities during diaper changing
- Doing pull-ups on walker
- Scooting, crawling, and climbing up and down an incline board
- Pushing bolster
- Care givers holding babies by waist or hands, walking them around
- Pushing a toy wagon
- Care givers encouraging babies to reach out or crawl for objects

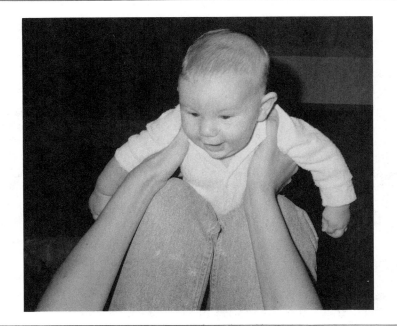

Figure 2-13
Infant interacts with care giver.

- Playing with pop-up pets
- Squeezing soft animals
- Care givers and babies playing pat-a-cake before mirror
- Watching overhead mobiles in cribs
- Care givers placing babies on tummy, raising them up and down
- Care giver and baby rolling ball while seated

Structured exercise programs in infant care centers that serve children age 6 weeks through age 1 are not necessary. An encouraging care giver (Figure 2–13) and a physical environment that permits freedom of movement and exploration are enough to help infants develop their natural abilities.

POLICIES OF THE INFANT CENTER

One soon realizes that nutritional care of the infant, especially the very young, is quite different from care of the preschooler. This is not only because of the infant's nutritional needs, but also because parents come with definite ideas on how, when, and what their babies should be fed. Their methods may not always be best for the infant.

Center policies regarding feeding are best understood when put in writing and explained to parents. In addition, the child's pediatrician or the health clinic should be notified of the established practices. However, a policy should not be arbitrary; it should have a foundation in the nutrition literature and be necessary for the health and well-being of the infant. This chapter has cited numerous references to assist the care giver. It is important that parents see the center working with other community agencies and resources as an extension of the primary health care given to their infant. Parenthood is often frightening and sources of information are varied and confusing. The center should not be an additional source of frustration to the parents.

The written feeding policy should include statements regarding basic nutrition for the infant. It should say when and how food will be introduced, where children will be fed, and who will feed them. Likewise, the availability of breast-feeding facilities (see "Center Assistance for Breast-feeding Mothers") for mother and infant and policies regarding illness and formula preparation should be included. If possible, the mother or father who decides to bottle-feed their infant should also be given the opportunity to come to the center and feed the baby.

The center should be equipped to keep records on each child so that care givers are well aware which child is receiving supplementation and what the supplement contains. If the supplementation is not in line with good nutritional principles, the parent should be consulted as well as the health agency or pediatrician. If regular vitamin and mineral preparations are provided, they should be given by parents. Forms for recording routines and feeding schedules are presented in Chapter 9.

SUMMARY

- Height, weight, skinfold thickness, hemoglobin, and hematocrit, along with dietary intake, are measurements used to evaluate nutritional status of young children in community settings. Appropriate use and interpretation of results are important for the care giver.
- It has been recommended that breast-feeding with supplementation is the preferred method of feeding infants from birth to 12 months of age.
- Iron-fortified formula given through the first year of life supplies the birth to 12-month-old child with all known essential nutrients (except fluoride) without the addition of vitamin and mineral supplements. For the infant who is not "at risk," there is no convincing evidence from the research that feeding whole cow's milk after 6 months of age is harmful, but adequate supplementary feedings must be given.
- Solid foods should be introduced when the child is developmentally ready to chew and when the need for formula exceeds 1 quart per day.
- Use of foods, eating utensils, and the eating situation as educational tools should begin during infancy.
- Iron-deficiency anemia, lactose intolerance, food allergies, obesity, constipation, diarrhea, and nursing bottle caries are nutrition-related problems experienced during infancy.
- Exercise and fitness routines for infants are looked upon as activities that most mothers have done naturally for centuries.
- Policies should be written and communicated to parents by care givers.

DISCUSSION QUESTIONS

1. If a child in your care appears overweight, what would you do?
2. Why should a mother be encouraged but not "forced" to breast-feed her child?
3. What might be the consequences of introducing solid foods before 4 months of age?
4. What is one of the most reliable sources of iron after 6 months of age?
5. Consider two nutrition-related problems of infancy. How might these problems be managed?
6. What can care givers do to stimulate movement activities for infants?

REFERENCES

1. Morrison, G. S.: Early childhood education today, ed. 4, Columbus, OH, 1988, Merrill Publishing Co.

2. National Center for Health Statistics: NCHS growth charts, monthly vital statistics report 25, Suppl. 3 (HRA) 76-1120, Rockville, MD, 1976, Health Resource Administration.

3. Hammill, P. V. V., and Moore, W. M.: Contemporary growth charts: needs, construction, and application, Public Health Currents (Ross Laboratory), 1976.

4. Frisancho, A. R.: Triceps skinfold and upper arm muscle size norms for assessment of nutritional status, Am. J. Clin. Nutr. 27:1052–1058, 1974.

5. U.S. Public Law 94-105, Oct. 7, 1975.

6. Simko, M. D., Cowell, C., and Gilbride, J. A.: Nutrition assessment: a comprehensive guide for planning intervention, Rockville, MD, 1984, Aspen Publishers.

7. Martinez, G. A., and Krieger, F. W.: 1984 Milk-feeding patterns in the United States, Pediatrics 76:1004–1008, 1985.

8. Martinez, G. A.: Ross Laboratory mother's survey, Columbus, OH, 1987, Personal correspondence.

9. American Academy of Pediatrics and American College of Obstetricians and Gynecologists: Guidelines for perinatal care, Elk Grove Village, IL, AAP, 1983, pp. 170–177.

10. Lawrence, R.: Breastfeeding: a guide for the medical professional, St. Louis, 1985, the C. V. Mosby Co.

11. Schoensiegel, B. B.: The expanded role of the dietitian as lactation educator or consultant, Top. Clin. Nutr. 2:21–30, 1987.

12. Marmet C., and Shell, E.: Training neonates to suck correctly, Mat. Child. Nutr. 9:401–407, 1984.

13. American Academy of Pediatrics, Committee on Nutrition: The use of whole cow's milk in infancy, Pediatrics 72:253–255, 1983.

14. American Academy of Pediatrics, Committee on Nutrition: Pediatric nutrition handbook, ed. 2, Chicago, 1985, American Academy of Pediatrics.

15. Fomon, S. J.: Breast-feeding and evolution, J. Am. Diet. Assoc. 86:317–318, 1986.

16. McMillan, J. S., Landaw, S. A., and Oski, F. A.: Iron sufficiency in breastfed infants and the availability of iron from human milk, Pediatrics 58:686, 1976.

17. American Academy of Pediatrics, Committee on Nutrition: Vitamin and mineral supplement needs, Pediatrics 66:1015–1020, 1980.

18. Paige, D. M., and Bayless, T. M.: Lactose digestion, Baltimore, 1981, The Johns Hopkins University Press.

19. Johns, S. B.: Allergy guide to brand name foods and food additives, New York, 1988, Nal Penguim Inc.

20. Scipien, G. M., Barnard, M. U., Chard, M. A., et al: Comprehensive pediatric nursing, New York, 1979, McGraw-Hill Book Co.

21. Santosham, M., Daum, R. S., Dillman, L., et al.: Oral rehydration therapy of infantile diarrhea, N. Engl. J. Med. 306:1070, 1982.

22. Broadribb, V.: Introductory pediatric nursing, Philadelphia, 1983, J. B. Lippincott Company.

23. Ideas that work with young children: What is curriculum for infants in family day care (or elsewhere)? Young children 42(5):59, July 1987.

24. Interviews and observation: Lessie Bates Davis Neighborhood House, E. St. Louis, IL, March 29, 1988.

APPENDIX 2-A Resources for Lactating Mothers

EDUCATIONAL MATERIALS

Health Education Associates, Inc.
211 S. Easton Rd.
Glendale, PA 19038
(215) 659-1149

La Leche League International
9615 Minneapolis Ave.
Franklin Park, IL 60131-8209
(312) 451-1891

Childbirth Graphic, Ltd.
1210 Culver Rd.
Rochester, NY 14609-5454
(716) 482-7940

ICEA Bookstore
P.O. Box 20048
Minneapolis, MN 55420-0048
(800) 328-4815

Lactation Institute and Breastfeeding Clinic
16161 Ventura Blvd., Suite 223
Encino, CA 91436
(818) 995-1913

Healthy Mother Coalition
Directory of Educational Materials
U.S. Dept. of Health and Human Services
200 Independence Ave. SW
Room 740-G
Washington, DC 20201

WIC Supplemental Food Section
Dept. of Health Services
WIC Warehouse
1103 N. B St., Suite E
Sacramento, CA 95814
(916) 324-6352

BOOKS FOR PROFESSIONALS

Arango, J.: Promoting breastfeeding: a guide for health professionals working in the WIC and CSF programs, Washington, DC, 1984, USDA Food and Nutrition Services, National Health Information Clearinghouse.

Lawrence, R. A.: Breastfeeding: a guide for the medical professional, St. Louis, 1985, Times Mirror/Mosby Co.

Olson, C., Psiaki, D., and Kaplowitz, D.: Current knowledge on breastfeeding, Ithaca, NY, 1982, Cooperative Extension Distribution Center.

Riordan, J.: A practical guide to breastfeeding, St. Louis, 1983, Mosby Company.

Worthington-Roberts, B. S., Veremeersch, J., and Williams, S. R.: Nutrition in pregnancy and lactation, St. Louis, 1985, Times Mirror/Mosby Co.

BOOKS FOR CONSUMERS

La Leche League International: The womanly art of breastfeeding, ed. 3, Franklin Park, IL, 1981.

McDonald, L.: The joy of breastfeeding, Pasadena, CA, 1978, Oaklawn Press.

Pryor, K.: Nursing your baby, NY, 1973, Pocket Books.

Satter, E.: Child of mine: feeding with love and good sense, Palo Alto, CA, 1983, Bull Publishing.

Sears, W.: Creative parenting, NY 1982, Dodd Mead.

White, A.: The total nutrition guide for mother and baby: from pregnancy through the first three years, NY, 1983, Ballantine Books.

In 1972 Congress authorized the Special Supplemental Food Program for Women, Infants and Children (WIC).* WIC provides participants with specific nutritious supplemental foods and nutrition education, at no cost. WIC participants are eligible low-income persons who are determined by health professionals (physicians, nutritionists, nurses, and other officials) to be a "nutritional risk" because of inadequate nutrition, health care, or both. Federal funds are available to participating state health departments or comparable state agencies. Indian tribes, bands, groups, or their authorized representatives who are recognized by the Bureau of Indian Affairs, U.S. Department of the Interior, or the appropriate area office of the Indian Health Service, U.S. Department of Health and Human Services, may also act as state agencies. These agencies distribute funds to the participating local agencies. The funds pay for supplemental foods for participants and pay specified administrative costs, including those of nutrition education.

ELIGIBILITY FOR THE PROGRAM

Pregnant, postpartum, and breast-feeding women and infants and children up to 5 years of age are eligible if they (1) meet the income standards (a state agency may either set a statewide income standard or allow local agencies to set their own); (2) are individually determined to be at nutritional risk and in need of the supplemental foods the program offers; and (3) live in an approved project area (if the state has a residency requirement) or belong to special population groups, such a migrant farm workers, Native Americans (Indians), or refugees.

FOODS INCLUDED IN THE WIC PROGRAM

The program allows infants up to 3 months of age to receive iron-fortified formula. Older infants (4 through 12 months) receive formula, iron-fortified

* U.S. Public Law 94-105, Oct. 7, 1975.

infant cereal, and fruit juices high in vitamin C. An infant may receive non-iron-fortified or special therapeutic formula when it is prescribed by a physician for a specified medical condition. Participating women and children receive fortified milk and/or cheese; eggs; hot or cold cereals high in iron; fruit and vegetable juices high in vitamin C; and either peanut butter, dry beans, or peas. WIC provides breast-feeding women with a food package to meet their extra nutritional needs. Women and children with special dietary needs may receive a package containing cereal, juice, and special therapeutic formulas. For a participant to receive this package, a physician must determine that the participant has a medical condition that precludes or restricts the use of conventional foods.

The state agency administering the program may use one or all of the following food delivery systems: (1) retail purchase, where participants use vouchers or checks to buy foods at local retail stores authorized by the state agency to accept WIC vouchers or checks; (2) home delivery, where the food is delivered to participants' homes; and (3) direct distribution, where participants pick up the food from a warehouse.

NUTRITION EDUCATION IN WIC

Nutrition education is available to parents or care givers of infant and child participants, and, whenever possible, to the child who participates. This nutrition education is designed to have a practical relationship to participants' nutritional needs, household situations, and cultural preferences and includes information on how participants can select food for themselves and their families. The goals of WIC nutrition education are to teach the relationship between proper nutrition and good health, to help the individual at nutritional risk to develop better food habits, and to prevent nutrition-related problems by showing participants how to best use their supplemental and other foods. The WIC program also encourages breast-feeding and counsels pregnant women on its nutritional advantages.

LEARNING OBJECTIVES

Students will be able to

- **State the physical and psychosocial characteristics of the toddler that may affect eating habits**
- **State the nutrient, energy, and food needs of the toddler**
- **Describe the care giver's activities related to foods and the eating environment**
- **Describe the management of nutrition-related problems**

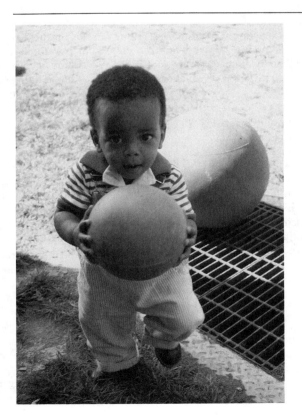

3

The Toddler
(1 to 3 Years)

If you could look back to your own development, you would realize that the toddler stage was a time when you became your own person. During the years from 1 to 3, you began to take on a unique personality with individual characteristics. This, coupled with a newfound ability to move about freely, gave your care giver some anxious moments. But, in turn, you provided those around you with a delightful array of surprises as you mastered one new task after another. Many of the new tasks you learned were associated with food and eating. If you and your family enjoyed consuming a wide variety of foods, today you probably select a nutritionally adequate diet (Figure 3–1).

PHYSICAL CHANGES

During the toddler years the rate of growth declines [1]. Never again after the first year should the child triple its weight in 12 months. The infant takes on the appearance of a young child, with the increase in height or length often exceeding the weight gain. It is estimated that at 18 to 24 months for girls and 24 to 30 months for boys, about 50% of adult height has been achieved. However, increase in weight is only beginning. The median weights and heights of children from 1 to 3 years are shown in Table 3–1; the gain in weight is approximately 5 pounds (2.25 kg) per year.

As discussed in Chapter 2, height and weight recorded over time are two of the best indicators of the child's growth pattern. Charts used to record the monthly height and weight for infants, shown in Chapter 2, can be used during the toddler years. If the child remains in the center through the preschool years,

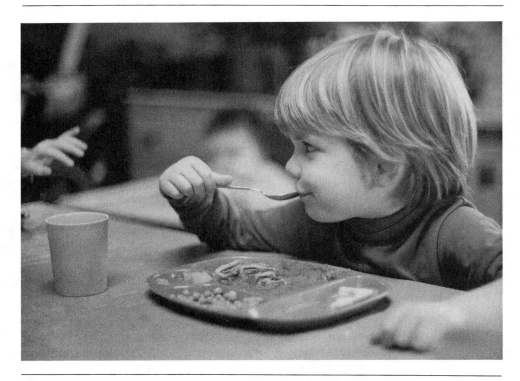

Figure 3-1
The toddler enjoys a wide variety of foods.

you could switch to the charts used for prepubertal girls and boys (found in Appendix VI at the back of this book). However, we recommend that you continue to use the charts labeled "Birth to 36 months" for the most accurate assessment of toddler growth.

The National Center for Health Statistics charts for children to 36 months are based on recumbent length and require that the toddler be lying down on a surface with an immovable head piece and a movable foot piece (Chapter 2). In practice, however, the child of 2 years will want to stand for measurements. For the charts marked for prepubertal boys and girls, the measurements are properly taken with the child in a standing position.

Standing height is best measured by a fixed rather than a freestanding measuring device. The child is positioned with the back against the measuring device and the feet close together and touching the device. The back should show as little curvature as possible. The whole body should be carefully centered and the head held erect with the gaze straight forward. The movable board should contact the top of the head (Figure 3-2). Three measurements should be taken and averaged, when possible.

Table 3–1
Weights and lengths (50th percentile) of girls and boys 1 to 3 years old

Age	Girls		Boys	
	Weight (pounds)	Height (inches)	Weight (pounds)	Height (inches)
1 year	21.0	29.3	22.2	30.0
2 years	26.3	34.1	27.7	34.5
3 years	30.7	37.6	32.1	38.0

Source: National Center for Health Statistics, Health Resources Administration, Department of Health, Education and Welfare, Hyattsville, MD. Data from the Fels Research Institute. Yellow Springs, OH, 1977.

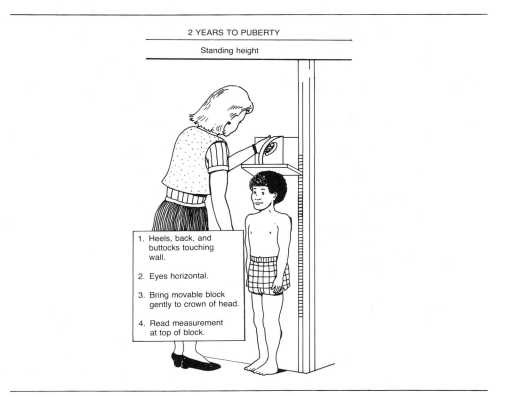

Figure 3–2
Technique for measuring standing height (*Source:* Reprinted with permission from *Maternal and Child Health Program Manual*, Maternal and Child Health Branch, North Carolina Division of Health Services, Raleigh, NC, 1978.)

Weight is best measured using a beam-balanced scale with nondetachable weights. As little clothing as possible should be worn. However, with serial measurements the same amount of clothing should be worn at each measuring.

What do the measurements, height (length) and weight, mean? In referring to the weight and length areas of the chart, single measurements at the 5th or 95th percentile should arouse some concern. Weight for height, or stature, is the most meaningful measure. Using the prepubertal weight-for-height chart (ages 2 to 10), Figure 3–3 plots the growth of three toddler girls. Note that one child represented in Figure 3–3 weighs 35½ pounds (16 kg) and is 40½ inches (101 cm) tall. These measurements correspond with the 50th percentile. Two additional measurements have been plotted using heights and weights that indicate possible problems. The one denoted with a circle between the 90th and 95th percentile indicates that with a height of 40½ inches and a weight of 41 pounds (18.5 kg), the child may weigh too much. Likewise, the triangle shows a child of similar stature with weight less than 30 pounds (13.5 kg). This, too, could present a problem, since the weight for stature is less than the 5th percentile.

Before referral to a health agency for further evaluation, the following factors must be taken into consideration: (1) birth weight, (2) nationality, and (3) heights and weights of biological parents. The premature or low birth weight child may take several years to catch up with the child who was in the normal range for height and weight at birth. Likewise, height and weight may be strongly influenced by the biological parents [2], and attention to parental body structure may help determine if the pattern of growth is actually abnormal for the child. Nationality of the child may also play a role; certain groups have longer legs and a shorter body structure, whereas others have shorter legs and a longer body structure.

If not attributable to these factors, a child's weight may still vary from month to month because of:

Faulty equipment
Error in measurement
Recent over- or underconsumption of food
Recent acute illness (for example, upper respiratory infection or diarrhea)
Chronic illnesses

If none of these conditions exist and losses or gains fall a pound or more above or below expected ranges, seek a more thorough examination from a health professional. The pediatrician or dietition can help the care giver and parents plan any modification in diet and exercise patterns.

Along with the toddler's decrease in rate of growth comes a decreased interest in and need for food. This phenomenon may be interpreted by the parent as illness or a sign to begin supplementing the diet with vitamins and minerals. It is merely a natural development of this period.

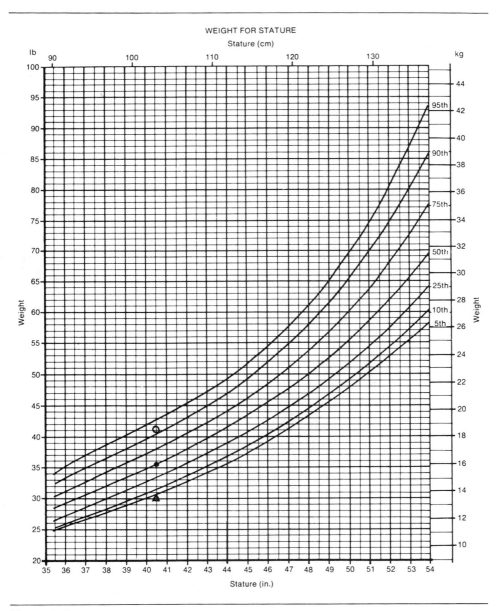

WEIGHT FOR STATURE

Figure 3-3
Weight for stature of three toddler girls, plotted on chart for 2- to 10-year-olds (*Source:* U.S. Department of Health, Education and Welfare, National Center for Health Statistics, 1979.)

DEVELOPMENTAL SKILLS

The toddler is gaining control of the body by practicing large muscle movements over and over [3]. Fine muscle control also is developing, allowing the child to master such tasks as drinking through a straw, eating with a spoon, and attempting to eat an ice-cream cone (Figure 3–4). Developmental scales provide a quick reference for parents who want to ensure that their child is feeding and eating according to developmental readiness. Table 3–2 lists developmental abilities that can be expected during the toddler years.

Having mastered hand-to-mouth coordination, the child can eat independently. Toddlers are still curious babies, and every new object must be handled and explored, probably with the mouth as well as the hands. Any solid or liquid, including poisons, becomes an item for exploration and a potential safety hazard.

To further help with the process of eating, teeth erupt; the front teeth begin erupting at about 6 months of age, and the molars at about 1 year. All 20 primary (baby) teeth have usually erupted by 2½ to 3 years of age. Often it is believed that children can be given foods to chew only after the teeth have erupted; however, most chewing can be done with the gums. We have observed that, if given proper stimulation, children can chew many foods although they do not have a large number of teeth (Figure 3–5).

Developmentally, the child is ready for a wide range of foods from the family table. However, these are new food tastes for the child. The commercially pre-

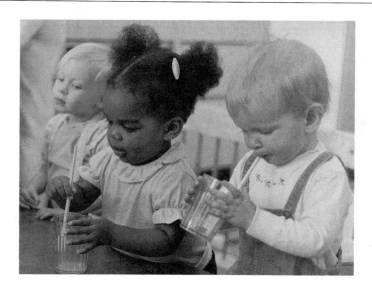

Figure 3–4
Toddlers learn to drink through straws.

Table 3-2
Stages of development for toddler years*

Stage	Physical	Nutrition	Intellectual
Toddler I: *1 year*	Loses subcutaneous fat. Mild lordosis and protuberant abdomen appear. Eight more teeth erupt.	Growth continues at a rapid pace (physical and brain). Appetite good with bite-size foods tolerated.	More words appear; words combined into phrases and short sentences. Thought can sometimes be substituted for action.
Toddler II: *2 years*	Slow but steady gain in height and weight.	Tolerates regular foods well. Growth begins to slow with some decrease in appetite.	Perception of self as distinct from others very prominent; child very assertive.

Stage	Gross Motor	Fine Motor	Oral/Motor
Toddler I: *1 year*	Climbs on and off furniture. Sits in a small chair with no lateral support. Walks well and rises to standing without assistance.	Opposition or thumb/forefinger grasp. Wrist extended and deviated to ulnar side for accurate prehension (12–14 months).	More refined cup-drinking (Stage II, Stage III). Chewing. Refined spoon-feeding by 2 years.
Toddler II: *2 years*	Runs. Ascends and descends stairs independently. Backs self into a small chair for sitting. Squats in play. Rides and steers a tricycle well.	Gradual progression of three jaw chuck position occurs.	By 3 years sucking through straw.

Stage	Speech and Language	Social/Behavioral
Toddler I: *1 year*	13–18 months: Rapid receptive growth. Slow expressive development. 18–24 months: The naming stage. Holophrases. Jargoning. Echolalia. Two- and three-word phrases.	Eats at table with family. More social and verbal. Negativism emerges.
Toddler II: *2 years*	By 2 years, uses 40% sentences. Rapid syntactic development. Early-developing consonants emerge.	Temper tantrums and refusal of food common. Toilet training in process if not already completed.

Source: Modified from Harvey-Smith, M., et al.: Feeding management of a child with a handicap: a guide for professionals, Memphis, 1982, University of Tennessee Center for the Health Sciences.

*This chart provides the health professional with a standard tool for assessing feeding levels.

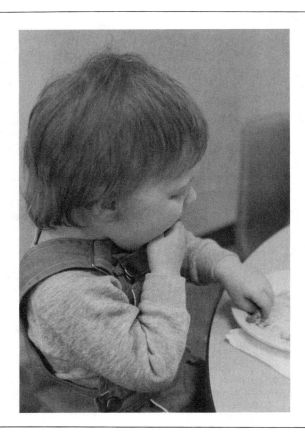

Figure 3-5
A young toddler eats.

pared ground or chopped foods probably eaten until now taste and feel quite different from the same foods served at the family table. The toddler may need time to adjust to new flavors and textures.

PSYCHOLOGICAL AND SOCIAL CHARACTERISTICS

Another characteristic of this period is sudden changes in mood, from the cooperative child who is a helper to the child who responds with only "no, no, no." Any question beginning with "do you want" may be answered "no," including questions regarding food and eating. Often care givers avoid confrontation by offering the child a choice between two equally acceptable alternatives.

The child wants and needs to become independent and must demonstrate the need for autonomy by doing things alone. Erikson [4] described the situation as autonomy versus shame. Attempting to accomplish tasks beyond the toddler's ability causes frustration and feelings of shame and doubt. The child's skill may outrun judgment, and the child must be restrained from certain activities that can be harmful [5]. Wanting to help the care giver chop vegetables with a knife instead of breaking them, to pour water from the large rather than small container, and to mix the fruit salad or bread dough with a large spoon in a large bowl are examples of how the child's curiosity and enthusiasm must be channeled into productive, but safe, activities (Figure 3-6).

Just at the time when the child is mastering the eating process and when almost all foods can be given directly from the family table, the toddler may experience a less than enthusiastic desire for food. This may be a result of

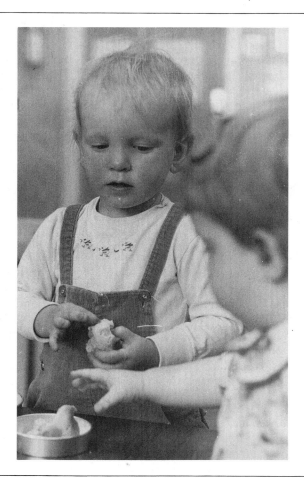

Figure 3-6
A young boy shapes small portions of bread dough.

physical, psychological, or social conditions. As previously stated, the child's rate of growth is slower during this period, with the child gaining less than ½ pound (0.22 kg) per month as compared to 1 pound (0.45 kg) or more per month during the first 6 months of life. In addition, the child may be too busy exploring the new environment, now viewed from an upright position, to be concerned about food. In any case, the care giver must be concerned that the nutritional needs of the toddler are met and be prepared to assure parents that the child is progressing at a normal rate of growth or, if necessary, to seek help from the health professional.

NUTRITIONAL NEEDS

Calories must count! Although the rate of growth slows and the child's appetite may decline, the needs brought about by continued growth and development remain. The additional activity of the toddler will increase energy needs. The infant and toddler have similar needs for nutrients but in different amounts (Table 3-3). In many cases the toddler will need more of each nutrient than the infant. The RDA may be used in planning diets for the toddler. However, it can be used only as a guide when looking at individual diets, since the nutritional status of a toddler whose diet is less than 100% of the RDA [6] may still be good.

Certain nutrients are of predominant concern in caring for the toddler and need special consideration in planning menus for children. These include protein, calcium, ascorbic acid, and iron.

Energy

As shown in Table 3-3, the caloric recommendation (RDA) for the toddler is 1300 kcal (approximately 45 kcal per pound of body weight). Any child's recommended allowance for energy can be calculated, given the weight and assuming moderate activity. (This child's energy needs may be viewed as about two thirds of what is recommended [RDA] for a woman 23 to 50 years of age [2000 kcal].) Remember, the energy allowance is only an estimate. Intake may range from 900 to 1800 kcal, and many children may eat more or less without a loss or gain in weight. The data obtained from taking heights and weights each month should be used as the best indicators of caloric needs.

Calculating Calories. If the child's eating pattern is determined to be typical and the weight in relation to height is within acceptable ranges, there is little need to recommend a change in energy allowance. However, the care giver should have some knowledge of the energy needs of the young child. Three methods are used to determine energy needs.

Table 3-3
RDA for toddler compared with that of infant

	Infant 6 to 12 Months (20 lb, 28 in. [9 kg, 70 cm])	Toddler 1 to 3 Years (29 lb, 35 in. [13 kg, 87.5 cm])
Food energy (kcal)	kg × 105	1300
	(lb × 47.7)	(lb × 44.8)
Protein (g)	(kg × 2.0)	(kg × 1.8)
Vitamin A activity (IU)	2000	2000
Vitamin D (IU)	400	400
Vitamin E activity (IU)	5	7
Ascorbic acid (mg)	35	45
Folacin (μg)	45	100
Niacin (mg)	8	9
Riboflavin (mg)	0.6	0.8
Thiamin (mg)	0.5	0.7
Vitamin B_6 (mg)	0.6	0.9
Vitamin B_{12} (μg)	1.5	2.0
Calcium (mg)	540	800
Phosphorus (mg)	360	800
Iodine (μg)	50	70
Iron (mg)	15	15
Magnesium (mg)	70	150
Zinc (mg)	5	10

Source: Based on Food and Nutrition Board, National Academy of Sciences—National Research Council: Recommended dietary allowances, revised 1980.

The simplest way to estimate energy needs is to start with a base of 1000 calories and add 100 calories for each year of age (method 1). When energy needs are presented in this text, the recommended amount is calculated based on body weight (method 2).

Birth to 6 months	115 kcal/kg (52.3/lb)
6 months–1 year	105 kcal/kg (47.7/lb)
1–3 years	100 kcal/kg (44.8/lb)
4–6 years	85 kcal/kg (38.6/lb)

To calculate the needs of an actual child in the center, using the RDA for energy based on *height* may be most meaningful (method 3):

1–3 years	37.1 kcal/in. (14.4/cm)
4–6 years	38.6 kcal/in. (15.2/cm)

With this method, energy needs increase as the child grows taller, thus taking into consideration individual growth patterns. A comparison of method 1 and method 3 in Table 3–4 shows that calculating kilocalories based on height yields higher values.

Protein

The recommended amount of protein is 1.8 g per kilogram or 0.8 g per pound of body weight (Table 3–3). A 29-pound (13 kg) child will need only about 23 g protein—less than that found in three glasses (24 ounces) of milk (8 ounces = 8 g protein) and 2 ounces of meat (1 ounce = 7 g protein). This is excluding the protein in vegetables and bread. The amount (23 g) is not what is actually required but is recommended by the National Research Council. An intake of 20 g may be adequate. As stated previously, protein intake is perhaps overemphasized; national studies [7] have shown that few children consume less than the recommended levels. However, extra servings of milk and meat help to meet some of the following nutrient requirements.

Minerals

Calcium. With the development of bones and teeth, calcium becomes crucial. A glass of milk contains approximately 300 mg calcium. Two to three glasses of milk per day along with other foods will supply the amount of calcium necessary to meet the needs of the 1- to 3-year-old child.

Milk and milk products are the main sources of calcium, but other sources include dried beans and dark green vegetables. Table 3–5 provides calcium equivalents. It becomes obvious that milk is by far the best source of calcium. Children who do not drink milk should have the diet supplemented with other calcium-containing foods. A wide variety of dairy foods can be used in the center to encourage adequate milk intake, and supplements are rarely indicated.

Table 3–4
Comparison of two methods for calculating energy values

Age	Method 1 (1000 kcal + age)	Method 3 (kcal/height [in.])
2	1200	1260 (34 in.)
3	1300	1370 (37 in.)
4	1400	1540 (40 in.)
5	1500	1660 (43 in.)

Table 3-5
Calcium values (mg) in common foods

Dairy products		Legumes	
Buttermilk, 1 C	296	Pork and beans, in sauce, 1 C	138
Cheese, American, pasteurized, process, 1 oz	198	Garbanzo beans, cooked, 1 C	150
Cheese, cheddar, 1 oz	204	Soybeans, cooked, 1 C	131
Cheese, cottage, creamed and low fat 2%, ½ C	77	Tofu, processed with calcium sulfate, 4 oz	145
Cheese, ricotta, part skim, ½ C	337	Fruits and vegetables	
Cheese, Swiss, 1 oz	272	Bok choy,½ C	126
Cheese food, American, 1 oz	163	Collards, raw, ½ C	179
Sour cream, 1 tbsp	14	Kale, raw, ½ C	103
Ice cream, vanilla, ½ C	88	Spinach, ½ C	84
Milk, chocolate, 1 C	284	Broccoli, stalk, ½ C	68
Milk, evaporated, 1 C	635	Turnip greens, raw, ½ C	126
Milk, evaporated, 1 part to 1 of water, 1 C	318	Orange, 1 medium	54
Milkshake, vanilla, 11 fl. oz	457	Grains	
Milk, low fat, 2%, 1 C	297	Bread enriched white, 1 slice	19
Milk, skim, 1 C	302	Bread, whole wheat, 1 slice	22
Yogurt, plain, low fat, 1 C	415	Corn bread, 2½″ square	94
Pudding, chocolate, ½ C	133	Pancakes, 4″ diameter (2)	116
Meat, fish, eggs, and nuts		Tortilla, corn, 6″ diameter	60
Almonds, ¼ C	83	Waffle, 7″ diameter	179
Brazil nuts, ¼ C	65	Combination foods	
Egg, scrambled, 1 large	47	Spaghetti, meatballs, and tomato sauce, 1 C	124
Meat loaf, 3 oz	68	Macaroni and cheese, ½ C	181
Oysters, raw, 7-9	113	Pizza, cheese, ¼ of 14″ pie	332
Salmon, red, with bones, 3 oz	167	Taco, beef, 1	174
Sardines, with bones, 3 oz	372	Other	
Shrimp, canned, 3 oz	99	Cake, devil's food, ¹⁄₁₆ of 9″ cake	41
		Chocolate bar, milk, 1 oz	65
		Molasses, blackstrap, 1 tbsp	137
		Sherbet, orange, ½ C	52

Source: Ohio State University Data Base, NDDA Laboratory, Southern Illinois University at Carbondale, 1984.

Iron.   The baby uses iron stored during the first months of life. However, stores may be low by the age of 1 year, particularly if the child was given whole milk and table foods by 6 months of age. For this reason, iron-fortified formula is often recommended for the child to 1 year of age and iron-fortified infant cereal to 18 months of age.

In practice, the early sources of iron—fortified formula and infant cereal—are usually terminated by the toddler stage. Thus, it is especially important that other good sources, such as meat, green vegetables, and enriched or whole-grain cereal products, be eaten by the child.

The amount of iron available to the body depends on the body's need for iron, the form of iron, the composition of the meal, and bulk in the diet. A child in need of iron will absorb more iron than a child who has normal levels in the body. The absorption of iron is greatest from meat (for example, beef or pork) and poorest from grains and vegetables. If meat, fish, or poultry is eaten with vegetables, the absorption of iron from the vegetables is enhanced. Consumption of foods high in vitamin C along with iron-rich foods will also help the body absorb iron. Excessive bulk in the diet, especially bran, may interfere with iron absorption.

It is difficult to provide the recommended 15 mg of iron for the 1- to 3-year-old or even to provide 10 mg, the allowance for the 4- to 6-year-old. Table 3–6 indicates the quantities of certain foods that a youngster would have to eat to obtain from 1 to 5 mg of iron. Note that only small quantities of formula and infant cereal are required to supply 1 and 5 mg of iron.

Fluoride.   Children younger than 3 years of age do not need supplemental fluoride if (1) they brush their teeth (as they should in the center) and (2) fluoride is present in the drinking water. If fluoride is not present in the water at home or in the center, the child's parents should consult the pediatrician or dentist for recommendations on supplementation. Children are prone to swallow much of the toothpaste used in brushing their teeth. If they brush more than twice a day this may be at least 1 to 3 mg.

Other Nutrients

A balance of all nutrients is important, and a daily source of vitamin C (ascorbic acid) is recommended, with sources of vitamin A every other day. The recommended amount of vitamin C, 45 mg, is supplied by less than 4 ounces (½ cup) orange or grapefruit juice or foods rich in vitamin C. Likewise, 2000 IU of vitamin A is relatively easy to acquire if the child eats a wide variety of foods including green and yellow vegetables such as carrots or spinach, fortified margarine, butter, and other fortified dairy products.

Supplementation

The toddler's decreased interest in food may be interpreted by the parent as illness or a sign to begin supplementing the diet with vitamins and minerals. In

Table 3-6
Approximate iron equivalents of selected foods

Foods	Iron (1 mg)	Iron (5 mg)
Meat and Meat Alternatives		
Beans, dry (cooked)	>3 tbsp	1 C
Beef round steak	1.0 oz	5.0 oz
Black walnuts	>¼ C	1⅓ C
Cashews	>3 tbsp	1 C
Egg yolk, medium	1¼ egg yolks	6¼ egg yolks
Lentils, dry (cooked)	¼ C	1¼ C
Liver, beef	<½ oz	2 oz
Liver, pork	<¼ oz	<1 oz
Oysters (raw)	1 medium	5 medium
Peanuts, roasted	⅓ C	1½ C
Peas, dry (cooked)	5 tbsp	>1½ C
Pecans	⅓ C	1½ C
Pork loin chops	1.0 oz	5.0 oz
Breads and Cereals		
Enriched cream of wheat, cooked*	1 tbsp	⅓ C
Enriched bread	1½ slices	7½ slices
Infant cereal (dry)	¾ to 1 tbsp	4 to 5 tbsp
Iron-rich formula	⅓ C	1½ C
Oatmeal (cooked)	⅔ C	3½ C
Ready-to-eat cereal, iron enriched (100% U.S. RDA)	>2½ tsp†	4½ tbsp†
Wheat germ	2 tbsp	½ C + 2 tbsp
Whole wheat bread	1¼ slices	6¼ slices
Fruits and Vegetables		
Asparagus (canned)	2½ spears	13 spears
Dried apricots	5 medium halves	25 medium halves
Dried prunes	3	15
Oranges, small	2	10
Raisins	3 tbsp	1 C
Spinach (cooked)	¼ C	1¼ C

Source: NDDA Laboratory, Southern Illinois University at Carbondale, 1984.

*40% U.S. RDA.

†Serving size indicated on box. If the serving size is 1 C (16 tbsp), the amount provided would be 18 mg/C or more than 1 mg/tbsp.

reality, it is a natural development of this period. By the time the child reaches 1 year of age, an adequate diet can be obtained through use of a variety of foods. It is generally believed that if the child receives sufficient nourishment from foods, vitamin and mineral supplementation are unnecessary. No particular benefit is seen from a multivitamin and mineral preparation. For a complete discussion of supplementation see Chapter 4.

Table 3-7
Recommended food intake according to food group and average serving size (ages 1 up to 3 years)

Food Group	Servings/Day	Average Serving*	
		Ages 1 up to 2	Ages 2 up to 3
Fruits and Vegetables	At least 4 including:		
Vitamin C source (citrus fruits, berries, tomato, cabbage, cantaloupe)	1 or more (twice as much tomato as citrus)	¼ C	¼ C
Green vegetables	1†	1–2 tbsp	2–3 tbsp
Other vegetables (potato and other green or yellow vegetables and/or other fruits)	2	1–2 tbsp	2–3 tbsp
Meat and Alternates	3–4 including:		
Lean meat, fish, poultry, and eggs‡	2	1 oz	1 oz
Nutbutters (peanut, soynut)		2 tbsp	2 tbsp§
Cooked dried beans or peas	1–2 ‖	2 tbsp	4 tbsp
Nuts		—	½ oz
Breads and Cereals (Whole Grain)	At least 4		
Bread		½ slice	½ slice
Ready-to-eat cereals, whole grain, iron fortified		¼ C or ⅓ oz	¼ C or ⅓ oz
Cooked cereal including macaroni, spaghetti, rice, etc. (whole grain, enriched)		¼ C	¼ C
Infant cereal (until 18 mo.)		6–8 tbsp	—
Milk and Milk Products	At least 4	¾ C	¾ C
Whole or 2% milk (1.5 oz cheese = 1 C milk) (C = 8 oz or 240 g)			
Fats and Oils			
Butter, margarine, mayonnaise, oils	3	1 tsp	1 tsp

*Additional servings of food may be needed to meet energy needs. See Appendix 3-A for nutrient composition.

†Allow a minimum serving of 1 tbsp/year of age for cooked fruits, vegetables, cereals, and pasta until the child reaches 8 years or ½ C portion size.

‡To enhance overall nutrient content of diet include eggs two to three times a week and liver occasionally.

§As recommended by Illinois State Board of Education, Department of Child Nutrition: Child Care Food Program—required meal patterns, Springfield, IL, June 1986, The Board.

‖Include nutbutters, dried (cooked) beans, or peas at least once a day to meet nutrient recommendations. Use additional servings of meats when legumes, beans, and nuts are omitted.

BASIC FOOD GUIDE FOR THE TODDLER

The Modified Basic Food Plan (Chapter 1) is the practical guide for planning food needs of adults as well as children. Table 3–7 specifies the recommended food intake in each food group with average serving sizes for the toddler years. Using this guide and the Child Care Food Program guidelines (Chapter 6), care givers and parents can plan nutritious meals that meet RDA standards. Figure 3–7 shows the nutrient composition of a diet (not shown), planned from Table 3–7. It is difficult to plan diets that meet the RDA without including fortified infant cereal in the 12- to 18-month period. For the older toddler, fortified cereals also help provide the RDAs. Although the RDAs are not requirements, they serve as guides in planning diets. Note also that the recommended food intake guide in Table 3–7 will help in choosing foods needed by the toddler, but additional foods should be included to meet energy needs.

Fruits and Vegetables

Fresh fruits and vegetables are the major sources of vitamin C. This group also contributes significant amounts of vitamin A, magnesium, and fiber to the diet.

```
PERCENT ENERGY DISTRIBUTION


         PROTEIN     23%           FAT     33%        CARBOHYDRATE    44%

NUTRIENT   %RDA 0%            20%      33%   40%            60%   66%        80%              100%
----------------I----------------I---------I-----I----------------I-----I---------I----------------I
ENERGY      69%  X X X X X X X X X X X X X X X X X X X X X X X X X X X X X X X X
PROTEIN    221%  X X X X X X X X X X X X X X X X X X X X X X X X X X X X X X X X X X X X X X X X X X X X X X X X X X
VITAMIN A  117%  X X X X X X X X X X X X X X X X X X X X X X X X X X X X X X X X X X X X X X X X X X X X X X X X X X
VITAMIN D   75%  X X X X X X X X X X X X X X X X X X X X X X X X X X X X X X X X X X X X X X
VITAMIN E  154%  X X X X X X X X X X X X X X X X X X X X X X X X X X X X X X X X X X X X X X X X X X X X X X X X
VITAMIN C   95%  X X X X X X X X X X X X X X X X X X X X X X X X X X X X X X X X X X X X X X X X X X X X X X X
FOLACIN    138%  X X X X X X X X X X X X X X X X X X X X X X X X X X X X X X X X X X X X X X X X X X X X X X X X X
NIACIN     126%  X X X X X X X X X X X X X X X X X X X X X X X X X X X X X X X X X X X X X X X X X X X X X X X X X
RIBOFLAVIN 247%  X X X X X X X X X X X X X X X X X X X X X X X X X X X X X X X X X X X X X X X X X X X X X X X X X
THIAMIN    135%  X X X X X X X X X X X X X X X X X X X X X X X X X X X X X X X X X X X X X X X X X X X X X X X X X
VITAMIN B₆  95%  X X X X X X X X X X X X X X X X X X X X X X X X X X X X X X X X X X X X X X X X X X X X X X X
VITAMIN B₁₂ 155% X X X X X X X X X X X X X X X X X X X X X X X X X X X X X X X X X X X X X X X X X X X X X X X X X
CALCIUM    145%  X X X X X X X X X X X X X X X X X X X X X X X X X X X X X X X X X X X X X X X X X X X X X X X X X
PHOSPHORUS 134%  X X X X X X X X X X X X X X X X X X X X X X X X X X X X X X X X X X X X X X X X X X X X X X X X X
IRON       101%  X X X X X X X X X X X X X X X X X X X X X X X X X X X X X X X X X X X X X X X X X X X X X X X X X
MAGNESIUM  122%  X X X X X X X X X X X X X X X X X X X X X X X X X X X X X X X X X X X X X X X X X X X X X X X X X
ZINC        53%  X X X X X X X X X X X X X X X X X X X X X X X X X X

----------------I----------------I---------I-----I----------------I-----I---------I----------------I


     108.9 MG CHOLESTEROL    2.4-3.6 GM DIETARY FIBER    944.4 MG SODIUM    1840.7 MG POTASSIUM
```

Figure 3–7
Nutrient analysis of toddler's diet derived from Table 3–7 (Source: NDDA Laboratory, Southern Illinois University at Carbondale.)

Children may have poor acceptance of this group because parents or care givers do not eat or like a wide variety of fruits and vegetables. Preparation methods of the care givers may also contribute to a child's rejection of certain foods. Vegetables or foods poorly consumed should be introduced when the child is hungry. Offer vegetables first while the other foods are being prepared for the toddler's tray. The hungry toddler will explore with interest a small serving of cooked vegetables (for instance, 1 inch of asparagus, one flowerette of broccoli, one green bean, one slice of carrot, or 1 tablespoon of cabbage).

Chopped or sliced foods are preferred for this age group because they require less chewing and may be used as finger foods. This does not mean that toddlers should be given only chopped or peeled foods. Toddlers approaching the age of 2 can handle a raw apple or at least a large section of one. To prevent choking, raw foods in large pieces may be safer than small chunks of foods (such as apples or pears) since the child can hold and chew the larger piece. Children should *always* be closely supervised when eating (Figure 3–8).

Preparation time presents a good opportunity to let children try a new food— perhaps cooked or raw broccoli, green beans, or greens. Fresh foods rather than canned, especially fruits and vegetables, have more appeal. A good rule to follow is never prepare frozen when you can buy fresh, and never prepare canned if you can buy frozen. Because overcooked vegetables are likely to lose nutritional

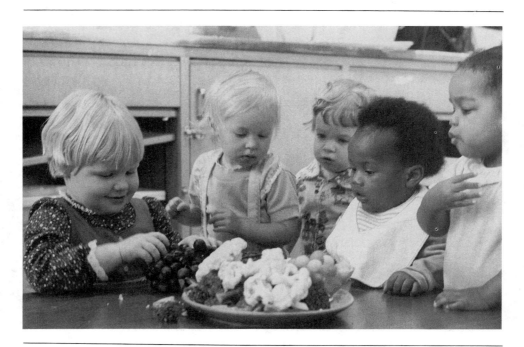

Figure 3–8
Toddlers eat raw vegetables and fruit.

value and be less accepted by children, food service personnel and teachers should keep cooking times brief. Vegetables should be slightly crunchy when served (Chapter 6).

The Modified Basic Food Plan recommends four different servings of fruits and vegetables each day. Care should be taken to include a vitamin C source daily, a vitamin A source three to four times per week, and a dark green vegetable daily, if possible. Vitamin A and C sources were reviewed in Chapter 1.

A good rule to follow for serving size is a minimum of 1 tablespoon per year of age for cooked vegetables. The 2-year-old child would receive the equivalent of 2 measuring tablespoons of cooked vegetables or cooked fruit and about twice this much of raw foods (Figure 3–9).

Meat and Meat Alternates

Most parents encourage the use of meats and meat products. However, meat alternates, beans, peas, and nutbutters can also provide a good protein source,

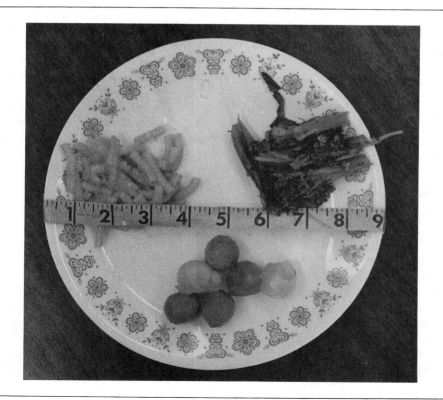

Figure 3–9
Small servings of food work best for the toddler.

especially when taken with a small amount of meat, milk, and cheese or when combined with grain (such as rice or wheat). Peas and beans should be included in the diet at an early age: when cooked in a soup, these foods are generally well accepted. Use caution when serving nuts, which could become lodged in a child's throat.

Meats and alternates should be cooked until tender and prepared for finger- or spoon-feeding. Cooked meat may be cut into meat sticks, which are easy to chew and to manipulate with fingers. Generally, gravies and sauces are too high in fat and low in nutritional value to be included in the child's diet, except maybe "milk gravies" or cheese sauces.

Luncheon meats, hot dogs, and other highly processed meats, which are salty and spicy, are generally well liked by children, and most care givers choose them because of their quick preparation. The debate on the relationship of diet— including the effect of sodium, saturated fat, and cholesterol—to heart disease continues. Excessive use of these substances may or may not affect the health of the child later in life. However, regardless of the possible consequences, most foods (convenience luncheon meats, hot dogs, and packaged dinners) are used in the home. The preschool or toddler center should provide the child with *new learning experiences involving foods.* Convenience foods, although a necessity in some centers, limit the child's involvement in food and nutrition activities.

Beans should be cooked until they can be mashed with a fork. Flatulence seems to be less of a problem if beans are served on a regular basis (two to three times per week). It appears that there is a change in the intestinal flora with frequent use of the product. A general rule to follow is ¼ cup of cooked beans in exchange for 1 ounce of meat.

Meat alternates, beans, peas, and nutbutters help to provide magnesium, zinc, folacin, iron, and B_6 (Chapter 1) to the young child's diet and should be eaten each day. Include a serving of these foods along with 2 ounces of meat.

Breads and Cereals

The easiest foods to chew and the easiest to abuse are from the bread and cereal group. A cracker or cookie has soothed many tears and has replaced foods served at regular mealtime.

Most commercially prepared breads and cereals are enriched or whole grain. Enriched flour has had the wheat bran and germ removed and some of the nutrients added after the flour has been milled. The enrichment process adds iron and several B vitamins, but other nutrients (vitamin E, vitamin B_6, folacin, and magnesium) are lost. Whole-grain cereals have retained the nutrients originally found in the grains of flour. Certain specialty cereal products need not be enriched, and local bakeries need not use enriched flour. However, any bread sold across state lines must be enriched.

Labels from bread and cereal products (bread, crackers, pastas, and so on) should always be checked to determine whether the product is prepared with enriched or whole-grain flours. Some manufacturers of cereals that contain 100% of the U.S. RDA for iron caution that their product is not recommended for children under 4 because of a chance of excessive iron intake. This is unlikely unless cereal becomes one of few foods eaten by the child. Each serving of ready-to-eat cereal fortified with 100% of the U.S. RDA for iron contains 18 mg of iron, which will meet the iron recommendation (15 mg) for toddlers.

Unlike fruits and vegetables, breads and cereals retain nutrients during preparation; since little preparation is necessary for many of the products, this food group is popular in the American diet. However, many bread and cereal products consumed by children (for example, cakes, sweet rolls, some cookies, and sugar-coated cereals) are prepared with a high sugar and fat content and cannot be counted as part of the bread and cereal servings. (It would be diffi-cult for a care giver to justify these foods for the child-care center menu.) Table 3–8 shows the sugar content, cost, and iron content of commonly eaten cereals.

A toddler needs four servings per day from the bread and cereal group. One-half slice of bread can be considered a serving for the young toddler, and approxi-mately 3 tablespoons of cooked cereal or ¼ to ⅓ cup of dry cereal, depending on the type, equals one bread or cereal serving. To meet 100% of the RDA for iron, approximately ¾ cup dry fortified infant cereal must be eaten.

Milk and Milk Products

If the toddler is using the bottle, milk consumption may be excessive (over 3 cups per day); if recently weaned, the child may need a reminder to drink milk or eat foods with appreciable amounts of calcium. The milk group contributes excel-lent sources of most nutrients, but it contains small quantities of iron and vitamin C (Chapter 1).

Milk is often consumed in large quantities at the expense of other foods, espe-cially if a bottle is taken between meals. Milk intake should be curtailed if more than 24 ounces (3 cups or 720 ml) is consumed per day, unless all foods are readily eaten and the child is not overweight. It is easy for an 18-month-old to drink a lot of milk and be unwilling to eat other foods. On the other hand, a child who only drinks scant amounts of milk may need to begin the meal with milk and be offered milk for snacks. Dairy products such as American cheese, cottage cheese, and yogurt are substitutes for milk (for calcium values see Table 3–5). If dairy products are not eaten, large quantities of other foods must be included in the diet to ensure adequate amounts of essential nutrients.

Dairy foods with added sugar are not recommended. Ice cream, pudding, and sugar-sweetened yogurt have small amounts of calcium compared with caloric value and, thus, have limited use in the preschool menu. Cream cheese, butter, and margarine cannot be used as milk substitutes. Three cups of milk or substi-tute servings of other dairy products meet the calcium allowance of 800 mg for the toddler.

Table 3-8
Sugar content, iron content, and cost of popular cereals

Cereal	Cost* (cents/serving)	Iron (mg/serving)	Sugar (g/serving)
Sugar Smacks	.14	1.8	15
Apple Jacks	.19	4.5	14
Smurfberry Crunch	.20	4.5	14
Super Sugar Crisp	.16	2.7	14
Chocolate Chip	.20	4.5	13
Fruit Loops	.18	4.5	13
Cocoa Pebbles	.17	1.8	13
Trix	.20	4.5	12
Cap'n Crunch	.14	4.5	12
Sugar Corn Pops	.17	1.8	12
Cocoa Puffs	.20	4.5	11
Lucky Charms	.18	4.5	11
Alpha Bits	.15	2.7	11
Honeycomb	.16	2.7	11
Cocoa Krispies	.18	1.8	11
Frosted Flakes	.13	1.8	11
Raisin Bran	.13	18.0	10
Crispy Wheats 'n Raisin	.16	4.5	10
Golden Grahams	.17	4.5	9
King Vitamin	.19	8.1	6
Life	.13	8.1	6
100% Bran	.11	2.7	6
Frosted Mini Wheats	.15	1.8	6
Bran Chex	.12	4.5	5
Product 19	.18	18.0	3
Total	.17	18.0	3
Corn Chex	.16	8.1	3
Kix	.19	8.1	3
Special K	.12	4.5	3
Grape-nuts	.10	2.7	3
Rice Krispies	.14	1.8	3
Rice Chex	.17	8.1	2
Corn Flakes†	.10	1.8	2
Cheerios	.15	8.1	1
Cream of Wheat	.08	8.1	0
Puffed Wheat	.22	.3	0

*Costs are based on prices listed at retail stores in Carbondale, IL, spring 1988.
†Some brands include higher amounts of iron.

EATING AND CARE GIVER'S ROLE

Beginning in infancy and continuing through the toddler stage, the development of good food habits is crucial. If given only a few selected food items, the child will have a limited range of food experiences as well as a limited number of foods from which to receive the necessary nutrients (Figure 3–10).

The care giver's role is supportive. You do not feed the toddler; the toddler eats! Messy as it may be, this is the time to allow the toddler to be an independent person. Food is put on the spoon with fingers, or fingers are used in place of a spoon, even for such foods as applesauce and scalloped potatoes. Sometimes foods are just squashed or crumbled to see how they feel. Care givers can cover

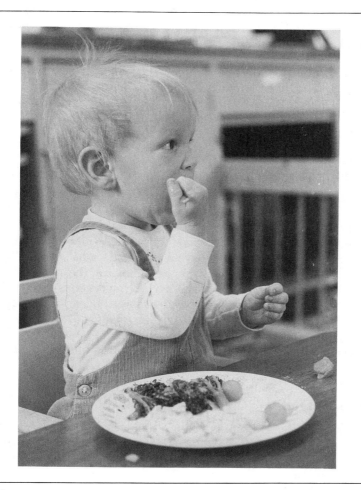

Figure 3–10
Toddler learns to eat a variety of foods.

the floor with newspapers, an old shower curtain, or a vinyl tablecloth, which can be discarded or cleaned.

Mealtime should not be rushed in order to "put the toddler down for a nap." If facilities and resources permit, it is ideal for the care giver to eat with the toddler while carrying on a conversation about the food and eating situation. Encouraging a toddler to try broccoli is much easier if the care giver is eating broccoli.

Bottle or Cup

You would be hard pressed to find research that supports a particular time when toddlers must abandon bottle or breast. For most toddlers weaning occurs as a natural part of development when the child begins to rely on a cup and more regular feeding periods. However, there is support for the strong recommendation that the child not be allowed to fall asleep at the breast or bottle or to drink more than 24 ounces (720 ml) of milk or formula when other essential foods are omitted.

The bottle presents a dilemma for many parents. It is easy to lull baby to sleep with the bottle, and baby can usually hold the bottle while drifting off to sleep at nap time. If the bottle is given, you should hold the toddler and not allow the child to fall asleep until drinking is completed (see the discussion of dental caries).

Commercial Toddler Foods

Although commercially prepared toddler foods are available and convenient, these are not practical from an economic viewpoint, especially in a group-care setting. However, they are now prepared without additional salt and are nutritionally acceptable when plain vegetables and meats are used.

Many of the commercially prepared foods called "junior" or "toddler" foods, like the "strained" infant foods, are really combinations of foods. Spaghetti and meat sauce and vegetables with meat are examples of these products. It is tempting to buy the combination foods, and they may serve a useful purpose for parents at home or when traveling, but they are more expensive and lack the nutrient density of plain meats, vegetables, and cereal products. During the toddler stage, child-care centers should encourage all children (1 year or older) to consume a wide variety of table foods prepared with limited quantities of salt, fat, and sugar.

Serving Food to the Toddler

Foods should be served in small portions, and less desired foods may be offered first while other foods cool or are being prepared; 1 tablespoon per year of age is the general rule for the serving size for cooked foods. One to three measuring tablespoons (15 mg), not the "serving" tablespoon, are intended (Figure 3–11). Serving small quantities permits the child to ask for additional servings. Milk

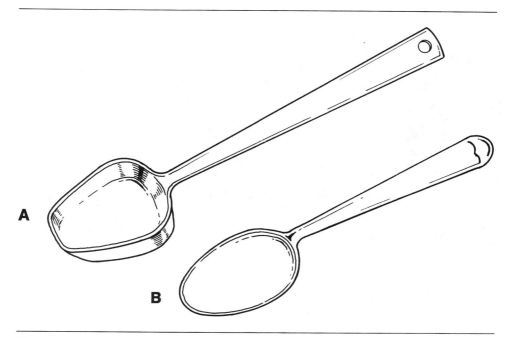

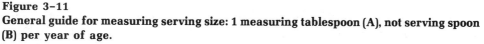

Figure 3-11
General guide for measuring serving size: 1 measuring tablespoon (A), not serving spoon (B) per year of age.

should be given in a small cup (4 to 6 ounces) filled one fourth to one half full (2 to 3 ounces).

Food should be given at five to six intervals throughout the day with at least 2 to 2½ hours elapsed between eating periods. The number of feeding periods may vary, depending on the appetite of the child and length of stay in the center; however, calorie and nutrient consumption tends to increase when the frequency of eating increases. Food and energy intake are positively affected by allowing the toddler to eat more than three times per day.

Serving family style at an early age helps develop the child's capacity to make choices. However, for the very young toddler the plate may need to be prepared in the kitchen because the child's ability to wait for other children to serve themselves is too limited. On the other hand, the young toddler may come to the serving area after food has been served onto the plate. By 18 to 24 months the child can definitely begin participating in the meal service at least by watching older children serve themselves.

Time and schedules usually run child-care centers, especially centers in which children spend only part of the day. However, the meal service should be expected to take at least 30 minutes if the care giver is using the environment as

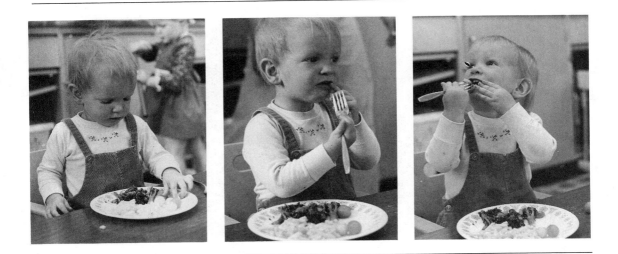

Figure 3–12
A 12-month-old experiments with the use of a fork.

an educational tool. Discussing the eating process and the foods the child eats is important. This time is also needed to practice the use of a fork and spoon (Figure 3–12). All activities surrounding food can be used to stimulate language development (Chapters 7 and 8).

Equipment

High chairs* for the very young are useful, but quickly the child can graduate to small tables and chairs. The child's feet should touch the floor, or a wooden box can be provided on the floor so that the child's feet do not dangle. Papers may be spread on the floor to prevent excessive cleanup.

Small flatware—spoons, knives, and forks—can be introduced by the toddler stage. The plate or bowl for the young toddler should have a curved edge so that the child can push the food against the edge in filling the spoon. In case you think this is unnecessary, we suggest you try eating peas from a flat plate, left-handed (if you are right-handed). Glasses or cups with heavy bottoms help to prevent spills. Filling a glass only partially full not only gives the child the opportunity to ask for more, but also limits the amount you need to clean up if accidents occur. Clear glasses (plastic) allow the care giver and the child to judge how much milk has been poured.

* Some states prohibit the use of high chairs in child-care facilities.

Eating Behavior

By the time the toddler stage is reached, the child may show strong preferences for particular foods. Although you may have taken care to give the infant a variety of nourishing foods without the addition of sugar or salt, the toddler may, even with limited exposure, demand these foods over other foods when available. Food may be refused at mealtime because children may not be hungry, may be exerting their independence, may be too busy exploring the environment, or may simply be tired and need to rest.

When food is not eaten by an individual child, especially the very young child, at mealtime, many care givers become anxious and supplement with snacks between meals. There is nothing wrong with snacks chosen from the basic food groups, but many times the snacks do not match up nutritionally to the meal or they replace important nutrients provided by the meal. Often energy needs are met with foods containing a high proportion of carbohydrate or fat or both with few other nutrients.

What if the child does not eat? The first word of caution is not to punish the child for refusing foods; on the other hand, center activities can be managed so that the child will learn to readily accept most, if not all, foods. Through positive experiences with food, the child can learn to like most foods. Research is explicit in stating that children dislike foods that are unfamiliar to them and those that their parents dislike [8]. Clearly, the responsibility for providing opportunities in which a variety of foods will be introduced to the child over and over rests with the care giver and food service personnel. The child becomes familiar with new foods only after frequent experiences with such foods.

The effect of various methods of encouraging the child to eat or try new foods has been reviewed by Satter [9]. The frequency of exposure has been shown to be important at least during the toddler stage [10]. The more a child is exposed to a food, the more likely the child will try the food. However, quality of exposure can also affect food preferences. Preschoolers who are enticed with a reward to try new foods were less likely to go back to that food than those who were simply exposed to it and allowed to try it on their own [11]. Foods that are presented in a positive situation or along with a rewarding situation (for example, a birthday or holiday) tend to be preferred [12]. Once the care giver has offered the foods and presented a positive and encouraging environment, the child should be allowed to enjoy the mealtime along with the care givers [13].

When the care giver is faced with a child who will not eat, there may be little the center can do but discuss the child's behavior with the family or, if available, a social service professional. The care giver may have little influence over children from dysfunctional families that are too controlling, over-organized, and too cohesive [14]. The parent-child relationship at home may affect the food intake and preferences. Nevertheless, the following questions may help the care giver understand the child who won't eat. Is the child

- Developmentally ready for the foods and equipment presented?
- Hungry?

- Exerting some independence?
- Too busy "on the go" exploring the environment?
- Tired and in need of sleep more than food?
- Expected to eat foods not eaten by other family members or care givers?
- Using utensils, chair, and table of right size?
- Served portions that are an appropriate size?
- Eating enough?
- Becoming ill or recovering from an illness?

Teachers use many techniques to resolve eating problems. Imitation is still one of the best means by which children learn. Children like to imitate adults as well as other siblings. Placing the picky eater at the table next to a child who

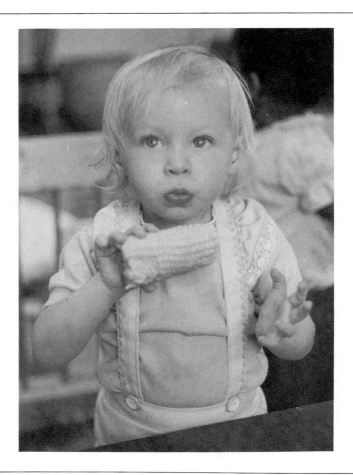

Figure 3-13
A toddler experiments with tasting.

has learned to enjoy all foods often helps encourage the child to try a variety of foods. Offering the new food first, while the child is hungry, also encourages the child to become acquainted with it (Figure 3–13). If schedules and policies permit, allow the toddler to prepare food or watch you or the food service personnel prepare foods. The child will want to explore by tasting each ingredient (for example, vegetables for the soup). Involving the food service staff in educational activities often improves the acceptance of food by children and teacher and may improve the quality of food service.

Another technique often used when a child refuses to eat is ignoring the behavior by walking away from the "whiny" child, especially if the child is using food to get attention. A frustrated and fatigued child should be allowed to rest before eating; you then avoid a tug-of-war over food.

NUTRITION-RELATED PROBLEMS

The major health problems that are nutrition related and may be affected by diet during childhood are anemia, obesity, dental caries, and cardiovascular disease. Lactose intolerance and food allergies are discussed in Chapter 2.

Anemia

The transition from infant feeding regimens, which often include fortified formulas and infant cereals, to whole milk and family foods can affect the iron content of the diet and subsequently the iron status of the child. Anemia is a condition in which the concentration of hemoglobin (measurement of the color of the red blood cells) and the hematocrit (measurement of the quantity of red cells) are below a certain standard. One of the most common causes of anemia is an iron deficiency in the diet.

Recent reports indicate an improvement of nutritional status related to iron among infants and children of high- and low-risk backgrounds [15,16]. The Women, Infants and Children (WIC) Supplemental Food Program has helped lower the prevalence of anemia in low-income families, and researchers also note a decline in prevalence of anemia among middle income children seen in private practices. This is considered a pediatric success story!

Before the toddler years, children in the WIC program (Chapter 2, Appendix 2–B) receive iron-rich formulas instead of whole milk. Toddlers also can receive iron-rich infant cereals until 18 months or longer followed by iron-fortified cereals through the WIC program.

Although the incidence of anemia appears to be declining with the use of iron-rich foods and medical attention, certain groups are still at high risk for anemia [17]. Children in these groups are characterized by:

1. Low socioeconomic background
2. Regular use of cow's milk started before 6 months

3. Use of formula without iron
4. Low birth weight

Unfortunately, discontinuing iron-fortified formulas at 6 months and inappropriately applying adult dietary guidelines to diets of very young children may reverse the decrease in anemia seen recently. Although low-fat, high-fiber foods are beneficial for the whole family, overuse of these foods is not best for very young children. As mentioned earlier, too much fiber may inhibit iron absorption. Also, while legumes, breads, iron-fortified cereals, and certain vegetables and fruits are good sources of iron, iron from "red" meats—which some families may be avoiding—is more readily available to the body than that supplied from plant products. Serve a diet with some readily available sources of iron, such as red meat, and a vitamin C source along with the high-fiber grains and legumes for optimal benefit.

In summary, nutrition guidelines to prevent iron deficiency include:

1. Prolong breast feeding to 6 months or more.
2. Use iron-fortified formula after weaning and for infants not breast-fed.
3. Delay starting regular cow's milk until 12 months.
4. Use infant cereals fortified with iron and ascorbic acid as one of the first solid foods introduced after 4 to 6 months.
5. Combine iron-rich and ascorbic acid–rich foods when meals of solid foods are given. For example, iron-fortified cereals, beans, and peas should be given with vitamin C–containing foods such as orange juice.
6. Give the young child some meat, fish, or poultry along with whole grains, legumes, beans, and nutbutters.
7. Limit intake of whole cow's milk to no more than 32 ounces per day.

Obesity

Recent data show that 25 to 29% of 6- to 11-years-olds are obese [18]. In addition, the number of preschool children considered obese is increasing [19].

Assessing a child's weight-for-height status is discussed in detail in previous chapters. Using the height-for-weight grids, measurements greater than 95th percentile usually indicate obesity. These measurements are best confirmed by the health professional with skinfold measurements in excess of the 85th percentile.

Recommending dietary restrictions for the young child based only on height and weight grids is not advisable. These measurements do not take into consideration the family history of obesity, environment, and physical activity patterns. The Committee on Nutrition of the American Academy of Pediatrics [20] estimates that for most obese children, unlike adults, lean body mass accounts for as much as 50% of the obese child's excess weight. The committee states that the weight-for-height grids will indicate false positives with heavy muscular children and false negatives with lighter children who have a relative excess of body fat. The grids also tend to underestimate adiposity (fatness) in chidren less than 3 years old.

Although techniques are available to assess and help prevent obesity, success has not been easy to achieve. In fact, research indicates that childhood family environment alone as seen in adoptive homes has little if any apparent influence on fatness in adults. There is, however, a clear relationship between the body mass of the biological parents and the weight class of their children. Although children favor the weight of their biological parents, not their adoptive parents, fatness is not necessarily determined at conception. The genetic tendency toward fatness can be fully expressed or repressed depending on environmental factors such as food supply and emphasis on exercise [2].

What should be done? "Prevention" is the obvious quick and easy response given to parents concerned that their child may be becoming obese. Peck and Ullrich [21] have addressed the current attitudes and practices involved with actual and potential weight-related problems of children and have detailed several recommendations for action. Their recommendations, based on the child's age and the severity of the weight problem, are given in Table 3-9.

A conservative approach to treating overweight children is recommended because no one has enough information to predict which children will spontaneously lose their excess fat, which will do so with some treatment, and which will always be fat. No action should be taken unless both care giver and counselor are aware of the history of growth, family eating patterns, and family attitudes toward food, body size, and physical activity.

In a recently published study of 6- to 11-year-olds, time spent viewing television emerged as the most powerful predictor of obesity in adolescence, even when controlling for other known variables associated with childhood obesity [22]. Therefore, one definite action every parent can take, even for toddlers, is limiting the number of television viewing hours. True, other activities may have to substitute for the television. Parents may find the substitute activity to be more educational for the child. Teaching a child to complete household activities at an early age may prove helpful as the child gets older and both parents find themselves working outside the household.

The history of one child's weight gain is presented in Figures 3-14 to 3-16. Note that the goal in working with an overweight child is maintaining current weight or curtailing weight gain, not reducing weight. As the child continued to grow taller (Figure 3-14), his weight remained the same for 6 months (Figure 3-15). During the next year he gained only 4 pounds (1.8 kg). At 2½ years the boy weighed 36 pounds (16.2 kg) and was 36 inches (90 cm) tall. The child was above the 95th percentile (weight for stature) as seen in Figure 3-16. By 36 months the child had grown to 37 inches (92.5 cm), but held his weight constant. This was accomplished by changing his activity patterns and following a plan agreed on by the care giver and the parents. At age 3½ years he was 39 inches (97.5 cm) and weighed 37½ pounds (16.9 kg). As the child reached 4 years, his height was 40½ inches (101.3 cm), and he weighed 40 pounds (18 kg), but his weight for height was now below the 90th percentile.

Table 3-9
Recommended actions for weight problems by degree of severity and age

		Degree of Overweight*		
		Mild**	Moderate**	Severe
Weight for Height Percentile		75–89	90–94	95 and above
Developmental Stage	*Age Range*	*Levels of Activities*		
Infant	0–12 mo	Action 1	Action 1	Action 1
Toddler	1–2 yrs	Action 1	Action 1	Action 2
Preschool	3–5 yrs	Action 1	Action 2	Action 2
Schoolage	6–9 yrs	Action 1	Action 2	Action 3
		Mild	Moderate	Severe
Percent overweight for height, age, sex		120–139	140–159	160 and above
Preadolescent	varies	Action 1	Action 2	Action 3
Adolescent	15–18	Action 1	Action 2	Action 3

Levels of Activity Related to Prevention and Treatment

Action 1
A. Ascertain history of the child's physical growth by use of National Center for Health Statistics growth charts if possible. If there is a marked change from the child's usual pattern of growth, move to Action 2.

* Based on NCHS growth charts.
** Mild and Moderate may be actually heaviness due to factors other than fat, i.e., muscularity and/or heavy body frame. Skinfold measurements can substantiate fatness.

Activity pattern can be modified by planning more gross motor activities and remembering that the child must have success at these activities. The obese, nonactive child may stay obese because gross motor activities have not been particularly rewarding for him in the past.

If all foods are consumed with equal gusto, then portion size has to be limited or the child diverted from second helpings. This can be done by keeping the child busy with table serving or cleanup activities or running to the kitchen for catsup, flatware, or napkins, by slowing all the children in their eating activities by asking them to chew every bite completely and to put down their spoon between bites, and by encouraging second helpings of low-calorie vegetables. If the child is a "milk drinker," milk can be given in smaller amounts. Providing a snack (low calorie) 30 minutes before mealtime may also help curtail the child's appetite.

If the center has an overweight child, there should be *no* food served that has a low nutritional density in proportion to calories. This principle is advisable in all centers, but especially in the center where some of the children are obese.

Table 3–9
continued

B. Ascertain family history of obesity: Neither parent obese—low risk of child becoming more obese; may need to explore other causes of obesity; one parent obese—moderate risk of child becoming more obese; Two parents obese—high risk of child becoming more obese. If moderate or high risk automatically move to Action 2.

C. Ascertain caretakers' or individual's knowledge, attitudes, and practices related to the following items and provide education where needed: Normal growth patterns; Body size and shape; Nutrient and food needs; Normal psychosocial development, especially in relation to food intake, discipline and control; Physical activity.

Action 2

A. A thorough assessment of the problem by a health practitioner who has an understanding of the many aspects of the problem and is capable of recognizing when referral is required, i.e., dietitian-nutritionist, pediatriican or other M.D. or nurse with special expertise in this practice.

B. Intervention program based on individual need for a period of time (6–12 months) to bring about change in behavior of caretaker and or child. If unsuccessful move to Action 3.

Action 3

A health assessment and the development of an intervention program by a multidisciplinary team at a specialized clinic. This program could then be carried out by a team of local professionals if the clinic is a distance from the home community.

Source: Peck, E. B., and Ullrich, H. D.: Children and weight: a changing perspective, 1985, Nutrition Communications Associates, Berkeley, CA 94708.

Finally, these activities must be coordinated with the home situation. Parents and care givers must cooperatively plan the best strategy for the child. The child's pediatrician should be notified of dietary modifications. Each week the child should be weighed and measured, and this weight and height measurement should be recorded and given to the parents along with information on the child's educational progress. If the child has been evaluated and parents and care givers both recognize the problem, the center's consulting dietitian or nutritionist should be asked to assist with the planning.

Specific steps can be taken to learn more about the problem before action is taken:

1. Record the eating behavior of the child in the center and the home, asking the parents to keep a dietary record (Appendix VI).
2. Record the activity patterns of the child in the center and the home, asking the parents to note the kind of exercise or activity and the time spent in exercise or activities.

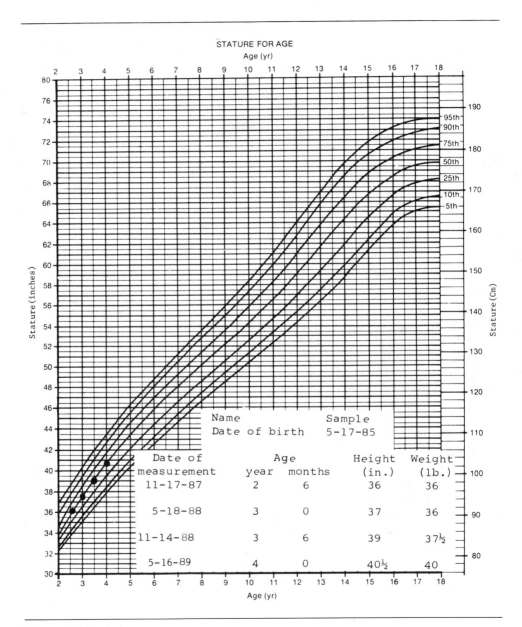

STATURE FOR AGE

Age (yr)

Date of measurement	Age year	months	Height (in.)	Weight (lb.)
11-17-87	2	6	36	36
5-18-88	3	0	37	36
11-14-88	3	6	39	$37\frac{1}{2}$
5-16-89	4	0	$40\frac{1}{2}$	40

Name   Sample
Date of birth   5-17-85

Figure 3–14
Height for age of preschool boy plotted against 50th percentile (*Source:* Department of Health, Education and Welfare, National Center for Health Statistics, 1979.)

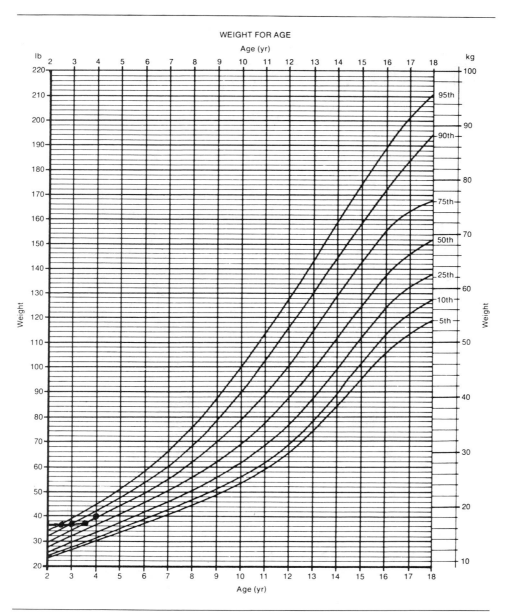

WEIGHT FOR AGE

Figure 3–15
Weight for age of preschool boy, plotted on chart for 2- to 18-year-olds (*Source:* U.S. Department of Health, Education and Welfare, National Center for Health Statistics, 1979.)

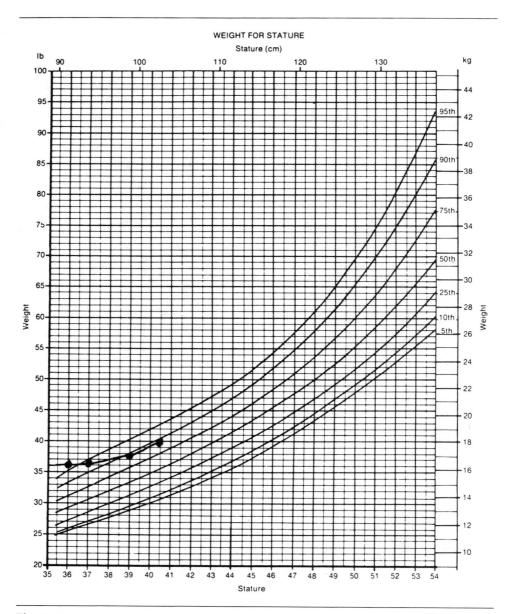

Figure 3–16
Weight for stature of preschool boy, plotted on chart for 2- to 11½-year-olds (*Source:* U.S. Department of Health, Education and Welfare, National Center for Health Statistics, 1979.)

3. Parents and care giver with dietitian or nutritionist can:
   a. Evaluate eating and activity patterns.
   b. Develop a weight-control management program for home and center to control excessive weight gain.
   c. Follow child's progress.

Dental Caries

Conditions that affect the incidence of dental caries begin during the toddler years. Dental caries consist of localized, progressive decay of teeth, initiated by demineralization of the outer surface of the tooth. This process is caused by organic acids produced locally by bacteria that ferment deposits of dietary carbohydrates; sucrose, or table sugar, is the primary carbohydrate. While many common foods can be cariogenic, some foods, such as aged cheddar cheese, can help decrease acid conditions and prevent carie formation.

After the toddler eats, care givers can clean the teeth as soon as practical by wiping the mouth with fine gauze wrapped around the finger. You can introduce a toothbrush by 12 to 15 months when the teeth have erupted, and by 18 months the routine can be well established. Toothpaste may be used, but it is not necessary.

Nursing bottle caries, or *nursing bottle syndrome,* refers to the destruction of the anterior (front) teeth as a result of contact with carbohydrate-containing solutions fed through the bottle. When the child is allowed to take a bottle to bed at naptime or in the evening, sucking and swallowing are infrequent, saliva flow is minimal, and sugar remains in contact with the teeth for a long time. This is especially true if the child is taking liquids with sucrose or glucose [4].

Bottles at bedtime should not be allowed in the center. If the child is drinking from a bottle, it should be given when the child is fully awake and upright. All sweetened fluids, including formula, should be given by cup and teeth brushed after the feedings, if possible.

Although frequent eating periods are advocated for the toddler, these feedings should not include sugary, calorie-dense foods (sugar, honey, corn syrup, candies, jellies, jams, sugared breakfast cereals, cookies, cakes, chewing gum, and sweetened beverages). Snacks, as well as meals, should include selections from the basic food groups—fruits and vegetables (avoid the sugar-sweetened varieties), breads and crackers with margarine or peanut butter, cheeses, milk, and meats.

Fluoride has a beneficial effect in decreasing the incidence and severity of dental caries. However, excessive intake of fluoride may cause mottled discoloration of teeth. Child-care centers located in areas where water is unfluoridated should alert parents whose children remain in the center all day to the need for supplementing the child's intake of fluoride.

Cardiovascular Disease

There is controversy over whether older children should be given a diet that is limited in total fat, saturated fat, and cholesterol [23, 24]. Although at home the child will likely be consuming a diet similar to the parents, the center should not aim to restrict the young child's intake of red meats, dairy products, and eggs. These foods provide high-quality protein, iron, calcium, and other nutrients necessary for the growth of children. A complete discussion of diet and cardiovascular disease for children is included in Chapter 5.

Lactose Intolerance

Lactose, the disaccharide or carbohydrate found in milk and milk products, is broadly consumed in its natural form and in a variety of manufactured and processed products. The adequacy of lactose digestion and absorption has important implications for care givers in centers that have a predominantly nonwhite population. Throughout the world *lactose intolerance*, a lack of sufficient quantities of the digestive enzyme lactase, is far more common than tolerance. Tolerance of lactose and large quantities of milk is peculiar to northern European and white American ethnic groups; most adults in the world cannot tolerate large quantities of milk because of lactose intolerance [25].

Studies of black children in the United States show a progressive decrease in lactose absorption with age. Most infants at birth can tolerate the high percentage of lactose found in breast milk or can tolerate formulas that contain lactose. However, at 1 or 2 years of age, 27% of black children have evidence of lactose malabsorption, and at ages 5 to 6 years, 33% may be malabsorbers [25]. This progressive increase in the prevalence of malabsorption with age has been noted for black children in both high and low socioeconomic groups.

It is important to recognize that lactose intolerance is not an all-or-none phenomenon. Rather, the availability of the enzyme lactase slowly declines, and this decline can be influenced by transit time (how fast the food moves through the intestinal tract), the food (cheese, milk, yogurt) in which the lactose is consumed, and intake of additional foods.

A child may not be able to tolerate a glass of milk when arriving at the center, but after or when eating other foods, tolerates milk well. Likewise, cheese may be tolerated when cow's milk causes gastric distress. Although a child may have been given a test that involves a tolerance dosage of lactose, there is a difference between an individual's ability to tolerate a large challenge dose of lactose and the ability to use the lesser amounts of lactose found in commonly consumed amounts of milk.

Because milk is an important food source for many vitamins, minerals, and protein, lactase can be purchased under various trade names and added to dairy products to predigest the milk sugar. Milk with lactaid is now available in some grocery stores. In addition, the care giver and parents can try cured cheese and yogurt, in which much of the lactose is broken down in the fermentation process. Finally, one can substitute other foods for the calcium in milk by referring to Table 3–5 for alternate calcium sources. Supplementation with calcium may be necessary in some cases.

EXERCISE AND PHYSICAL FITNESS

Concerned parents often begin pressuring care givers to provide more energy expenditure through exercise for children in this age span. This is the result of a constant barrage of fitness survey reports that are reported over and over on television and in magazines and newspapers. National studies of youth fitness over a period of 27 years have revealed that children in the United States are underexercised [26]. Interestingly, these surveys were conducted with children aged 6 years to 17 years. Still the message is loud and clear. Our kids are overweight and out of shape.

There is a mounting concern among young parents that something needs to be done and it needs to be done early. Many parents of toddlers are beginning to react by seeking out early childhood programs that offer fitness as part of

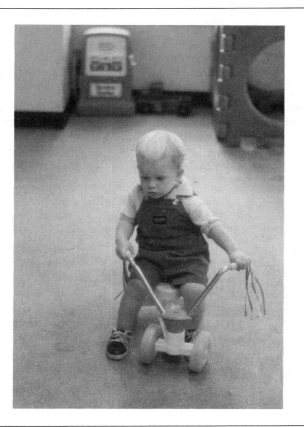

Figure 3-17
A toddler enjoys a four-wheeled toy.

their curriculums. Some national child-care chains are offering "muscle rooms"—large rooms with balance beams, tumbling mats, climbing cubes, and an obstacle course that can be travelled by the children [27].

Home programs are also on the market. Matchbox Toys manufactures a do-it-yourself kiddie exercise kit called Baby-Cise. The kit costs $100 plus for an instructional video, plastic barbells, a baby balance beam, and a clutch ball for developing hand-eye coordination [28].

Over the past 15 years a number of fitness programs targeted specifically for children aged 3 months through 4 years have begun. One such program, Gymboree, began with one center in 1976 and expanded to 326 franchises spread throughout the country by 1988. Gymboree has also expanded to offer a retail line of fitness wear and equipment designed for movement and growth.

The hallmarks of the majority of the franchise programs are songs and games and stretching and climbing exercises in which the children participate with one or both parents. Activities are designed to foster the development of both gross and fine motor skills. Classes are priced $8 to $12 a week for 12 weekly sessions.

The concerns of these parents are valid; however, again we refer you to the cautions regarding exercise programs that were given in Chapter 2.

The early childhood environment should be well stocked with climbers, large cardboard boxes, slides, barrels, large blocks, large balls, puzzles, four-wheeled toys, and push-and-pull play materials (Figure 3–17) [29].

Exercise will occur naturally as the toddlers climb, crawl, pull, walk, bend, and jump. These movements will provide an abundance of exercise for all muscles. Since toddlers are excited and happy about these new movement skills, they will spend much time practicing them over and over both indoors and out of doors. There is no need for a structured exercise program.

SUMMARY

- The toddler, age 12 to 36 months, is growing proportionately more slowly than the infant; however, continued attention to the child's height and weight, developmental skills, and dietary intake is important.
- Although the toddler's demand for energy is proportionately lower, 45 kcal per pound compared with 48 for a 6- to 12-month-old infant, the need for essential nutrients is still great. The food eaten must contain essential nutrients without excessive energy or calories.
- The care giver's task is to interest the child in food and eating when the child is hungry and to acquaint the child with a wide variety of food experiences.
- Foods from the food groups should be carefully chosen to encourage the child to self-feed using fingers and small-sized flatware, and a variety of new and interesting combinations of foods along with familiar foods should be introduced.

- Some nutrition-related problems develop during the toddler stage. Iron-deficiency anemia may become acute if the infant was not given iron supplements or a diet high in iron during the 6- to 12-month period. Obesity may persist or become evident in the toddler years. Dental caries may develop as a result of frequent consumption of foods that contain large quantities of sticky carbohydrates, nursing bottle syndrome, or consumption of an unfluoridated water supply without the addition of fluoride supplements. A few toddlers who could tolerate milk during infancy may develop an intolerance to milk during the toddler and preschool years as a result of the condition known as lactose intolerance.
- Many parents become overly concerned about exercise for children during the toddler years.

DISCUSSION QUESTIONS

1. List preparation methods which could be used with specific foods to stimulate a toddler to use fingers, spoon, and fork.
2. A child is anemic. How would you help the mother choose foods that would increase the iron supply in the child's diet?
3. A toddler's height for weight is above the 95th percentile. Which factors would you take into consideration before discussing the perceived problem with the parents and health professionals?
4. What are the energy and nutrient needs of the toddler compared with those of the infant?
5. What type of exercises occur naturally during the toddler period?

REFERENCES

1. Grand, R. J., Sutphen, J. L., and Dietz, W. H.: Pediatric nutrition theory and practice, Boston, 1987, Butterworth Publishers.
2. Stunkard, A. J., Sorensen, T. I. A., Hanis, C., et al.: An adoption study on human obesity, N. Engl. J. Med. 314:193–198, 1986.
3. Anselmo, S.: Early childhood development: prenatal through age eight, Columbus, OH, 1987, Merrill Publishing Co.
4. Erikson, E. H.: Childhood and society, ed. 2, New York, 1963, W. W. Norton & Co., Inc.
5. Stone, L. J., and Church, J.: Childhood adolescence: a psychology of the growing person, ed. 3, New York, 1973, Random House, Inc.
6. National Research Council, Food and Nutrition Board: Recommended Dietary Allowance, ed. 9, Washington DC, 1980, National Academy of Science.
7. National Center for Health Statistics, U.S. Department of Health and Human Services, Public Health Service: Dietary intake source data: United States, 1976–80. DHHS Publication No. (PHS) 83–1681, Hyattsville, MD, 1983.

8. Burt, J. V., and Hertzler, A. A.: Parental influence on the child's food preference, J. Nutr. Educ. 10:127–128, 1978.

9. Satter, E. M.: The feeding relationship, J. Am. Diet. Assoc. 86:352–356, 1986.

10. Birch L. L., and Marlin, D. W.: I don't like it; I never tried it: effects of exposure on two-year-old children's food preferences, Appetite: J. for Intake Research 3:353–360, 1982.

11. Birch L. L., Marlin, D. W., and Rotter, J.: Eating as the "means" activity in a contingency: effects on young children's food preference. Child Dev. 55:431–439, 1984.

12. Birch, L. L., Zimmerman, S. I., and Hind, H.: The influence of social-affective context on the formation of children's food preferences, Child Dev. 51:856–861, 1980.

13. Satter, E. M.: Child of Mine: feeding with love and good sense, Palo Alto, CA, 1986, Bull Publishing Co.

14. Kinter, M., Boss, P. G., and Johnston, N.: The relationship between dysfunctional family environments and family member food intake, J. Marriage Family 43:633, 1981.

15. Yip, R., Walsh, K. M., Goldfarb, M. G., and Blinkin, N. J.: Declining prevalence of anemia in childhood in middle class children: a pediatric success story? Pediatrics 80:330, 1987.

16. Yip, R., Blinkin, N. J., Fleshood, L. and Trowbridge, F. L.: Declining prevalence of anemia among low-income children in the United States, J.A.M.A. 258:1619–1623, 1987.

17. Dallman, P. R.: Has routine screening of infants for anemia become obsolete in the United States? Pediatrics 80:439, 1987.

18. Gortmaker, S. L., Dietz, W. H., Sobol, A. M., Wehler, C. A.: Increasing pediatric obesity in the United States, Am. J. Dis. Child. 141:535–540, 1987.

19. Ginsberg-Fellner, F., Jagendorf, L. A., Carmel, H. et al.: Overweight and obesity in preschool children in New York City, Am. J. Clin. Nutr. 34:2236–2241, 1981.

20. American Academy of Pediatrics, Committee on Nutrition: Nutritional aspects of obesity in infancy and childhood, Pediatrics 68:880–883, 1981.

21. Peck, E. B., and Ullrich, H. D.: Children and weight: a changing perspective, Berkeley, CA, 1985, Nutrition Communications Associates.

22. Dietz, W. H., and Gortmaker, S. L.: Do we fatten our children at the television set? Obesity and television viewing in children and adolescents, Pediatrics 75:807–812, 1985.

23. American Heart Association, Nutrition Committee and the Cardiovascular Disease in the Young Council: Diet in the healthy child, Circulation 67:1411, 1983.

24. American Academy of Pediatrics, Committee on Nutrition: Prudent lifestyle for children: dietary fat and cholesterol, Pediatrics 78:521, 1986.

25. Paige, D. M., and Bayless, T. M.: Lactose digestion, Baltimore, MD, 1981, The Johns Hopkins University Press.

26. The President's Council on Physical Fitness and Sports, National School Population Fitness Survey, HHS—Office of the Assistant Secretary for Health Research Project No. 282-84-0086, University of Michigan Press, 1986.

27. Ward, A.: Born to jog: exercise programs for preschoolers, The Physician and Sports Medicine 14:163, 1986.

28. Kantrowitz, B., and Joseph, N.: Building baby biceps, Newsweek 107:79, May 26, 1986.

29. Mena, J. G.: Toddlers: what to expect, Young Children 42:50, 1986.

LEARNING OBJECTIVES

Students will be able to

- **State the physiological characteristics of the preschooler that may affect eating habits.**
- **State the nutrient and energy needs of the preschool child**
- **Evaluate the diet using food groups**
- **List acceptable snack foods from each food group**
- **Describe the vegetarian diet and its use in the preschool center**
- **State common nutrition-related problems**

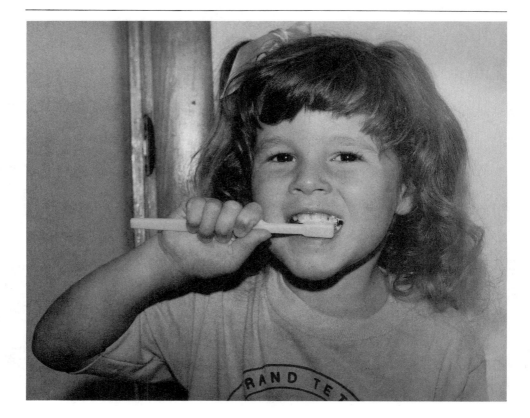

4

The Preschooler
(3 to 5 Years)

The preschool child is often called the "runabout." However, the run for the table is not simply to practice running, but for a specific purpose—to join friends at lunch. The child between 3 and 5 years of age is usually a physical child, and although the toddler moved around excessively, the preschooler often surpasses the toddler in activity. As new skills develop, those learned during the toddler stage become refined, and the preschooler gains sophistication in motion control. Long gone are the days when the child practiced gaining head control, the upright posture, and the basic abilities. The beauty of this particular age is that the child no longer has to struggle with learning to suck, swallow, chew, and use a spoon, fork, and knife. If the parents or care givers have regularly eaten with the child and the child has practiced using utensils, only the use of a knife for cutting and spreading may need some refinement. Thus, this is the first real opportunity for the care giver and child to actively participate together in the food and nutrition program (Figure 4-1).

Up to now the challenges for the teacher have been to acquaint the child with a wide variety of food tastes and choices and to teach the basic use of utensils. If this is done successfully before 3 years of age, any food can be used as an educational experience. However, if the child has been encouraged to eat only a small number of foods and many foods of poor nutrient quality, the task of introducing a wide variety of foods into the child's diet will be added to the responsibilities of the nutrition program at the child-care center.

Physically, though, the child will want to participate in most activities in the center. This means that preparing food, setting the table, serving the food, cleaning up, and occasionally going to the market can become a regular part of the child's activities. The child at this point can use scissors to cut out pictures and

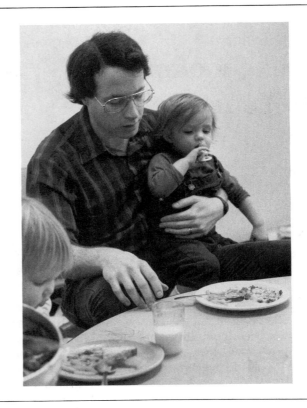

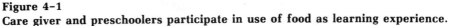

Figure 4-1
Care giver and preschoolers participate in use of food as learning experience.

can color. These skills can be used to make placemats for the tables and can be incorporated into other activities that will make meals a special learning time. Psychosocially, the child struggles to develop a sense of initiative and takes an eager and inquisitive approach to the surroundings. Size, form, color, shape, time, and space take on a new meaning and can be related to foods and mealtime.

WEIGHT AND STATURE

The relative state of health of the child influences growth. Ordinary illnesses such as upper respiratory tract infections or the childhood diseases usually are not severe or prolonged enough to interfere with growth. Chronic, repeated, or severe illness, however, may cause the body to conserve resources, and the rate of growth may slow.

Table 4-1
Weight and stature by sex and age for 3- to 5-year-olds

Age (years)	Girls		Boys	
	Weight (pounds)	Stature (inches)	Weight (pounds)	Stature (inches)
3	31.0	37.0	32.2	37.4
4	35.1	40.0	36.7	40.5
5	37.0	42.7	41.1	43.3

Source: Modified from charts showing smoothed percentiles of weight and stature by sex and age developed by National Center for Health Statistics, U.S. Department of Health, Education and Welfare, PHS, Hyattsville, MD, 1977, The Center.

Watching the stature and weight charts can be important, and any prolonged slowdown in growth should be noted. Stature and weight of the preschool child should be taken on a monthly basis and recorded on charts for boys and girls ages 2 to 18 years (Appendix VI). The physical growth of the preschooler can be monitored through the use of a scale and measuring stick as described in Chapter 3.

The preschooler's height and weight do not increase as rapidly as they did during the first 12 months. The 4-year-old probably will weigh five times as much as at birth. Therefore, the 7½ pound (3.8 kg) baby can now be expected to weigh about 37 pounds (16.7 kg). This is a general rule, and individual weights will vary. Between 3 and 5 years of age the child will probably not gain more than 4 pounds (1.8 kg) per year or approximately ⅓ pound (0.15 kg) each month (Table 4-1).

The preschooler's weight may vary up to a pound or two from one month to another. Although this fact should cause some concern, a recent illness or increased food or beverage consumption may cause weight to change.

If the child has gained a pound or two in less than a month, look for the reasons. Weight gain may be a result of overeating, error in measurement, or faulty equipment. Losses or gains of a pound or two each month over a 2- or 3-month period without a change in height should cause concern. After ensuring proper use of eating equipment, take time to talk with the parents about any changes in the child's physical or eating behavior. Then, if necessary, check with the physician or dietitian/nutritionist who will review height, weight, skinfold, dietary, and health history.

CHILD DEVELOPMENT SKILLS

Although discussed later, the language skills are emphasized here to remind the care giver that the child is now ready for verbal exchange regarding the eating period. The child is eager to help the care giver and parents with preparation,

Table 4-2
Stages of development for preschool and early elementary years*

Stage	Physical	Nutritional	Intellectual
Preschool: 3 to 4 years	Slowed steady height-weight gain; lordosis and prominent abdomen disappear; face grows faster than cranial cavity; jaw widens	Assertion of independence increases; appetite declines with picky food habits	Concept of "conservation" begins (i.e., some features of objects remain the same despite changes in other features)
Elementary I: 5 to 6 years	Steady average weight gain 3 to 3.5 kg/yr and height gain of 6 cm/yr; growth of head slows	Rate of growth stabilizes, accompanied by more regular appetite; likes to be included in food-related activities	Child can begin to take others' viewpoints; school begins

Stage	Gross Motor	Fine Motor	Speech and Language
Preschool: 3 to 4 years	Stands and hops on one foot; jumps heights and distances	Minute degrees of flexion and extension of inter-phalangeal joints in three jaw chuck position	Sentence length and complexity increase; uses language for a variety of purposes (to satisfy needs, pretend, argue, etc.); other consonants emerge
Elementary I: 5 to 6 years	Rides a bicycle; begins organized play activities and perfects game skills	Refinement of individual finger coordination (i.e., piano playing); ability to use one upper extremity for one task, one for a different task	Receptive and expressive language develop in relation to cognitive growth

Stage	Social/Behavioral
Preschool: 3 to 4 years	Moves from parallel to cooperative play; able to conform
Elementary I: 5 to 6 years	Acceptable table manners; peers becoming more important

Source: Modified from Harvey-Smith, M., et al.: Feeding management of a child with a handicap: a guide for professionals, Memphis, 1982, University of Tennessee Center for the Health Sciences.

*This chart provides the health professional with a standard tool for assessing feeding levels.

service, and cleanup of food. However, it should be remembered that because of the child's quickness in movement and occasional inattentiveness, there may be spills or broken dishes. Mishaps are inevitable, but generally these are not intentional. The child simply misjudges situations, and these miscalculations, combined with the haste of a preschooler to accomplish a task, cause accidents. During the preschool period the rate of growth stabilizes and appetite is regular. The child likes to be included in food-related activities (Table 4-2).

ENERGY AND NUTRIENT NEEDS

Energy

The energy needs of children of the same age, sex, and size can vary due to differences in physical activity or the efficiency with which children utilize energy.

The RDA can be the guide for energy needs for the 4- to 6-year-old. It can be seen in Table 4–3 that the energy requirements per pound or per kilogram of body weight have decreased since the toddler years. At birth the child required about 52 kcal per pound; between 1 and 3 years approximately 45 kcal per pound; and by 4 years the child requires only about 39 kcal per pound.

Total calories increase as the child grows taller and gains weight. For this age group it may be easier to base energy needs on an individual basis and consider allowing 38 to 39 calories per inch (Chapter 3). If the child is very active, additional energy will be required.

Table 4–3
RDA for ages 1–3 and 4–6

	1 to 3 Years (29 lb, 35 in. [13 kg, 87.5 cm])	4 to 6 Years (44 lb, 44 in. [19.8 kg, 110 cm])
Food energy (kcal)	1300 (lb × 44.8)	1700 (lb × 38.6)
Protein (g)*	23	30
Vitamin A activity (IU)	2000	2500
Vitamin D (IU)	400	400
Vitamin E activity (IU)	7	9
Ascorbic acid (mg)	45	45
Folacin (μg)	100	200
Niacin (mg)	9	11
Riboflavin (mg)	0.8	1.0
Thiamin (mg)	0.7	0.9
Vitamin B_6 (mg)	0.9	1.3
Vitamin B_{12} (μg)	2.0	2.5
Calcium (mg)	800	800
Phosphorus (mg)	800	800
Iodine (μg)	70	90
Iron (mg)	15	10
Magnesium (mg)	150	200
Zinc (mg)	10	10

Source: Based on Food and Nutrition Board, National Academy of Sciences—National Research Council: Recommended dietary allowances, revised 1980.

*Assumes protein equivalent to human milk.

In any case, given an energy allowance of 1300 to 2300 kcal (for 4- to 6-year-olds) and a need for a wide variety of nutrients, the diet should contain foods of high nutrient density. Foods that supply few nutrients in addition to energy should not be included in the diet. Children often prefer sweet grain products; however, adding foods such as cakes and pies adds many kilocalories without adding necessary nutrients.

Once again, the energy needs are not fixed for the child and depend on whether the child is maintaining a proper height-weight gain. The monthly record of height, weight, and skinfold measurements is the best health indicator available to the pre-school care giver.

Protein

The recommended amount of protein is 1.5 g per kilogram (RDA for the 4- to 6-year-old). Therefore, for a 45-pound (20 kg) 4-year-old child, 30 g of protein is recommended. You are reminded that this is the recommended amount, not the amount actually required by the child (Chapter 1). To meet this need the child should drink between 2 and 3 cups (16 to 24 ounces) of milk (16 to 24 g of protein). This is not only to supply protein, but also to help meet the calcium, riboflavin and other vitamin and mineral needs of the child. Two cups of milk supply 16 g of protein (half the allowance). Two ounces of meat (7 g of protein per ounce of meat) supply 14 g of protein and, along with the 16 g from milk, will supply the recommended 30 g of protein. This excludes the protein in vegetables and bread, which would increase the total protein intake. Contrary to what many people believe, studies have indicated that the average intake of protein for the 1- to 5-year-old child from both high- and low-income families meets the recommended allowances [1].

In addition to meat, it is important to consume nuts, legumes, and beans, which contain protein. Requirements for magnesium, zinc, folacin, and vitamin B_6 are difficult to meet without a wide variety of high-protein sources. Although high-protein foods may be included on a menu in amounts sufficient to meet protein needs, a higher intake of these foods helps the child meet other nutrient needs. Therefore, consuming a variety of protein foods is important.

Minerals/Vitamins

Calcium. Calcium is one of the nutrients found in less than the recommended amounts in some diets. Three cups of milk readily provide the necessary 800 mg of calcium (1 cup supplies approximately 280 mg calcium). If the child likes milk, there is usually little concern that this mineral is taken in quantities necessary for building bones and teeth. However, obtaining enough calcium without consuming dairy products is difficult (Chapter 3). Dried beans and green vegetables are sources of calcium, but the quantity of these foods necessary to meet the child's calcium needs is large and not a practical option during the growing years. If the child cannot drink fresh, fluid milk, then canned (processed) milk, dry milk, yogurt, and cheese (excluding cream cheese) should be tried. These products contain comparable quantities of calcium and may be more easily tolerated.

Iron. About 95% of the children 1 to 5 years of age have iron intakes below the standard, and by the age of 3 many children are believed to have iron-deficiency anemia [2]. The RDA for iron for 1- to 3-year-olds (Table 4–3) is 15 mg. At 4 to 6 years the RDA for iron is 10 mg.

Milk is a poor source of iron, and consuming it in large quantities (more than 3 to 4 cups) may replace foods with higher iron content, especially iron-rich cereals. Discontinuing fortified infant cereals and iron-rich formula also contributes to iron-deficiency anemia in the toddler years. In some cases the toddler may still be eating cooked iron-fortified cereal or iron-fortified infant cereal. But by the preschool years the cooked cereals (for example, Cream of Wheat, Malt-O-Meal) have given way to sugar-coated dry cereals, some of which are not iron fortified.

The preschool child's RDA for iron is less than that of the toddler (10 mg as opposed to 15 mg), and the child is able to chew meat products more readily than at the earlier age. Some of the iron may not be available from plants because of the phytate and fiber components that naturally occur in plants. It has been reported that phytate and fiber bind some of the iron into a complex that the body cannot use [2, 3]. However, the evidence is not conclusive and does not warrant the discontinuation of the use of plant foods as a source of iron.

As indicated, it is difficult to consume enough iron if the energy intake is wasted on food with low nutrient density. Good sources of iron with a high nutrient density are meat, greens, and enriched or iron-fortified whole-grain cereal products (see Chapter 3). In addition, egg yolk, beans, and nuts are good sources of iron. Molasses and dried fruits are good sources of iron, but these products are seldom eaten.

Liver is often cited as one of the best sources of iron, and indeed it is. One ounce of beef liver supplies almost 2 mg of iron, whereas 1 ounce of ground beef supplies only 1 mg. Likewise, 2 tablespoons of wheat germ, ¾ cup of oatmeal or rolled oats, two rye wafers, or 3 tablespoons of cooked spinach supply 1 mg of iron. See Chapter 6 for ways to include iron in the menu.

Vitamin C. A balance of all nutrients is as important for the 3- to 5-year-old as it is for the younger child. A daily source of vitamin C is important, since there is evidence that vitamin C enhances iron absorption.

The question of whether to add vitamin C to the child's diet to prevent the common cold is often raised. Studies have indicated that vitamin C does not reduce the number of colds, but it can make one or more cold symptoms less severe. The greatest effect seems to be to reduce total sick days rather than to actually prevent the common cold [4–6]. See Chapter 1 for a further discussion of vitamin C.

Zinc. Zinc, like iron, is needed in small amounts. The RDA is 10 mg for the preschooler. Zinc is part of the insulin molecule and is necessary for the passage of glucose from the blood into many body cells. The energy of glucose cannot be released until this passage is accomplished. Zinc is an essential nutrient found in many food sources, including organ meats, oysters, egg yolk, beans, and nuts. Milk, meats, legumes, beans, whole-grain cereals, and wheat germ supply more than 1 mg per serving. Many of these foods are also good protein sources.

Many other nutrients must be included in the diet. We have singled out those nutrients that have been found to be consumed in less than recommended amounts or are often presented on child-care centers' menus in less than recommended quantities. These nutrients are difficult to supply without careful planning of menus.

FOOD NEEDS

To determine a child's acceptance of food and the child's nutritional needs, use the dietary history along with physical measurements of growth and development. You may use the 24-hour dietary recall method described in Chapter 1 or a dietary questionnaire listing frequency of foods eaten (Appendix IV). Because many preschoolers are on the go constantly and are now more self-sufficient than during the toddler stage, they can open refrigerator doors, climb onto kitchen cabinets, and open jars to find their favorite foods. This means, for example, that cookies may be stuffed into little pockets when the child enters the center at 7:00 AM. The care giver should realize that the parents may not be able to provide complete information on the kinds and amounts of food the child has eaten.

A good dietary history taken by the care giver may reveal that the amounts of food consumed by the child are less than recommended. Looking further into the family's food intake will reveal that there are numerous occasions when the child may have acquired food without the parents' knowledge.

Parents and care givers should expose children to a variety of foods without rewards or punishments [7–9]. If only a limited diet is served, the child learns to enjoy only a few foods. Given the dietary record, the basic food guide is once more used to evaluate the nutrient intake.

Table 4–4 shows the daily food pattern for a preschooler; actual foods consumed by one 4-year-old are given in Table 4–5. As shown in Table 4–5, the diet provides adequate amounts from each food group. It also meets or exceeds the recommended dietary allowance of most essential vitamins and minerals (Figure 4–2). However, the diet provides less than the recommended kilocalories for a child weighing 40 pounds (energy needs are approximately 1600 kcal, 39 kcal per pound). Additional energy or calories may be needed for some children.

A child needs the same foods as an adult but in smaller portions. This child consumed four servings of milk, three different foods from the meat/meat alternate group, four from the fruit and vegetable group, four servings of whole-grain

Table 4–4
Recommended food intake according to food group and average serving size (ages 3 up to 6 years)

Food Group	Servings/Day	Average Serving (ages 3 up to 6)
Fruits and Vegetables	At least 4 including:	
Vitamin C source (citrus fruits, berries, tomato, cabbage, cantaloupe)	1 or more (twice as much tomato as citrus)	¼–½ C
Green vegetables	1*	4–6 tbsp (⅓ C)
Other vegetables (potato and other green or yellow vegetables and/or other fruits)	2	4–6 tbsp (⅓ C)
Meat and Alternates	3–4 including:	
Lean meat, fish, poultry, and eggs†	2	2 oz
Nutbutters (peanut, soynut)		3 tbsp§
Cooked dried beans or peas	1–2‡	⅜ C
Nuts		¾ oz
Breads and Cereals (Whole Grain)	At least 4	
Bread		¾–1 slice
Ready-to-eat cereals, whole grain, iron-fortified		½ oz
Cooked cereal including macaroni, spaghetti, rice, etc. (whole grain, enriched)		¼ C
Milk and Milk Products	At least 4	¾ C
Whole or 2% milk (1.5 oz cheese = 1 C milk) (C = 8 oz or 240 g)		
Fats and Oils		
Butter, margarine, mayonnaise, oils	3	1 tsp

*Allow a minimum serving of 1 tbsp/year of age for cooked fruits, vegetables, cereals, and ʲasta until the child reaches 8 years or ½ C portion size.

†To enhance overall nutrient content of diet include eggs two to three times a week and liver occasionally.

‡As recommended by Illinois State Board of Education, Department of Child Nutrition: Child Care Food Program—required meal patterns, Springfield, IL, June 1986, The Board.

§Include nutbutters, dried (cooked) beans, or peas at least once a day to meet nutrient recommendations and decrease the fat content of the diet. Use additional servings of meats when legumes, beans, and nuts are omitted.

cereals, and three servings of fats and oils. A preschooler would need to consume only one half to three fourths of a slice of whole-grain bread; however, one slice has been allowed in the example. Once again, the rule for minimum serving size is 1 tablespoon (measuring) per year of age. The diet emphasizes frequent use of legumes and nuts as substitutes for meat and meat products, whole-grain

Table 4–5

Diet for a preschooler (4 years) compared with recommended servings from basic food groups

Food (amounts)	Milk	Protein	Fruits/ Vegetables	Whole-Grain Products*	Fats/Oils
7 AM					
Orange, ½			1		
Cereal, iron fortified, ½ oz				1	
Milk, 2%, ¾ C	1				
10 AM					
Peanut butter, 1½ tbsp		½			
Whole wheat bread, 1 slice				1	
Margarine, 1 tsp					1
12:30 PM					
Hamburger (2 oz)		1			
Whole wheat bun, ½				1	
Cooked beans		½			
Mayonnaise, 1 tsp					1
Lettuce					
Broccoli, ⅓ C			1		
Milk, 2%, ¾ C	1				
5:30 PM					
Broiled fish, 2 oz		1			
Whole wheat pasta, ¼ C				1	
Apricots, ⅓ C			1		
Margarine, 1 tsp					1
Milk 2%, ¾ C	1				
8 PM					
Milk 2%, ¾ C	1				
Banana, ½			1		
TOTAL	4	3	4	4	3
RECOMMENDED SERVINGS	3	3–4	4	4	3

*Iron-fortified cereal may be included to meet recommended needs. Add additional servings to meet energy needs.

cereals and breads, fruits and vegetables, specifically the dark green varieties and those with a high vitamin C content, and milk and milk products.

Fruits and Vegetables

You will remember that the care giver perhaps had more success at introducing a new food when the child was still a toddler. You were urged to present new foods, especially vegetables, when the child was hungry, while other foods were in preparation. However, the care giver has less control over the eating environ-

```
PERCENT ENERGY DISTRIBUTION

              PROTEIN    22%              FAT    37%          CARBOHYDRATE    41%

NUTRIENT   %RDA 0%             20%      33%    40%            60%    66%     80%            100%
----------------I----------------I---------I-----I----------------I-----I---------I----------------I
ENERGY        77%  X X X X X X X X X X X X X X X X X X X X X X X X X X X X X X X X X X
PROTEIN      250%  X X X X X X X X X X X X X X X X X X X X X X X X X X X X X X X X X X X X X X X X X X X X X X X X X X X X
VITAMIN A    294%  X X X X X X X X X X X X X X X X X X X X X X X X X X X X X X X X X X X X X X X X X X X X X X X X X X X X
VITAMIN D     75%  X X X X X X X X X X X X X X X X X X X X X X X X X X X X X X X X X X X X X
VITAMIN E    375%  X X X X X X X X X X X X X X X X X X X X X X X X X X X X X X X X X X X X X X X X X X X X X X X X X X X X
VITAMIN C    281%  X X X X X X X X X X X X X X X X X X X X X X X X X X X X X X X X X X X X X X X X X X X X X X X X X X X X
FOLACIN      182%  X X X X X X X X X X X X X X X X X X X X X X X X X X X X X X X X X X X X X X X X X X X X X X X X X X X X
NIACIN       227%  X X X X X X X X X X X X X X X X X X X X X X X X X X X X X X X X X X X X X X X X X X X X X X X X X X X X
RIBOFLAVIN   260%  X X X X X X X X X X X X X X X X X X X X X X X X X X X X X X X X X X X X X X X X X X X X X X X X X X X X
THIAMIN      169%  X X X X X X X X X X X X X X X X X X X X X X X X X X X X X X X X X X X X X X X X X X X X X X X X X X X X
VITAMIN B₆   173%  X X X X X X X X X X X X X X X X X X X X X X X X X X X X X X X X X X X X X X X X X X X X X X X X X X X X
VITAMIN B₁₂  232%  X X X X X X X X X X X X X X X X X X X X X X X X X X X X X X X X X X X X X X X X X X X X X X X X X X X X
CALCIUM      142%  X X X X X X X X X X X X X X X X X X X X X X X X X X X X X X X X X X X X X X X X X X X X X X X X X X X X
PHOSPHORUS   177%  X X X X X X X X X X X X X X X X X X X X X X X X X X X X X X X X X X X X X X X X X X X X X X X X X X X X
IRON         165%  X X X X X X X X X X X X X X X X X X X X X X X X X X X X X X X X X X X X X X X X X X X X X X X X X X X X
MAGNESIUM    160%  X X X X X X X X X X X X X X X X X X X X X X X X X X X X X X X X X X X X X X X X X X X X X X X X X X X X
ZINC          84%  X X X X X X X X X X X X X X X X X X X X X X X X X X X X X X X X X X X X X X X X X X X X
----------------I----------------I---------I-----I----------------I-----I---------I----------------I

        160.4 MG CHOLESTEROL    7.6-11.4 MG DIETARY FIBER    1193.0 MG SODIUM
```

Figure 4-2
Nutrient analysis of preschooler's diet in Table 4-5 (*Source:* NDDA Laboratory, Southern Illinois University at Carbondale.)

ment of the preschooler, who eats with the other children at the table and who selects foods from serving bowls.

Many preschoolers do not readily consume vegetables and some fruits. Fruits and vegetables introduced in the child-care center may be strange to the child, and vegetables may not be properly prepared. Both situations can easily be remedied if the menus are part of the educational curriculum (Chapter 6). Obviously, you will have to pay particular attention to introducing vegetables and fruits with high nutritional content, especially the dark green vegetables and the iron- and vitamin C–rich foods (Table 4-6). To help the child gain familiarity with new foods, the picky eater should be encouraged and allowed to participate in preparing and serving vegetables and fruits.

During service, small pieces of broccoli and cauliflower should be placed in the serving bowls so a child need take only one flower of broccoli, one asparagus spear, or one brussels sprout. Cooked cabbage is often served to the preschooler in large chunks and spinach greens served with a spoon instead of tongs; therefore, the child *cannot* take a small serving. Sometimes the greens are overcooked and mushy. Chopped greens or spinach, not overcooked, may be easier to serve. A child should be allowed to serve only a teaspoonful of a particular

Table 4-6
Contributions of vitamin C and iron made by fruits and vegetables

Item	Serving	Energy (kcal)	Vitamin C (mg)	Iron (mg)
*Fruits**				
Apricots	2 halves (dried or cooked)	18	>1	0.4
Blackberries	½ C	42	15	0.3
Cantaloupe	¼ fruit	48	54	0.6
Grapefruit	½ C	36	34	0.4
Grapes	1 oz	19	1	0.1
Mango	½ C	55	29	0.3
Orange	1 small fruit	64	66	0.5
Papaya	½ C	28	39	0.2
Peaches	½ C	39	7	0.5
Pineapple	½ C	45	13	0.4
Plums	5 small fruits	33	0	0.3
Prunes	⅛ C	52	1	1.6
Raisins	1 oz	82	>1	0.8
Raspberries, black	½ C	49	11	0.6
Raspberries, red	½ C	38	16	0.6
Strawberries	½ C	28	44	0.8
Tangerine	1	34	27	0.4
Vegetables				
Acorn squash	½ C, mashed	57	14	1.2
Asparagus	½ C, cooked	22	25	1.0
Broccoli	½ C, cooked	24	70	0.6
Brussels sprouts	½ C, cooked	24	63	0.6
Cabbage	½ C, shredded	15	75	0.2
Cauliflower	½ C, cooked	28	35	0.5
Collards	½ C, cooked	32	49	0.7
Green beans	½ C, cooked	16	8	0.4
Green peppers	½ C, raw	8	51	0.3
Kale	½ C, cooked	22	51	0.9
Lima beans	½ C, cooked	111	11	2.4
Mustard greens	½ C, cooked	16	34	1.3
Potatoes, white	½ C, no skin	51	13	0.4
Pumpkin	½ C, canned	40	6	0.5
Spinach	½ C, cooked	21	25	2.0
Sweet potatoes	½ C, mashed	146	22	0.9
Swiss chard	½ C, leaves	16	14	1.6
Tomato, raw	1 small	19	20	0.4
Tomatoes	½ C, canned	26	21	0.6
Turnip greens	½ C, cooked	15	50	0.8
Turnips	½ C, cubed	18	17	0.3
Zucchini	½ C, cubed	13	10	0.4

*Fresh unless specified.

item. This gives the child an opportunity to successfully taste the food without being responsible for a large portion and perhaps being forced to leave some on the plate.

Vegetables should not be overcooked, since they are less well accepted by the preschooler and tend to lose some nutritional value (for example, vitamin C and fiber). Steaming fruits and vegetables *briefly* in a small amount of water is a good way to avoid overcooking. Vegetables should be slightly crunchy when served. Too often we have entered centers at 10:00 AM for noon food service and found the frozen vegetables already boiling on the stove. By 11:00 AM they are in a "holding pattern" for 11:30 or noon meal service. Broccoli and asparagus should be firm enough to be used as finger foods.

When the center can afford to buy fresh, rather than canned, it is advised that they do so. If fresh is not available, buy frozen, and if frozen is not available or economically feasible, the last resort should be canned vegetables and fruits.

Casseroles or combination dishes have been scorned by preschool operators as unpopular foods. Check to see how they are prepared. If you use fresh or frozen vegetables that can be identified in the combination dishes and meat that has been freshly cooked and not allowed to stand in the refrigerator, the casserole will be welcomed. From our experience most canned vegetables baked in a casserole are overcooked by the time the casserole is served. If the vegetables are to be easily identifiable, frozen or fresh should be used.

Meats and Meat Alternates

Most preschoolers accept some meat products readily. For example, hamburgers and hot dogs seem to be favorites. Meats are an important part of the preschool center menu, since they are the best source of the iron as well as protein. However, meat alternates or protein foods including lentils and legumes (such as peas, beans, and nuts) also provide iron as well as folacin, magnesium, vitamin E, vitamin B_6, and zinc and should be included frequently. Meat alternates are emphasized in the sample menu in Table 4–5.

Meats and meat alternates should be cooked until tender and prepared so that the children can easily serve themselves from bowls on the table. This means that one half of a hamburger, a small pork chop, or a piece of roast beef will be on the serving plate. Meat does not have to be chopped fine or legumes cooked until they appear as puree, but meats should be soft and moist enough to cut with table knives or to allow the child to eat them as finger foods.

Ordinary gravies and sauces are too low in nutritional quality to be included in the preschool diet. However, cheese sauces and milk gravy made with meats, fat drippings, and whole milk are nutritious and acceptable in the preschool menu.

Should you serve luncheon meats, hot dogs, Polish sausage, and spiced sausage, which are salty and high in fat, but are generally well-liked by children and care givers? The nutritional content of the food as well as the potential a food or combination of foods has for providing educational experiences must be taken into account. For example, a wiener roast may be planned as part of the curriculum, making hot dogs an appropriate part of the child-care menu. The final decision regarding food choices may rest with the center administrator who plans the menus. We recommend that use of foods with a high proportion of salt, fat, and sugar be limited.

Breads and Cereals

Items from the bread and cereal group are probably the easiest for the preschooler to ingest, and this food group is likely to be abused by both toddlers and preschoolers. Crackers and especially cookies are easy for the preschooler who wants to "eat and run." They satisfy the child's hunger and are not as messy as fresh fruit, milk, or some meat products.

Either whole-grain or iron-fortified "breakfast cereals" can be served in the child-care center. Because the nutrient density of whole-grain cereals is higher than that of some fortified cereals (Chapter 1), whole-grain cereals should be encouraged. However, some cereals advertised as whole grain may also include a high sugar content along with 100% of the U.S. RDA for iron. This presents a dilemma for the care giver and parents who wish to limit the child's sugar intake. A few cereals that contain high amounts of iron do not contain sugar (see Table 3–8 in Chapter 3 for a list of the iron and sugar content of cereals).

Wheat germ adds iron and other nutrients to cereal products. One teaspoon of toasted wheat germ can replace each teaspoon of uncooked cereal with good acceptance by preschoolers.

We believe the center should not serve rich cakes, sweet rolls, and most cookies, which have a high fat and sugar content, because these foods cannot be counted as part of the whole-grain bread and cereal food group. Birthdays without birthday cake are sometimes difficult to justify to parents. However, many parents welcome more nourishing substitutes in their children's diets. Watermelon or cantaloupe, hollowed out and filled with fruit, with candles around the edge, can substitute for birthday cake. Infrequently providing foods that have a low nutrient density (such as birthday cakes) will not harm the child; however, a center with 15 to 30 children could conceivably have many birthday celebrations.

Milk and Milk Products

During the toddler years, drinking from the bottle may have caused an overconsumption of milk; however, the preschool child, no longer taking milk from the bottle, may still be drinking more than 3 cups of milk a day. More than 3 cups of milk is too much if it replaces other foods and nutrients in the diet.

Imitation milk is a nondairy product, usually fortified with vitamins and calcium, but it is not approved by USDA Child Care Food Program, where reimbursement is allowed for milk and for meals served to children (Chapter 5). Whole milk, skim milk, or 2% milk can be served in the preschool center. Before the age of 5, it is recommended that whole or 2% be served.

The caloric contribution of skim milk is one half that of whole milk. Most whole milk contains 3.2% to 3.5% butterfat, whereas skim milk has less than 1% butterfat. Two-percent milk contains 2% butterfat. The difference in energy between a half cup of 2% and a half cup of whole milk equals about 15 to 16 kcal, making 2% milk an acceptable product for children.

To review, milk and milk products are primary sources of riboflavin, vitamin A, vitamin D, calcium, and protein. During the preschool period, milk may replace other nutrients in the diet, or the child may not be consuming enough milk.

Ice cream, puddings, and sweetened yogurt have little place on the menu of the child-care center. However, plain yogurt (unsweetened) or yogurt sweetened with fresh fruit can be a substitute for milk nutritionally, but current regulations by USDA (Chapter 5) require use of fluid milk in the center. Cream cheese, butter, and margarine cannot be used as milk substitutes.

SUPPLEMENTATION

A question frequently asked by the center staff is whether to supplement the diet of the preschooler with medicinal supplements such as vitamin or mineral pills. Supplementation is a real concern, and if a nutritionist or dietitian is available, a group meeting to discuss this issue is often helpful for parents. If a vitamin or mineral—including fluoride—must be added to the diet, it should be prescribed by the physician or public health clinic. This is especially true in the case of iron. Anemia is not always caused by iron deficiency but may be caused by lack of folacin or may be secondary to other disease states and should be further investigated by a health professional.

The strict vegetarian diet will need supplementation with vitamin B_{12} if animal products (milk, eggs, meat, and fish) are not included in the diet. Further discussion of the vegetarian diet is included in the section, "Special Concerns Related to Dietary Intake."

Too many vitamins, especially the fat-soluble vitamins A and D, may prove harmful. Because scientists do not completely understand the interaction between certain vitamins and minerals and the effect of megadoses, a word of caution is advised in providing vitamin and mineral supplementation.

Poor growth records are not a signal to start supplementation; instead they should signal the care giver to advise parents to seek a more thorough examination from a physician or other health professional. The supplement could mask a more serious medical condition.

EATING BEHAVIOR

At least 2½ hours should elapse between snacks and meals. Many preschool centers that operate half-day programs try to supply a snack and a meal or two meals. Care givers often rush to serve breakfast and then a snack or lunch before the children go home. If children are not in the center for more than 3½ hours, it is difficult or impossible to serve more than one meal unless children come to the center hungry and are given a snack immediately.

During the toddler stage, at least until 1½ to 2 years of age, the care giver is probably placing most of the food on the child's plate. However, the 2½-year-old enjoys being able to serve food. The care giver should fill the spoon for the child and be ready to assist, but the young preschooler should put the food on the plate (Figure 4-3). A child who is progressing normally will be capable of serving independently by 3½ years of age. This activity may seem like a small

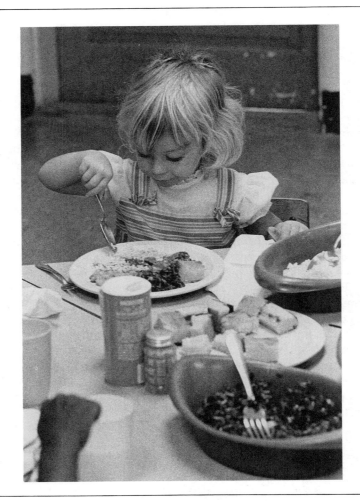

Figure 4-3
Preschooler places food onto plate.

accomplishment to the care giver or parents; however, the child is given the opportunity to make a decision about a very important activity: How much of a food will I eat?

The child should be expected to try each food that is served; however, the child may take only a small portion. Eating at least one green bean, one flower of broccoli, or one-half spear of asparagus is appropriate when becoming familiar with a new food. The child should taste all the food prepared and served. Having the opportunity to serve from the bowls of food or pour from the pitcher allows the child, not the teacher, to decide how much the child is going to eat. When the teacher decides how much food to serve onto the child's plate and then insists that the food be consumed, the battle has begun. The teacher is really telling the child, "I want you to eat the food that I have decided you should eat." If the situation is reversed, the teacher can give the responsibility to the child by asking the child to eat the food taken from the serving bowl. You cannot expect perfection during the child's first, second, or even third week in the center. However, after a month or two the child should begin to be able to make decisions regarding how much food to serve and to take responsibility for eating the food. There are exceptions, and some children overestimate portion sizes and must be monitored by the care giver.

As discussed in the menu chapter (Chapter 6), utensils should be used at mealtime. These may include a spoon, fork, and knife for spreading (Figure 4–4). Foods for the spoon include those that stick to the spoon (for example, fruit, plain yogurt). Foods that can be used with a fork include mashed potatoes and small pieces of meat and vegetables; margarine can be served to give the child an opportunity to use a knife for spreading. Allow the child to spread margarine onto one-half slice of bread and then cut the bread. These activities stimulate fine motor coordination. In addition, the child should be able to begin to cut pieces of vegetables and tender meat with a table knife (not a sharp knife). Serving foods, spreading margarine, and making sandwiches can be done more easily by the food service personnel in the kitchen, but if we are to use mealtime as a learning experience, the child should be allowed to fully participate in these activities.

Equipment

Equipment should be the proper size for young children. Eating utensils should be small. The chairs should be of child's proportion, allowing feet to be squarely placed on the floor. Buy sturdy chairs, since adults should sit on the children's chairs rather than having the children sit on adult chairs. Plates approximately 7 to 9 inches in diameter encourage the child to take smaller portions than do larger plates.

Avoid spilled milk and the accompanying frustration by checking the glass design and noting that a small glass (not larger than 4 to 6 ounces) is filled with only 2 to 4 ounces of milk. The glass should have a weighted bottom, making it less likely to tip. Use clear glasses so that the child can see how much milk is

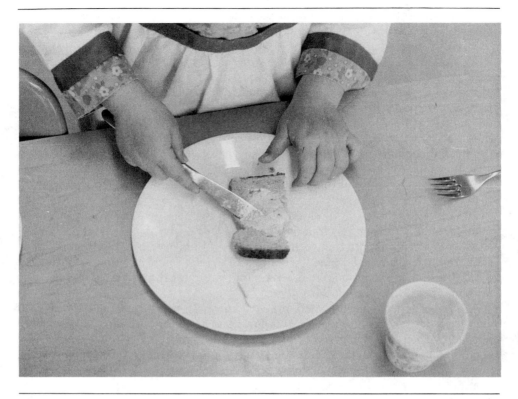

Figure 4-4
Preschooler learns to spread margarine.

being poured into the glass. The child can refill the glass from a small pitcher of milk on the table (Figure 4-5).

Table arrangements for young children are important. The table should be attractive and the chairs comfortable. Active or easily excitable children should be seated between quiet, calm children, and children who enjoy eating should sit next to children who tend to be picky eaters.

Six and possibly eight children may sit at one table with a care giver. It is important to allow enough room for children to pass the bowls of food from one child to another. Small groups of children allow for a small quantity of food to be placed in each bowl. If there are three or four items served at each meal, at least half of the children can begin serving themselves when food service starts. For example, one child can be pouring milk, one serving broccoli, one serving mashed potatoes, one serving meat, one serving the fruit dish, and one taking a slice of bread. Allowing children to serve food at the center takes 4 to 5 minutes after 4 to 6 weeks of practice. Do not attempt to encourage a child to serve all the foods during the first week at the child-care center. Begin with carrot and

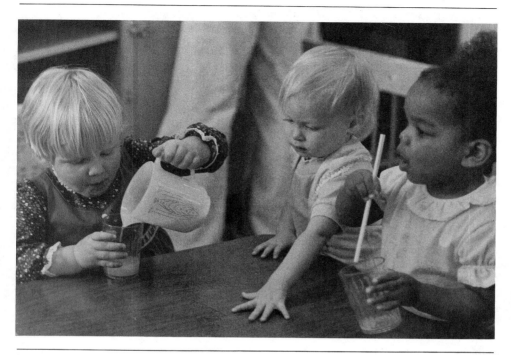

Figure 4-5
Child learns to pour juice from small pitcher.

celery sticks, and let the child serve these foods onto the plate. If your center has not begun this experience, start with only one serving bowl per table and progress slowly until children are serving all foods onto their plates.

Location

In some cases the gymnasium is the only location for food service; however, if at all possible carts should be purchased and food should be transported to the classroom or center or a place that is relatively quiet. Generally children and care givers can converse about food and food service with less confusion if they are in the center or in a room where they participate in other activities during the day. They may then relate food on the table to pictures of menu items discussed before the meal. They may also decorate tables for meal service or set tables and serve food.

SPECIAL CONCERNS RELATED TO DIETARY INTAKE

It is not the intention of this book to cover all the diet-related concerns of the preschool period. Diet-related problems discussed in Chapters 2 and 3 include obesity, dental caries, lactose intolerance, and food allergies. There may also be children in the center who have serious allergies, who require diabetic diets, or who have other conditions that require special dietary treatment. The administrator should have specific written instructions from physicians or nutritionists explaining the implications of specific diets. However, several areas of concern are often expressed by care givers and parents. These include the use or abuse of snack foods; use of salt, sugar, or sweetener; vegetarian diets; "natural" or organic foods; additives; and hyperactivity.

Snack Foods

Snack foods with low nutrient density include snack cakes, soft drinks, or even breakfast cereals, as well as some foods sold in fast food restaurants. These foods provide little nutritional value.

How do you combat the intake of foods with low nutrient density by children? Withholding these foods may be easier at the center than at home. Feeding only foods that appear in the basic food groups is perhaps idealistic. Grandparents, friends, and neighbors supply children with cake, cookies, candies, and snack chips, especially during holiday seasons.

Many of the snack foods currently on the market provide relatively few nutrients. Judging whether a food should be served as a snack depends on whether the food (1) can be classified as part of a basic food group and (2) contains sufficient nutrients to justify the caloric value. The USDA Child Care Food Program guidelines (Chapter 6) offer an excellent source for determining whether a food is an acceptable part of a program. Acceptable snacks can be chosen from each of the food groups. However, if snacks are chosen of low nutrient density, they should not preclude the selection of a well-balanced diet. Snack foods providing primarily energy often replace some of the foods from the food groups. If all the required foods are consumed in addition to high-calorie snacks, the child may have consumed too much energy.

Snack foods from the cereal group are presented in Table 4–7. It includes the energy and iron values for high and low nutrient density cereal products. The cereal group probably provides the easiest opportunity for selecting foods that are high in energy with relatively few nutrients. As stated earlier, meat— especially red meat—is probably the best source of iron, the nutrient often low in preschool diets; however, whole-grain or enriched cereal products provide some of the least expensive sources of iron. As can be seen from Table 4–7, the choice of whole wheat crackers over saltines can increase the iron content by at least five times.

Dairy products used as snack foods are included in Table 4–8. Using products with added sugar raises the energy value without providing extra calcium, the nutrient supplied most readily from milk or dairy products.

If all components of a nutritionally adequate diet are included in the preschooler's diet and additional energy is still needed, foods providing energy with low nutrient density probably are not harmful.

Table 4-7
Energy and iron value for snacks from bread and cereal group

Food Quantities	Iron (mg)	Energy (kcal)
Bread, 1 slice (25 g)	0.7	70
Cereals, ready-to-serve (1 oz)		
Special K, 1 C	4.5	108
Rice Krispies, 1 C	1.8	93
Sugar Frosted FLakes, 1 C	1.8	114
Total, 1 C	18.0	110
Buc Wheats, 1 C	8.1	110
Crackers		
Round, 1⅞ in., 4	0.08	60
Cheese, 1 in. square, 10	0.1	45
Saltines, 4	0.1	50
Oyster, 10	0.1	35
Graham, 2½ in., 2	0.2	60
Rye wafers, 2	0.5	45
Wheat rye thins, 2	0.6	71
Danish pastry, 4 in.	0.6	270
Muffin, 2½ to 3 in.	0.6	100–130
Rolls		
Brown and serve, white flour, enriched, 1	0.5	90
Hamburger or hot dog, white flour, enriched, 1	0.7	120
Cake, plain, 3 × 3 × 2 in., ⅑ of a cake	0.3	313
Fruitcake, 1/15 of a 1 lb loaf	0.4–0.8	120
Angel food, 1/16 of 9 in. tube pan	0.1	120
Devil's food, 2 × 2 × 4 in.	0.7	160
+ White icing	(trace)	280
Gingerbread, 3 in. square	1.14	200
Coffee cake, ⅙ of a cake	1.2	230
Pretzel		
Dutch, twisted, 1	0.2	60
Thins, twisted, 1	0.09	25
Sticks, 10	0.1	25
Pie, ⅙ of 9 in.		
Banana custard	0.8	336
Custard	0.9	331
Pumpkin	0.8	321
Apple	0.5	404
Chocolate meringue	1.1	383
Lemon meringue	0.7	357
Butterscotch	1.4	406
Peach	0.8	403
Raisin	1.4	427
Pecan	3.9	577

Source: Information as interpreted from manufacturers' labels by the NDDA Laboratory, Southern Illinois University at Carbondale, 1983.

Table 4–8
Nutritional values for snacks from milk group (with common additions)

Food	Energy (kcal)	Calcium (mg)
Milk, whole, 1 C	160	300
+ Chocolate syrup, 2 tbsp	+ 90	—
Buttermilk, 1 C	90	300
Half-and-half, 1 tbsp	15	16
Ice cream, school lunch, 3 oz	98	80
Ice cream, regular, ½ C	130	100
+ Fudge sauce, 2 tbsp	+ 120	—
+ Whipping cream, ¼ C	+ 220	+ 50
+ Coconut, ¼ C	+ 110	—
Ice milk, soft serve, 1 C	270	250
Yogurt, plain, 1 C		
Made from whole milk	150	250
Made from skim milk	120	300
+ Preserves or jam, 1 tbsp	+ 60	—
Cheese		
Cheddar, 1 oz (on pie)	110	200
Parmesan (on spaghetti), 2 tbsp	45	130
American, 1 oz	110	200
Pudding, ½ C		
Mix made with whole milk	160	135
Vanilla, home recipe	140	150
Chocolate, home recipe	195	125
Tapioca	110	85
Cottage cheese, ½ C		
Creamed	130	115
Uncreamed	85	90

Source: Approximate values from Agricultural Research Service, United States Department of Agriculture: Nutritive value of American foods in common units, Agriculture Handbook No. 456, Washington, DC, Nov. 1975.

Table 4–9 provides a general list of snack foods primarily from the fruit and vegetable group. The list includes opportunities for pouring (and drinking), for using fingers, and for practicing with a knife for spreading. Care givers can use snack time as well as mealtime to practice some of the fine motor skills of the eating activity.

Fast Foods

The question of whether to eat at fast food establishments is often asked of nutritionists, especially when the preschool center wishes to take the children "down the street" for a hamburger and french fries. Table 4–10 provides a listing of

Table 4–9
Snacks that provide educational opportunities for children

Activity	Snack
To pour and drink	Natural fruit juices, milk, protein shake (½ C milk, ½ C orange juice, ¼ C powdered milk), water
For fingers	Fruit:* Orange, grapefruit, tangerine, banana slices, apple, pear, peach slices, pineapple wedges, dried apricots, dates, raisins, grapes, plums, berries Ice pop made from fruit juice or pureed fruit, fruit puree, pudding (made with fluid milk), plain yogurt Vegetables: Cherry tomatoes and other vegetables, raw or cooked crunchy—cucumber, zucchini, potato, turnip, green beans, cauliflower, green pepper strips or wedges, asparagus, broccoli, brussels sprouts, peas (for older children), lima beans
To spread on	Peanut butter, yogurt dips, flavored margarine (make your own)
To use spoon, fork	Yogurt†, cottage cheese, cold meat cubes, whole-grain crackers and cookies (limit sugar and fat), whole-grain bread, whole-grain or fortified cereals with milk

*Most fresh or canned fruit (e.g., bananas cut in disks or pieces, oranges, grapefruit, pineapple) can be frozen on a tray, brought out 10 minutes before snack time, and enjoyed as a crunchy snack.
†Plain yogurt may be sweetened by adding fresh fruit.

several items from fast food establishments and their relative nutrient composition. A complete listing of the nutritional analysis of fast foods has been compiled by Young, Sims, Bingham, and Brennan [10].

As seen in Table 4–10, foods served at fast food restaurants can make a substantial contribution to the diet. A 275 kcal hamburger from Burger King would take 16% of the 4- to 6-year-old's energy allowance (1700 kcal) and provide 3 mg, or 30%, of the child's RDA for iron (10 mg). The hamburger also provides protein, B vitamins, and some minerals. With other hamburgers, the cooking method (frying) and the addition of salad-dressing sauces yields far more fat and, consequently kilocalories. (Differences in fat content may also be due to differences in portion size.) Certainly an occasional meal from a fast food establishment is not objectionable, but a diet composed primarily of these foods would be limited nutritionally.

Sweeteners

A question that you will be asked is, "Should I serve artificial sweeteners or sugar to preschoolers?" Nutritionists are often tempted to answer with a question, "Is either really necessary?" It is difficult to find extensive scientific

Table 4-10
Nutrient composition of fast foods*

	Weight (g)	Energy (kcal)	Protein (g)	Carbo-hydrate (g)	Fat (g)	Choles-terol (mg)	Vitamins A (IU)	B₁ (mg)	B₂ (mg)	Niacin (mg)
Arby's†										
Roast beef	147	350	22	32	15	39	x	.23	.43	7.6
Beef'n Cheddar	190	490	24	51	21	51	x	.12	.34	5.0
Burger King‡										
Hamburger	109	275	15	29	12	37	150	.23	.25	4.0
Cheeseburger	120	317	17	30	15	48	341	.23	.29	4.0
Church's Fried Chicken&										
White chicken (wing-breast cut)	97	303	22	9	20	—	—	—	—	—
Dark chicken portion (thigh)	93	306	19	9	22	—	—	—	—	—
Dairy Queen&&										
DQ cone, small	85	140	3	22	4	10	100	.03	.17	x
DQ sundae, small	106	190	3	33	4	10	100	.03	.17	x
Jack in the Box#										
Hamburger	98	276	13	30	12	29	50	.36	.24	3.2
French fries	68	221	2	27	12	8	x	.07	.03	1.2
Onion rings	108	382	5	39	23	27	x	.21	.12	1.8
Kentucky Fried Chicken##										
Original Recipe dinner										
Drum and thigh*	154	425	31.6	11.8	28.02	203	244	.14	.41	7.5
Extra crispy dinner										
Drum and thigh*	172	544	32.3	19.7	37.2	186	202	.14	.41	8.0
Long John Silver's**										
Fish with batter (2 pieces)	172	404	26	22	24	62	—	—	—	—
4 Piece Chicken Planks Dinner	—	1037	41	82	59	25	—	—	—	—
McDonald's††										
Egg McMuffin	138	340	18.5	31	15.8	259	591	.47	.44	3.77
Big Mac	200	570	24.6	39.2	35	83	380	.48	.38	7.2
Cheeseburger	114	328	15	28.5	16	40.6	353	.3	.24	4.33
Wendy's‡‡										
Single hamburger (white bun)	117	350	21	27	18	65	—	.22	.25	5.0
French fries	98	280	4	35	14	15	—	.15	.03	3.0

Source: Reprinted with permission of Ross Laboratories, Columbus, OH 43216, from Public Health Currents, Vol. 27, pp. 12-21, © 1987 Ross Laboratories.

Dashes indicate no data available. x, Less than 2% U.S. RDA.

†Arby's Inc, Atlanta, Georgia. Nutritional Analyses by Arby's Laboratory and other independent testing laboratories.

‡Burger King Corp Inc. Nutritional analyses by Hazelton Laboratory of America (formerly Raltech Scientific Services Inc), Madison, Wisconsin, and Campbell Laboratories, Camden, New Jersey.

&Church's Fried Chicken, San Antonio, Texas. Nutrient analyses of chicken by Texas Testing Laboratories Inc, San Antonio.

&&International Dairy Queen Inc, Minneapolis, Minnesota. Nutrient analyses by Hazelton Laboratory of America (formerly Raltech Scientific Services Inc), Madison, Wisconsin.

	Vitamins						Minerals							Moisture (g)	Crude Fiber (g)
B$_6$ (mg)	B$_{12}$ (μg)	C (mg)	D (IU)	Ca (mg)	Cu (mg)	Fe (mg)	K (mg)	Mg (mg)	P (mg)	Na (mg)	Zn (mg)				
—	—	x	—	80	—	3.6	—	—	—	590	—	—	—
—	—	x	—	80	—	5.4	—	—	—	1520	—	—	—
—	—	3.0	—	37	.06	2.7	235	23	124	509	2.4	—	—
—	—	3.0	—	102	.06	3.8	247	26	186	651	2.6	—	—
—	—	—	—	—	—	—	—	—	—	583	—	45	0
—	—	—	—	—	—	—	—	—	—	448	—	42	0
—	.36	x	—	100	—	.4	—	—	100	45	—	—	—
—	.36	x	—	100	—	.4	—	—	150	75	—	—	—
—	—	1.2	—	70	—	2.7	—	—	—	521	—	—	—
—	—	3.0	2	10	—	.5	—	—	—	164	—	—	—
—	—	3.0	3	30	—	1.4	—	—	—	407	—	—	—
—	—	4.0	—	40.4	—	1.647	—	—	—	786	—	—	—
—	—	4.0	—	61.3	—	1.816	—	—	—	1112	—	—	—
—	—	—	—	—	—	—	—	—	—	1346	—	—	—
—	—	—	—	—	—	—	—	—	—	2433			
—	—	1.4	—	226	—	2.93	—	—	—	885	—	—	—
—	—	3.0	—	203	—	4.9	—	—	—	979	—	—	—
—	—	2.1	—	169	—	2.84	—	—	—	743	—	—	—
—	—	—	—	32	—	4.5	—	—	—	410	—	—	—
—	—	12	—	x	—	1.1	—	—	—	95	—	—	—

#Jack in the Box Restaurants, Foodmaker, Inc, San Diego, California. Nutrient Analyses by Hazelton Laboratory of America (formerly Raltech Scientific Services Inc), Madison, Wisconsin.

##Kentucky Fried Chicken Corp. Nutrient analyses by Hazelton Laboratory of America (formerly Raltech Scientific Services Inc), Madison, Wisconsin.

*Edible Portion.

**Long John Silver's Inc, Lexington, Kentucky. Nutrient Analyses by Department of Nutrition and Food Science, University of Kentucky.

††McDonald's Corp, Oak Brook, Illinois. Nutrient Analyses by Hazelton Laboratory of America (formerly Raltech Scientific Services Inc), Madison, Wisconsin.

‡‡Wendy's International Inc, Dublin, Ohio. Nutrient Analyses: entree items, Hazelton Laboratory of America (formerly Raltech Scientific Services Inc), Madison, Wisconsin.

literature indicating that consumption of table sugar per se is detrimental to health for the preschooler. However, reduction of simple sugars is advisable for treatment of diabetes, treatment and prevention of obesity, and prevention of dental caries.

Fructose, sorbitol, and xylitol are also sweeteners with approximately the same caloric value as table sugar but are used by the body in a different way than table sugar is. Many "sugar-free" candies and gums that are sweetened with sorbitol and xylitol can cause diarrhea, especially in young children. Therefore, although candy or gum may be labeled sugar-free, it may still contain calories and in some cases cause the preschooler gastric distress and diarrhea. Read the labels! Those sweeteners commonly used in food preparation that contain nutrients and energy are listed in Table 4-11.

The care giver can evaluate the nutrient contribution of the various options. The energy and iron content of natural sweeteners show that the primary nutrient in each of the sweetening agents is carbohydrate and a small amount of iron. An exception is blackstrap molasses (first extraction), which, in addition to iron, contains calcium (1 tablespoon is equal to ½ cup milk) (Table 4-11).

Because iron is one of the nutrients that is apparently in short supply in the child's diet, the use of a sweetener other than granulated sugar would help, if only slightly, to provide more iron in the diet. Blackstrap molasses has an overall nutrient density for iron above the other products, considering the 3.2 mg iron, which contributes significantly to the 10 mg recommended. Only 2.4% of the kilocalories is required for 32% of the iron allowance. However, the flavor is not generally acceptable to child and care giver. Cooked with cereal products and baked beans, it may become an acceptable product on the child-care menu.

Table 4-11
Caloric and iron content of selected natural sweeteners

Sweetener (1 tbsp)	Kilocalories	Iron (mg)
Molasses, blackstrap		
Dark	43	3.2
Light	50	0.9
Syrup		
Corn (light and dark)	59	0.8
Maple	50	0.2
Brown sugar, dark (packed)	51	0.47
Honey	64	0.1
Granulated sugar	46	trace
Crystalline fructose	42	trace

Source: Calculated by NDDA Laboratory, Southern Illinois University at Carbondale, 1983.

Light molasses with the less pungent taste may be better accepted, but it has less iron.

Brown sugar might be the next choice. Note that the amount used is 1 table-spoon. Generally, a preschooler would use only about 1 to 2 teaspoons (½ table-spoon) in sweetening cereal. The amount of iron found in 1 tablespoon of packed brown sugar is equal to about one-half slice whole wheat bread (0.4 mg). However, one-half slice of bread in addition to supplying other nutrients has approximate-ly 30 to 35 kcal, whereas 1 tablespoon of brown sugar supplies 51 kcal.

Aspartame.   A low-calorie nutritive sweetener now available to the care giver is aspartame, commonly known as NutraSweet.* This sugar replacement is 180 times sweeter than sugar. Composed of two amino acids, it is used by the body as are other amino acids found in food. Research to date has shown that use of aspartame presents no risk of toxicity for healthy individuals [11]. However, a child with a condition known as phenylketonuria (PKU) should not use aspar-tame. Because this condition is so rare and the diet is very restricted in all pro-tein foods, the mother and dietitian would be working closely with the care giver and food service personnel and a problem would be unlikely. Nevertheless, the use of any sugar replacement or table sugar should be limited in the child-care center, thus allowing parents to decide when and how much of any sweetener the child can consume.

VEGETARIAN DIET

With an apparent increasing interest in the vegetarian diet and requests by some child-care centers to serve vegetarian meals, a discussion of the types and nutrient composition of each seems appropriate [12]. Vegetarian diets are classified as follows:

> Vegetarian diets differ in the extent to which they avoid animal products. Veganism, or total vegetarianism, completely excludes meat, fish, fowl, eggs, and dairy products. Lactovegetarianism is the avoidance of meat, fish, fowl and eggs, whereas ovo-lacto-vegetarianism involves avoidance of only meat, fish, or fowl. Semi-vegetarian patterns allow limited amounts of most animal foods [13].

According to the American Dietetic Association [14], when planning a vegetarian diet one should choose a wide variety of foods from the major food groups. The foods may include fresh fruits, vegetables, whole-grain breads and cereals, nuts and seeds, legumes, low-fat dairy products or fortified soy substitutes, and a limited number of eggs, if desired. Vegetarians are advised to limit their intake of foods with low nutrient density. Consuming a good food source of ascorbic acid with meals will further enhance absorption of available iron. Grains, vegetables, legumes, seeds, and nuts eaten over the course of the

*NutraSweet Company brand name for aspartame.

day complement one another in their amino acid profiles to form complete proteins, and precise planning and complementation of proteins within each meal, as urged by the recently popular "combined proteins theory," is unnecessary.

With the help of a registered dietitian or public health nutritionist, care givers should discuss the vegetarian diets of children with parents. Growth charts, especially heights for age, should be used to record and monitor height and weight in the center for children on modified diets as well as for all children.

Children's diets that are restricted in animal products should contain fortified soy milk through the preschool years. Another good protein alternate is tofu, the curd produced from clotting soy milk (soybean product). A good protein and calcium source, this custardlike product can be used in a variety of ways, and it appeals to many children.

The U.S. Department of Agriculture allows reimbursement for meals served to vegetarian children if a suitable protein substitute is included in the meal (for example, eggs, cheese, legumes, soy protein) in the amounts required. Care givers can plan meals for vegetarians by choosing from the allowed foods those items that supply essential nutrients and meet the energy needs of individual children. Combination dishes that have complementary proteins or include milk products and eggs and supplement the plant proteins are included in Figure 4–6.

Is the Vegetarian Diet Safe for Children?

The concern of many care givers is whether the vegetarian diet will retard growth and development of children. Use of a vegetarian diet that allows ample energy and adequate supplies of dairy products and eggs is safe for children. Researchers have found that preschool children raised in families using lac-

Baked beans and brown bread
Lentil soup with rice
Hopping John (beans and rice)
Split pea soup with bread
Cereal, hot or cold, with milk
Cereal cooked with milk
Pizza, cheese, with whole wheat crust
Cheese sandwich
Peanut butter sandwich
Tamale pie with beans and cheese
Toast and eggs
Granola with cereal, nuts, and seeds

Figure 4–6
Food combinations that supply complete protein (See Chapter 6 for combinations and quantities of foods that qualify for Child Care Food Program reimbursement.)

toovovegetarian diets have heights and weights similar to the norms for nonvegetarians.

On the other hand, multiple nutritional deficiencies have been found in infants raised in a strict vegetarian community without the use of fortified soy milk products [15]. Some groups who describe their diets as "macrobiotic" are vegetarians who do not include any egg and dairy products in their diets [12]. The growth curves, especially for height, for one group of macrobiotic vegetarian children were more depressed than those of other vegetarian children. Growth patterns among vegetarians vary; when diets were more restricted to animal foods, children's growth was consistently more affected [16]. Obtaining enough energy in the diet appears difficult for some vegetarian children. Although protein intake may fall within the normal range, energy levels for some vegetarian children may be below recommended levels.

NUTRITIONAL CONCERNS

Nutrients that are most difficult to acquire on a vegan or strict vegetarian diet are listed in Table 4-12 along with the animal and plant sources for the nutrients. The nutrients include protein, vitamin A, riboflavin, vitamin B_{12}, vitamin D, calcium, and iron. We concur with the American Dietetic Association, which states that vegetarian diets are adequate if "planned according to established scientific nutritional principles" [13, 14].

Natural? Organic?

Natural and organic foods are discussed frequently, and more and more centers are asked if they provide only "natural" foods. Words such as processed, natural, organic, and refined provide little solid nutrition information, unless they are defined in a quantitative framework. Today this is not possible. In the supermarket "natural" may mean absence of artificial colors, flavors, and additives in one food product and the absence of processing or refinement in another.

Although there is no clear definition, natural foods may also mean those products grown without use of chemical fertilizers and pesticides, but the term organic rather than natural has generally been applied to these foods. The plant cannot tell the difference between nitrogen, phosphorus, and potassium coming from organic (containing carbon), or natural, fertilizers and inorganic forms (chemical fertilizers). One serves equally as well as the other for converting the nutrients in the soil to "plant nutrients."

Everyone would agree that a fresh apple is a natural food, although perhaps not organically grown. What about cheese and yogurt, which are processed and prepared in the factory? Sugar derived from beets or sugar cane (often called refined) is really natural, although molasses, which undergoes a variety of processes and is derived from sorghum is called natural. It is wise to keep these

Table 4–12
Nutrients often limited in vegan or strict vegetarian diets

Nutrient	Food Sources	
	Animal	Plant
Protein–amino acids	Meat, poultry Fish Eggs Milk, cheese Yogurt	Legumes Nuts, seeds Soy milk Meat analogs
Vitamin A value	Liver Butter Whole milk Cheese Fortified low-fat milk	Orange vegetables and fruits Greens Fortified margarine
Riboflavin (B$_2$)	Liver Milk products Red meat	Fortified cereals Fortified soy milk
Vitamin B$_{12}$	Liver, meat Poultry, fish Milk products Eggs	Fortified soy milk, cereals, and meat analogs
Vitamin D	Fortified milk Fish oils	Fortified soy milk
Calcium	Milk, cheese Yogurt Sardines and salmon with bones	Calcium-fortified soy milk Greens Almonds, filberts
Iron	Liver Red meat	Fortified grain products Dried beans and lentils Whole wheat bulgar

Source: Modified from Vegetarian nutrition, Rosemont, IL, 1979, National Dairy Council.

thoughts in mind when considering whether to use all "natural" or "unprocessed" products.

Additives

The question of additives is often bothersome for the care giver, and parents may question the use of food with additives. Table 4–13 provides a list of some of the additives and their functions. Because of the use of additives, mainly preservatives, the marketplace is filled with a variety of products that would otherwise not be marketable. Without additives the shelf life of a loaf of bread, including whole wheat bread, would be a day or two instead of more than a week. The cost of such a product would be at least doubled or tripled, making bread an unobtainable product to the lower-income family who depends on it for many nutrients.

On the other hand, many of the products in which additives are used could be eliminated from the child's diet if the calories are not required for weight gain (for example, gelatin, cake mixes, jams, jellies, or foods that have a low nutrient density).

Diet and Hyperactivity

In the 1970s the Feingold diet [17] became popular for the treatment of hyperactivity. The diet is based on the idea that much of the hyperactivity associated with learning disabilities that occurs in school-aged children can be attributed to ingestion of food additives and salicylates (an ingredient commonly found in aspirin). Feingold asserted that hyperactivity could be treated effectively through dietary changes in up to two thirds of the children. Claims of the diet's success have had an impact on care givers and parents who have children with hyperkinesis (severe hyperactivity) in their care.

Since that time, the scientific community, the National Institutes of Health, the Food and Drug Administration, and the National Education Association have studied the issues and diet. Recommendations have been published, and those that are relevant to the care giver and parents are as follows:

1. There is no evidence to recommend a ban on foods containing artificial food colorings in federally supported food programs such as those served by care givers.
2. Because the diet has no apparent harmful effects and because the nonspecific effects of this dietary treatment are frequently beneficial to families, there is no reason to discourage families that wish to use the diet as long as other therapy is continued and the child's nutritional status is monitored [18].

More recently, studies of hyperactivity and sucrose and aspartame use showed that sucrose does not adversely affect behavior of children [19]. The dietary characteristics of hyperactive boys and a matched control group were similar, with refined sugar intake within the normal range for both groups. Parents of hyperactive children often attempted to control sugar intake but were unsuccessful. Attempting to impose restrictions may exacerbate already strained parent-child interactions [20].

EXERCISE AND PHYSICAL FITNESS

Three-, 4-, and 5-year-olds are beginning to gain control of fine muscles while the large muscles are still growing. They love to run, jump, throw, and catch, and need little encouragement for active movement. However, the care giver

Table 4–13
Role of some common additives in food

Additive	Function
Tocopherols	Inhibit rancidity in fatty foods, though not as effectively as BHA/BHT. One of the tocopherols is vitamin E, which prevents cell membranes from breaking down.
Benzoate of soda	Controls mold in syrups, margarine, soft drinks, and fruit products. Remains stable under the high temperatures used in canning.
BHA (butylated hydroxyanisole)	Prevents fats, oils, and dried meats from turning rancid; keeps baked goods fresh. Extends storage life of breakfast cereals. Stable even under high temperatures.
BHT (butylated hydroxytoluene)	Prevents rancidity in potato flakes, enriched rice, and shortenings containing animal fats. Stable even under high temperatures.
Diglycerides	Most common emulsifiers, derived primarily from vegetables oils. Prevent ice cream from separating while melting, and keep oil in peanut butter from separating. Make baked goods soft.
Disodium guanylate	Brings out flavor of meat and meat-based products.
EDTA (ethylene-diaminetetraacetic acid)	Prevents unappealing color changes in salad dressings, sauces, and canned vegetables. Stable under the high temperatures used in canning.
Guar gum	One of the most common vegetable gums, which, in some foods, are much more effective than starches as thickeners. Used in gravies, sauces, pet foods.

needs to be acutely aware of the necessity to include motor fitness into the total curriculum (Figure 4–7).

Javernick reports that "although most preschool programs purport to encourage gross motor development, we teachers often neglect this area of development and emphasize instead fine motor, cognitive and social development" [21].

Table 4-13
continued

Additive	Function
Modified food starches	Special starches with desired characteristics (heat-stable, freeze-thaw stable) "built-in." Give body to pie fillings, gravies, and sauces. Derived from cereal grains and potato.
Pectin	Jelling substance extracted from citrus rind; provides consistency of body in all jams, jellies, and preserves.
Potassium sorbate	Controls surface molds on cheese, syrups, margarine, mayonnaise.
Sulfur dioxide	Inhibits browning in fresh and dried fruits. Prevents undesirable color changes when wine is exposed to air.
Acetic acid	Commonly used to give tartness to dressing, sauces, relishes. The key ingredient in vinegar.
Ascorbic acid (vitamin C, sodium ascorbate)	Keeps fruit slices from darkening inhibits rancidity in fatty foods. Enhances nutrition value of beverages, beverage mixes.
Carrageenan	Improves consistency and texture of chocolate milk, frozen desserts, puddings, syrups. The most common stabilizer used in ice creams. Derived from seaweed.
Vitamin B_6	Needed to help body use protein, carbohydrate, and fat. Added to cereals, other foods.
Vitamin B_{12}	Helps all body cells function normally. Added to cereals, other foods.
Zinc	Mineral added to cereals to promote proper growth. Deficiency can cause dwarfism.

Javernick also cites Broadhead and Church [22], who wrote, "Without enriching experiences, children are often thought to be at risk educationally. Typically, intervention programs aimed at compensating for existing or expected problems are cognitively and socially oriented. There is little emphasis upon motor development."

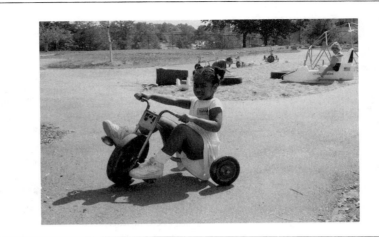

Figure 4-7
A preschooler exercises naturally.

In their position statement on Good Teaching Practices for 4- and 5-year-olds, the National Association for the Education of Young Children recommends that "children have daily opportunities to use large muscles, including running, jumping, and balancing. Outdoor activity is planned daily so children can develop large muscle skills, learn about outdoor environments and express themselves freely. Children have daily opportunities to develop small muscle skills through play activities such as pegboards, puzzles, painting, cutting, and other similar activities" [23].

Gallahue categorizes fundamental movement abilities developed through play as locomotor, manipulative, and stability abilities [24]. He feels that teachers should integrate into their daily program opportunities for movement activities that reflect preschoolers needs, interest and levels of ability (Figure 4-8).

Vannier and Gallahue [25] classify the fundamental abilities into three groups: locomotor, manipulative, and nonlocomotor. They define locomotor movement abilities (LMA) as those by which the body is transported in a horizontal or vertical direction from one point in space to another. Activities that are considered to be fundamental LMA are running, jumping (vertical or horizontal), leaping, galloping, skipping, hopping, sliding, and climbing.

Manipulative movement abilities (MMA) are those that involve giving force to objects or receiving force from objects. Activities are overhand throwing, catching, kicking, striking, dribbling, ball rolling, trapping, and volleying.

Nonlocomotor movement abilities (NLMA) are those where the body remains in place but moves around on its horizontal or vertical axis. Nonlocomotor movements place a premium on gaining and maintaining equilibrium in relation to the force of gravity. Axial movements such as reaching, twisting, turning, bend-

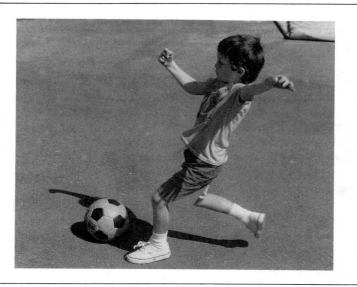

Figure 4-8
A preschooler makes the most of a movement opportunity.

ing, stretching, lifting, carrying, pushing, and pulling are fundamental nonlocomotor abilities.

The following suggestions will help you offer a better balanced fitness program:

1. Be aware that preschoolers are involved in developing and refining fundamental movement patterns in the three categories of movement. These movements are developed and refined through exploration and discovery. Plan your environment to facilitate such.
2. Follow the NAEYC's "Good Teaching Practices for 4 to 5-Year-Olds" [23] to provide a program that daily encompasses all areas of child development including physical development.
3. Get into the act. The teacher/care giver needs to participate enthusiastically but not to dominate or control motor activities. It will help you to become physically fit also.
4. Be aware that during ages 3 to 5 there should be no reason to provide formal periods of exercise. Under "normal" conditions (that is, in a balanced program), preschoolers will acquire movement skills through everyday activity.*

*In special situations with the handicapped child more structured motor experience may be necessary. See Cook, Ruth E, Tessier, Annette, and Armbruster, Virginia B.: Adapting early childhood curricula for children with special needs, 1987, Merrill Publishing Co.

5. Beware of unusual sounding movement activity programs that make extravagant but untested claims. (See Appendix 4–A for a listing of appropriate play materials for 3-, 4- and 5-year-olds.)

SUMMARY

- The preschool child should interact with other children and the teacher regarding food, food preparation, food service, and cleanup.
- Mealtime should be related to other educational activities in the center (for example, those fostering language development skills).
- Energy needs per kilogram are decreasing during the preschool years, although the actual amount of energy required has been increasing over the previous 3 years.
- Dietary intakes of the preschooler may be less than recommended for iron, calcium, vitamin C, and vitamin A.
- The care giver, along with the dietitian or nutritionist, can assess growth patterns and dietary intake patterns to ensure that growth is progressing within normal limits and that the dietary intake contains enough of the energy and nutrients known to be essential for the preschooler.
- Snacks should be offered from the basic food groups. They should contribute nutrients without supplying excessive energy to the diet.
- Children consuming vegetarian diets can be well nourished if their diets contain all the essential amino acids.
- When considering the use of sweeteners, care givers and food service personnel must take responsibility for preparing foods with a high nutrient density and without excessive calories from fat and sugar.
- Studies of the Feingold diet for hyperactivity have shown no evidence to recommend banning all additives, nor evidence that the diet is harmful. Therefore, there is no reason to discourage families from continuing its use.
- The early childhood environment provides numerous opportunities for both fine and gross motor development, yet teachers often neglect the gross motor, which results in an unbalanced program.

DISCUSSION QUESTIONS

1. List the reasons you may record a gain of 2 pounds or more per month for a 4-year-old.
2. How do the nutrient and energy needs of the preschooler compare with those of the toddler?
3. State how the food needs of the preschooler differ from and are similar to your own.
4. Describe the vegetarian diet and its use in the preschool center.

5. Should foods containing additives be eliminated from the preschool diet to control hyperactivity?
6. What do you feel can be done to ensure a balanced program that will include opportunities for total motor fitness?

REFERENCES

1. National Center for Health Statistics, U.S. Department of Health and Human Services, Public Health Service: Dietary intake source data: United States, 1976–1980, DHHS Publication No. (PHS)83-1681, Hyattsville, MD, 1983.
2. Williams, S. R.: Nutrition and diet therapy, ed. 4, St. Louis, 1981, the C.V. Mosby Co.
3. Gillooly, M., Bothwell, T. H., Torrance, A. P., et al.: The effects of organic acids, phytates, and polyphenols on the absorption of iron from vegetables, Brit. J. Nutr. 49:331, 1983.
4. Counsell, J. N., and Hornig, D. H. (eds.): Vitamin C (ascorbic acid), Englewood, NJ, 1982, Applied Science Publishers, Inc.
5. Karlowski, T. R., Chalmers, T. C., Frenkel, L. D., et al.: Ascorbic acid for the common cold: a prophylactic and therapeutic trial, J.A.M.A. 231:1038–1042, 1975.
6. Hodges, R. E.: Ascorbic acid, New York, 1976, The Nutrition Foundation, Inc.
7. Burt, J. V., and Hertzler, A. A.: Parental influences on the child's food preferences, J. Nutr. Educ. 10:127–128, 1978.
8. Birch L. L., and Marlin, D. W.: I don't like it; I never tried it: effects of exposure on two-year-old children's food preferences, Appetite: J. for Intake Research 3:353–360, 1982.
9. Birch L. L., Marlin, D. W., and Rotter, J.: Eating as the "means" activity in a contingency: effects on young children's food preference, Child Dev. 55:431–439, 1984.
10. Young, E. A., Sims, O. L., Bingham, C., and Brennan, E. H.: Fast foods update, Public Health Currents 27(3), 1987. Columbus, OH, Ross Laboratories.
11. Horwitz, D. L., and Bauer-Nehrling, J. K.: Can aspartame meet our expectations? J. Am. Diet. Assoc. 83:142–146, 1983.
12. American Dietetic Association: Position paper on the vegetarian approach to eating, J. Am. Diet. Assoc. 77:61–69, 1980.
13. American Dietetic Association: Position of the American Dietetic Association: vegetarian diets—technical support paper, J. Am. Diet. Assoc. 88:352–355, 1988.
14. American Dietetic Association: Position of the American Dietetic Association: vegetarian diets, J. Am. Diet. Assoc. 88:351, 1988.
15. Zmora, E., Gorodischer, R., and Bar-Ziv, J.: Multiple nutritional deficiencies in infants from a strict vegetarian community, Am. J. Dis. Child. 133:141, 1979.
16. Dwyer, J. T., Andrew, E. M., Berkey, C., et al.: Growth in "new" vegetarian preschool children using the Jenss-Bayley curve fitting technique, Am. J. Clin. Nutr. 37:815, 1983.
17. Feingold, B. F.: Why your child is hyperactive, New York, 1975, Random House, Inc.
18. Lipton, M. A., and Mayo, J. P.: Diet and hyperkinesis—an update, J. Am. Diet. Assoc. 83:132–134, 1983.
19. Wolraich, M., Milich, R., Stumbo, P., and Schultz, F.: Effects of sucrose ingestion on the behavior of hyperactive boys, J. Pediatr. 106:675–682, 1985.
20. Wolraich, M., Stumbo, P. J., and Milich, R., et al.: Dietary characteristics of hyperactive and control boys, J. Am. Diet. Assoc. 86:500–504, 1986.
21. Javernick, E.: Johnny's not jumping: can we help obese children? Young Children 43:21, 1988.
22. Broadhead, G., and Church, G.: Motor characteristics of preschool children, Research Quarterly for Exercise and Sport 56:208–214, 1985.

23. Good teaching practices for 4 and 5 year olds—a position for the National Association for the Education of Young Children, Washington, DC, 1986, National Association for the Education of Young Children.

24. Gallahue, D.: Understanding motor development in children, New York, 1982, John Wiley & Sons.

25. Vannier, M. H., and Gallahue, D.: Teaching physical education in elementary schools, Philadelphia, 1978, W. B. Saunders Co.

APPENDIX 4-A Equipment and Play Materials for Preschoolers

Equipment must be available in needed quantity and it must be varied according to children's needs. The following items* are suggested.

Balance boards

Balls of various sizes and materials

Barrels for creeping through, for rolling in, and for imaginative play

Bars firmly fixed and at varied heights for hanging, swinging, turning

Bats paddles, mallets

Batting tees these should be adjustable; they may be made of galvanized pipe and pieces of old garden hose

Bean bags

Benches these must be sturdy but light enough for children to carry; they can be used for jumping, as inclined planes, and for vaulting

Blocks, bricks, stones, and boards for building and for carrying, lifting, pushing, and pulling

Boards these should be well-cured, smooth and 6 to 8 inches wide; cleats underneath or hooks on the ends allow various attachments

Bounce board this may be purchased or constructed

Boxes sturdy wooden boxes and large corrugated cardboard boxes such as those refrigerators come in

Cargo nets (climbing nets) these may be obtained as Army-Navy surplus or from regular supply sources; they are useful for a variety of climbing activities

Climbing structures sturdy arrangements of metal tubing sometimes called towers, jungle gyms, etc. The larger ones are permanent fixtures; smaller structures are portable but also must be very sturdy

Flip-It Bowling Set a useful device easily cared for; it may be purchased or constructed

Hoops

Jumping standards these may be easily constructed and are now commercially available in suitable sizes

*Source: Sinclair, C. B.: Movement of the young child age two to six, Columbus, OH, 1973, Merrill Publishing Co.

Ladders to be used vertically, horizontally, and inclined at various angles; hooks on the end provide stable fixation

Logs short and long; poles with smooth surfaces

Mats small and washable for individual use; larger mats for small group activities; pads of foam rubber may be used temporarily

Obstacle course a wide variety of materials may be used to involve jumping, running, climbing, going over, under and through

Old bathtub when appropriately set up is fine for water play

Padded sawhorses, tables, and benches may be used for vaulting and many tumbling activities instead of more expensive apparatus

Parachute may be obtained as Army-Navy surplus

Pitchback net may be purchased or constructed; enables one child to play throw and catch

Pool portable plastic pool for wading and shallow water play

Portable metal stands these are light enough for children to carry but well constructed; they may be utilized with boards and ladders to make ever-changing apparatus

Reach and jump target strips of plastic graduated in length and suspended from a bar so that children may jump and reach to touch them

Record player and records readily available from many sources. Records selected should allow for creativity in movement

Rhythm instruments a sturdy drum is a must and should be used often by the teacher; rattles, drums, triangles, and many other instruments may be purchased or constructed.

Roller skates these are not usual in nursery schools but may be used if facilities and space permit

Rope ladder one or more of these offer an interesting challenge and they are easily stored

Ropes long ropes are useful for turning and as climbing equipment; they may be used on the ground to mark off areas to jump over, to define floor patterns, etc. Short ropes for individual use may be used in countless ways.

Rugs   for outdoor use a blanket or sheet of foam rubber may be used as a rug. Small woven rugs may be used as substitutes for mats.

Slides and swings   these should be selected, located and erected with professional advice.

Spades, rakes, shovels   these are available in small sizes and should be of strong construction.

Spools   large wooden spools are often discarded after utility contruction; they should be weather-proofed and used for jumping, climbing, and building. They may also be rolled about the area.

Stairways   five to seven steps should be provided for a realistic experience. Many children do not use stairways at home or school.

Stall bars   ladder-like bars erected close to a wall; these take up little space and are excellent for indoor use.

Suspended balls   good for hitting practice; require adequate space; should be pulled up after use.

Stools and tables   if strongly constructed these may be used for many purposes and old ones may be substituted for more expensive equipment.

Swinging bridge   made of rope and boards and suspended about head height.

Targets   fixed or portable; these may vary widely in type—an open frame, concentric circles painted on cloth or plastic, flags or traffic cones for markers, and many others.

Tires   bicycle, car, and truck; tubes and casings.

Traffic cones   these may be available without cost or can be easily constructed. They are useful as markers and goals and may also be used as supports for light objects.

Tree trunks and stumps   wonderful for climbing, vaulting, jumping; they may be used as or converted into ships, horses, trucks, houses, etc.

Trestles and sawbenches   these may be used as supports for boards, ladders, and bridges. When constructed of wood the tops can be padded and used for vaulting and tumbling.

Tricycles and bicycles

Tunnels   fabric and collapsible, concrete or ceramic.

Wagons, sleds, and wheelbarrows

Walking beam

Wands   smooth wooden sticks, also may be made of metal; the wooden ones are strong and inexpensive.

LEARNING OBJECTIVES

Students will be able to

- State the characteristics of the young child that may affect food intake
- Describe physical activities that can facilitate energy balance
- Describe acceptable foods for after-school snacks
- List steps in managing the low-fat diet to prevent cardiovascular disease and other nutrition-related problems
- State food needs related to nutrient and energy recommendations

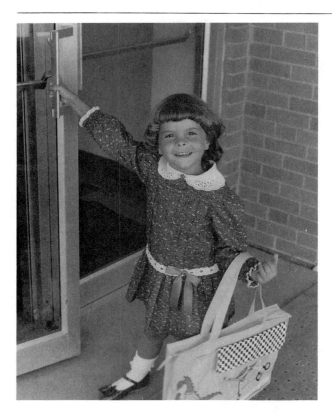

The 6- to 8-Year-Old

Middle childhood is generally defined as beginning at 6 years of age and ending at the onset of puberty. Whereas the young girl at 7 to 8 years may already have accelerated growth, rapid growth rate will not be seen in the young boy until 9 or 10 years at the earliest. For both girls and boys the period from 6 to 8 years is a relatively stable growth period and may even be called latent compared to the preschool years or what is still to come during adolescence.

The influence of school and extracurricular activities becomes more important during middle childhood. The significance of body image, especially for young girls, may be seen in what clothing is worn and what foods are eaten. School and community activities allow the child to use the increased physical ability. Attendance at school for a full day provides regularity for activities, including food service. Foods are generally accepted and appetite improves as the child participates in activities that cause increased energy expenditure. The routines and activities of full-day school seem to encourage systematic snacks and meals.

WEIGHT AND STATURE

Before 6 years boys may be taller and heavier than most girls, but by 8 to 9 years the girls are catching up and many weigh almost as much as the average boy in the same class. From infancy to 6 years, the percentage of body fat for both boys and girls decreases, while lean body mass increases. However, at about 6 years girls again begin to have a higher proportion of their weight as fat. Girls will continue into adolescence and adult years to have a higher proportion of their weight as fat. Children at this age gain approximately 2 to 3 inches in height and 4.5 to 6.5 pounds per year (Table 5–1).

Table 5-1
Weight and stature for 6- to 8-year-olds

Age (years)	Girls		Boys	
	Weight (pounds)	Stature (inches)	Weight (pounds)	Stature (inches)
6	42.9	45.1	45.5	45.7
7	48.0	47.5	50.3	47.9
8	54.6	49.8	55.7	50.0

Source: Modified from charts showing smoothed percentiles of weight and stature by sex and age developed by National Center for Health Statistics, U.S. Department of Health, Education and Welfare, PHS, Hyattsville, MD, 1977, The Center.

ENERGY AND NUTRIENT NEEDS

Dietary recommendations for the 6- to 8-year-old are found in two RDA groupings (Table 5-2). Decreased amounts of protein and energy are required as growth slows, but wide ranges in recommendations reflect the variation in individual growth and physical activity of children at this age. Current weight has been used (weight (lb) × kcal/lb) to assess recommended caloric intake in Table 5-2.

When using calories per inch to estimate needs, the 7- to 10-year-old will begin needing more per inch. The 6-year-old's energy need, according to the RDA, is still 39 calories per inch; by 10 years it will increase to 46 calories per inch. In addition, the energy allowance per inch is greater for the child who begins an early growth spurt. A child's height and weight should be plotted on the growth charts (Appendix VI) at regular intervals. Changes will alert the care giver to any abnormalities and the need to refer the child to a dietitian or other health professional for further evaluation.

Nutrients

The nutrient needs are increasing in proportion to the need for energy. Diets of children during this period have been found to supply sufficient amounts of most nutrients. Parents who have been concerned about their child's appetite earlier in life often find the child willing to eat more foods now.

Dietary Supplementation

According to the American Academy of Pediatrics [1], national dietary and health surveys have shown little evidence of vitamin or mineral inadequacies, with the exception of iron, for this age group. There is little basis for routine vitamin and mineral supplementation in healthy children, especially as the growth rate decreases after infancy. However, supplements may be indicated for some children, including those

Table 5-2
RDA for ages 4-6 and 7-10

	4 to 6 Years (44 lb, 44 in. [20 kg, 112 cm])	7 to 10 Years (62 lb, 52 in. [28 kg, 132 cm])
Food energy (kcal)	1700 (39 kcal/lb)	2400 (39 kcal/lb)
Protein (g)	30 (1.5/kg or .68/lb)	34 (1.2/kg or .55/lb)
Vitamin A (IU)	2500	3500
Vitamin D (IU)	400	400
Ascorbic acid (mg)	45	45
Folacin (μg)	200	300
Niacin (mg)	11	16
Riboflavin (mg)	1	1.4
Thiamin (mg)	0.9	1.2
Vitamin B_6 (mg)	1.3	1.6
Vitamin B_{12} (μg)	2.5	3
Calcium (mg)	800	800
Phosphorus (mg)	800	800
Iron (mg)	10	10
Magnesium (mg)	200	250
Zinc (mg)	10	10

Source: Based on Food and Nutrition Board, National Academy of Sciences—National Research Council: Recommended dietary allowances, revised 1980.

- From deprived families, especially children who suffer from parental neglect or abuse
- With anorexia, poor and capricious appetites, or poor eating habits
- On dietary regimens to manage obesity
- Consuming vegetarian diets without adequate dairy products (vitamin B_{12} is absent from vegetable foods)

FOOD NEEDS

Meeting the food needs of middle childhood requires consumption of food in slightly greater quantities than at earlier years. Because energy needs for these children vary widely, monthly heights and weights should serve as a guide to the need for additional energy. Serving portions will be similar to, and in some cases larger than, the adult serving size. Table 5-3 shows a recommended food pattern that meets the RDA for nutrients for the child 6 to 10 years of age. Energy allowances average 1800 to 2000 kilocalories, and more food should be included to meet additional energy needs.

Table 5-3
Recommended food intake according to food group and average serving size (ages 6 up to 10 years)

Food Group	Servings/Day	Average Serving (ages 6 up to 10)
Fruits and Vegetables	At least 4 including: 1 or more (twice as much tomato as citrus)	½ C
Vitamin C source (citrus fruits, berries, tomato, cabbage, cantaloupe)		
Green Vegetables	1*	½ C
Other vegetables (potato and other green or yellow vegetables and/or other fruits)	2	½ C
Meat and Alternates	3–4 including:	
Lean meat, fish, poultry, and eggs†	2	3 oz
Nutbutters (peanut, soynut)		4 tbsp‡
Cooked dried beans or peas	1–2§	½ C
Nuts		1 oz
Breads and Cereals (Whole Grain)	At least 4	
Bread		1 slice
Ready-to-eat cereals, whole grain		1 oz
Cooked cereal including macaroni, spaghetti, rice, etc. (use whole grain if possible)		½ C
Milk and Milk Products	At least 4	
2% or skim milk (1.5 oz cheese = 1 C milk) (C = 8 oz or 240 g)		1 C
Fats and Oils		
Butter, margarine, mayonnaise, oils	3	1 tsp

*Allow a minimum serving of 1 tbsp/year of age for cooked fruits, vegetables, cereals, and pasta until the child reaches 8 years or ½ C portion size.

†To enhance overall nutrient content of diet include eggs two to three times a week and liver occasionally.

‡Illinois State Board of Education, Department of Child Nutrition: Child Care Food Program—required meal patterns, Springfield, IL, June 1986, The Board.

§Include nutbutters, dried (cooked) beans, or peas at least once a day to meet nutrient recommendations and decrease the fat content of the diet. Use additional servings of meats when legumes, beans, and nuts are omitted.

WHAT INFLUENCES EATING PATTERNS?

Eating patterns can be influenced when specific foods are promoted by the media, especially television. The child in elementary school spends more time in front of a television set each year than in the classroom.

Some studies show preteens are influenced more by peer pressure than parental actions [2]. However, family income and economic status do influence the types and amounts of food that can be purchased and where foods will be eaten (restaurants or in the home). Family structure and employment patterns of parents may make preparing meals with a wide variety of foods difficult. For example, single-parent families use convenience foods and visit fast food restaurants more often than the general public [3].

Six- to 8-year-olds increasingly select their own meals, especially breakfast, from what is available in the kitchen. They alone can be responsible for choosing from 15% to 20% of their foods every day. With widespread use of microwaves and prepackaged frozen microwave items, children have a wider variety of foods from which to choose and can learn at an earlier age to prepare nutritious meals for themselves (Figure 5–1). Day-care providers can educate parents on alternative choices for quick nutritious food service at home. The varied diet that began in the preschool years should be continued with only minor modifications; larger portion sizes will provide the required energy and nutrient needs.

Parents are now less in control of what the child eats. Responsibility rests with the school system to provide at least ⅓ of recommended nutrients for the child participating in school lunches. An after-school care giver may provide another 150 to 300 calories (for example, with crackers or cookies and milk), 10% to 15% of energy and nutrients. Parents, therefore, may be responsible for less than 40% of total energy needs, serving the child only one meal per day.

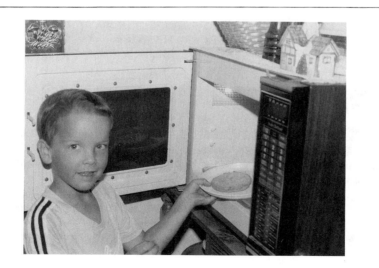

Figure 5–1
A child prepares a microwave snack.

Teachers' and coaches' advice on what to eat and their eating behavior also influence the child's food choices. An educator who eats a wide variety of foods, gets involved in the food programs at school, and demonstrates a positive attitude toward nutritious foods served at school will encourage children to become interested in eating an array of nutritious foods.

Snack Foods

As with younger children, sugary, and especially fatty, snacks should be avoided. By the time the child reaches 6 years the diet should contain no more than 30% of the calories from fat; thus, very few foods in the diet can have a composition that is high in fat.

Table 5–4 shows the fat and sugar content of snacks consumed by one group of children during a weekend period. Fat contributed more than 30% of the

Table 5–4
Energy from fat and sugar for favorite snacks

Food (serving size)	Total Kcal*	Fat		Total Sugars†	
		Kcal	%Kcal	Kcal	%Kcal
Milk chocolate with almonds (1 oz)	151	91	60	55	36
Reese's pieces (1 pkg)	240	90	38	112	47
M & M, peanut (1 pkg)	240	108	45	89	37
Chocolate chip cookies (1)	52	21	40	14	26
Oreo cookies (1)	51	20	40	14	27
Toaster pastry, blueberry frosted (1)	200	45	23	60	30
Pudding pops, banana (1)	94	23	25	57	60
Ice cream, 10% fat (1 C)	273	131	48	95	35
Soda pop, cola (12 oz)	144	0	0	144	100
Potato chips (1 oz)	161	102	63	0	0
Cheetos, puff (1 oz)	155	87	56	tr	tr
Popcorn/oil (1 oz)	128	56	44	tr	tr

*Kilocalories from protein, fat, and carbohydrates.

†Includes all mono- and disaccharides; excludes complex carbohydrates (starch and fiber).

Sources: Data from

FOOD VALUES OF PORTIONS COMMONLY USED, 14th Edition by Helen Nichols Church and Jean A. T. Pennington. Copyright © 1980, 1985 by Helen Nichols Church B.S. and Jean A. T. Pennington Ph.D. R.N. Reprinted by permission of Harper & Row, Publishers, Inc.

United States Department of Agriculture: Nutritive value of American foods in common units, Agriculture handbook No. 456. November 1975.

NDDA Laboratory, Southern Illinois University at Carbondale, 1988.

Matthews, R. H., and Pehrsson, P. R.: Provisional table on the sugar content of selected foods, October 1986, United States Department of Agriculture, Human Nutrition Information Service.

calories for 9 of 12 items chosen by the youngsters. Two items, fruit pastries and pudding treats, were within the acceptable range for fat. Some snack foods that seem to be low in fat and high in complex carbohydrates are just the opposite—popcorn cooked in oil and potato chips get more than 30% of their calories from fat. Restricting fat generally means avoiding calorie-rich foods that are often low in other nutrients.

The best snack foods are those in which complex carbohydrates and sugars, not fat, are the largest single source of energy (Table 5–5). Although some of the carbohydrate in these snacks is from simple sugars (monosaccharides), much is complex and is "packaged" along with other nutrients (as in saltines). Even though nutbutters and nuts are a rich source of many nutrients not readily

Table 5–5
Energy from fat and sugar for recommended snacks

Food (serving size)	Total Kcal*	Fat		Total Sugars†	
		Kcal	%Kcal	Kcal	%Kcal
Apple (1 medium)	81	4	5	55	68
Apple with ½ tbsp peanut butter	128	41	32	58	45
Banana (1 medium)	105	5	5	64	61
Grapes (1 C)	107	5	5	87	81
Orange (1)	64	3	5	43	67
Bagel with 2 tsp jelly	201	13	6	20	10
Whole wheat bread with fruit butter (2 tsp)	87	11	13	28	32
Saltine crackers (6)	78	19	24	tr	tr
Graham cracker (3 squares)	81	18	22	15	17
Wheat cracker (4 small)	64	20	31	—	—‡
Apple butter (2 tsp)	26	1	4	24	92
Yogurt, plain, low fat (1 C)	144	32	22	46	32

*Kilocalories from protein, fat, and carbohydrates.

†Includes all mono- and disaccharides. Excludes complex carbohydrates (starch and fiber).

‡No reliable data.

Sources: Data from

FOOD VALUES OF PORTIONS COMMONLY USED, 14th Edition by Helen Nichols Church and Jean A. T. Pennington. Copyright © 1980, 1985 by Helen Nichols Church B.S. and Jean A. T. Pennington Ph.D. R.N. Reprinted by permission of Harper & Row, Publishers, Inc.

United States Department of Agriculture: Nutritive value of American foods in common units, Agriculture handbook No. 456. November 1975.

NDDA Laboratory, Southern Illinois University at Carbondale, 1988.

Matthews, R. H., and Pehrsson, P. R.: Provisional table on the sugar content of selected foods, October 1986, United States Department of Agriculture, Human Nutrition Information Service.

available in other foods, the high fat content should be taken into consideration when planning and evaluating the child's diet.

NUTRITION-RELATED PROBLEMS

Nutrition-related problems for this age group include cardiovascular disease, lactose intolerance, dental caries, and persistent weight problems. A discussion of lactose intolerance and dental caries is included in Chapter 3.

Lactose intolerance may be seen in as many as 30% of children in this age group. Many children have learned that they can drink milk with meals but not alone for the afternoon milk break. Some children can tolerate flavored milk better than regular whole or skim milk. Once children reach this age, parents and teachers must include them in decisions regarding foods that can be tolerated.

The school personnel should reinforce the parents' and child's efforts to maintain good dental health. Children should have a regular routine established for care of teeth and gums at home and, if possible, brush after meals at school. They should be familiar with the dentist, participating in regular visits at least once a year. Many dentists apply sealants as new permanent teeth emerge to deter the development of caries.

Cardiovascular Disease and Diet Modification

The child 6 to 8 years old is generally healthy and at low risk for many of the nutrition-related problems occurring at earlier ages. Due to increasing media coverage of the risk factors associated with cardiovascular disease, care givers and parents want diets for their very young children that will protect the heart. There is general agreement that atherosclerosis may begin in youth and undergo progression through young adulthood, even though clinical manifestations usually do not appear until middle age or later.

The relationship between high levels of serum cholesterol and arteriosclerosis (hardening of the arteries) is strong, but the correlation between cholesterol taken in diet and cholesterol measured in the serum is less certain. Lowering total dietary fat appears to be somewhat effective in lowering serum cholesterol.

Whether to recommend diet restrictions for young children and at what age is still being debated. There appears to be agreement that lowering dietary fat during the primary school years is a good preventive measure without undue effects on growth and development. However, modification of diets in healthy children before 5 years of age has recently been advocated as a means of influencing plasma cholesterol levels [4]. The American Academy of Pediatrics takes a more moderate approach, providing the following recommendations for planning children's diets:

> Current dietary trends in the United States toward a decreased consumption of saturated fats, cholesterol, and salt and an increased intake of polyunsaturated fats should be followed with moderation. DIETS THAT AVOID EXTREMES ARE SAFE FOR

CHILDREN. THE SAFETY OF DIETS DESIGNED TO DECREASE CALORIC INTAKE, INCREASE CONSUMPTION OF COMPLEX CARBOHYDRATES, DECREASE INTAKE OF REFINED SUGARS, DECREASE CONSUMPTION OF FAT AND CHOLESTEROL AND LIMIT SODIUM INTAKE HAS NOT BEEN ESTABLISHED IN GROWING CHILDREN AND PREGNANT WOMEN. [5]

If cereal grains with high fiber content are chosen in place of animal protein, the intake of vitamins and minerals that have protective value—for example, iron—may decrease. Excluding these nutrients might pose health risks to children. Animal products are rich in protein and have many essential nutrients difficult to obtain from other foods.

More attention is now being focused on identifying risk factors in very young children for coronary heart disease (CHD) so that preventive measures can be introduced early. CHD risk factors in children are primarily hypertension and elevated plasma cholesterol. Modifying diets in these children seems appropriate.

The recommendations for lowering the risk of cardiovascular disease include cutting fat intake to 30% of calories and cholesterol to 100 mg/1000 kcal. Considering one egg has approximately 300 mg cholesterol and a 2- to 4-year-old needs less than 1500 kcal per day, this means that eggs and whole milk would be almost totally excluded from the diet.

In addition to decreasing fat and cholesterol intake, dietary measures that have been shown to be effective in promoting good health habits include: consumption of a variety of foods; maintenance of desired body weight; increased consumption of starch and fiber; decreased consumption of refined sugar; and decreased consumption of sodium [6].

In summary, menus that strictly interpret the Dietary Guidelines for Americans are generally not recommended for use with children until after 2 years. The older child, however, can benefit from moderate dietary modifications.

Calculating the Low-Fat Diet. Care givers may wish to determine how to plan a diet with 30% of calories from fat. What foods should be selected for the elementary school child to restrict fat intake? Figure 5–2 shows how to calculate a low-fat diet. The number of calories that would be supplied by fat in diets of various caloric levels is shown in Table 5–6.

The menu in Figure 5–3 shows the difficulty in meeting an actual child's energy needs and still keeping fat within 30% of calories without changing current eating patterns. Assuming the child needs 2000 kcal, the fat would be limited to 66 to 67 grams (30% of total calories from fat). This child still needs additional foods for energy, but fat content has already reached 30% (67 g) of calories. The food pattern in Table 5–3 (page 182) is a guide from which to choose foods for a nutritionally adequate, low-fat diet. Table 5–7 gives additional suggestions for planning low-fat meals.

Fabricated Foods. The use of fabricated foods should not be condemned nor advocated for young children. *Fabricated foods* are those which generally serve to substitute for cheese, eggs, milk, and other foods. Most were developed primari-

Steps

1. Find energy level (kcal) of diet (total calories needed—see Chapter 2).
2. Multiply energy (kcal) by percent fat allowed (kcal × .30 = fat kcal).
3. Divide fat kcal by 9 (Step 2 divided by 9 kcal/g fat) to get total grams of fat allowed in diet.
4. Find the serving of food you plan to eat using food tables (Appendix I) or food labels.
5. Note the number of grams of fat listed for a food and subtract from total grams of fat allowed in the diet (Step 3).

Example

Step 1. 2000 kcal (estimated total energy needs)
Step 2. .30 × 2000 = 600 kcal from fat
Step 3. 600 ÷ 9 = 66–67 g fat
Step 4. 6 oz hamburger = 19 g fat
Step 5. 67 − 19 = 48 g of fat remain from allowance

Figure 5–2
Calculation of diet with 30% of calories from fat

ly to reduce the dietary energy and fat intake. An increased effort is needed to evaluate the nutritional adequacy of these foods in animal and clinical studies before advocating widespread use, particularly in children [1].

Obesity

The treatment for childhood obesity has been reviewed by Peck and Ullrich [7] and included in Chapter 3. The persistence of adolescent obesity into adulthood and its resistance to current successful treatment programs provide valid reasons for developing school programs that focus on prevention and treatment [8]. Some successful programs have included behavior modification, nutrition education, and physical activity. In one 10-week school-based program for 5- to 12-year-olds, 95% of the children lost weight and reversed a trend to steady weight gain [9]. School food service programs can be an asset in prevention of obesity [10].

Table 5–6
Fat as 30% of calories in various diets

Total Calories	Fat (kcal)	Fat (g)
1500	450	50
1600	480	53
1800	540	60
2000	600	67
2200	660	73
2400	720	80

Foods	Fat (g)	Kcal (approx.)
6 oz hamburger (lean)	19	400
1 oz American cheese	9	110
½ C broccoli	trace	25
½ C peaches	trace	35
1 large baked potato	trace	150
1 C whole kernel corn	1	150
3 slices whole wheat bread	3	225
½ C spaghetti	trace	110
2 tsp mayonnaise-type salad dressing	4	45
½ tbsp margarine (served with vegetables)	6	53
1 oz potato chips (1 serving)	11	161
1 C whole milk* (at school)	9	160
1 C 2% milk (at restaurant)	5	120
1 C skim milk (at home)	trace	90
TOTAL	67†	1834

*Note difference in fat content between whole and skim milk.

†Fat is calculated for 30% of 2000 kcal, or 67 g. Although fat intake has reached this level, the child needs additional energy.

Figure 5-3
Grams of fat in menu pattern for 6- to 8-year-old

Table 5-7
Specific recommendations to lower fat intake

Use	Include Less Often
Skim milk	Whole milk
Yogurt, skim cottage cheese*	Dairy dips with sour cream
Fruit ices, sorbets, and sherbets	Ice cream, prepared pudding
Low-fat meats	High-fat meats
Margarine (sparingly)	Butter and palm and coconut oil
Low-fat cheese*	High-fat cheese
Low-fat dressings	Regular oil- or fat-based dressings
Legumes, beans, and peas	High-fat nuts
Fruits and vegetables	Deep fried vegetables and fruits

*Check labels for fat content.

EXERCISE AND PHYSICAL FITNESS

Children 6 to 8 years old have gained better control of small muscles and can coordinate hand and eye to an increasing degree. This is a time when children become immersed in games and physical activities. To continually develop and refine locomotor and nonlocomotor skills, they must have many opportunities to test and retest their abilities [11]. It is during this age span that the green light is given to begin more structured physical fitness activities both at home and at school.

Components of Fitness

The American Academy of Pediatrics Committee on Sports Medicine and School Health defines the components of fitness to include muscle strength and endurance, flexibility, body fat composition, and cardiorespiratory endurance [12].

Frequency of Physical Education Classes

In their position statement regarding integrated components of appropriate and inappropriate practice in the primary grades, the National Association for the Education of Young Children recommends that physical education be integrated into the curriculum each day [13]. The American Academy of Pediatrics stresses that physical education classes be held at least three times weekly in the primary grades and that such classes are critical to developing and maintaining physical fitness in young children [12].

Parents often feel that their children get plenty of exercise in their school's gym classes and at recess. The fact is that many students get as little as one hour of physical education a week. In addition, schools have traditionally emphasized sports that promote agility and specialized skills (baseball, basketball, football) rather than cardiovascular fitness (bicycling, swimming, running, fast walking, aerobic exercise, tennis). Most of a typical primary child's physical activity occurs outside of physical education classes (Figure 5-4) [14]. In light of these facts, in 1987 the American Academy of Pediatrics issued a policy statement urging parents and pediatricians to appeal to their local school boards to maintain, if not increase, physical education programs [14].

As indicated in Chapter 2, numerous fitness surveys have indicated that children in the U.S. are underexercised. Society's current emphasis on academics has resulted in an unbalanced curriculum that lacks opportunities for children to develop and refine motor skills. Nevertheless, the United States has more physical educators, more gyms, more swimming pools, and more recreational opportunities than any country in the world. Some would say we also have the best medical science system in the world, yet we lead the world in degenerative diseases [15]. Regularly scheduled physical education classes, incorporating lifelong cardiovascular fitness skills, rather than those that promote game skills that are often not carried into adulthood, must be provided. Without such pro-

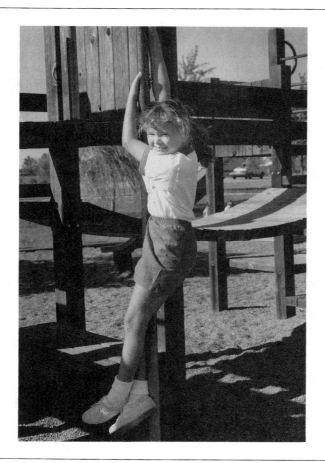

Figure 5–4
Physical activity often occurs outside of physical education classes.

grams the risk of latent disorders such as obesity, elevated blood pressure, and high cholesterol level, all of which can lead to coronary heart disease, will continue to threaten our children.

The President's Council on Fitness and Sports recommends that the cardiovascular system be stressed for at least 30 minutes a day through vigorous activity. Without this activity, children can progressively decondition with the final result being alarmingly poor cardiac condition [15].

Parent's Role

As with all societal problems, the schools can't do it all. Parents can do much to instill awareness of fitness in the primary aged child. We caution, however, that parents must remember that if it is not fun, children won't do it. The American Academy of Pediatrics suggests that parents:

1. Incorporate fitness activities into the family lifestyle.
2. Introduce children to a variety of athletic activities; they are easily bored.
3. Become involved with your children's activities by either playing a sport with them or coaching a team.
4. If safe, encourage your child to walk to school or take a shorter bus ride and walk part way.
5. Encourage after school activities and limit TV viewing during this time.
6. Set a good example. [12]

The 6- to 8-year-old has everything to gain by being physically fit. Exercise boosts self-image and improves physical strength and stamina as well as scholastic performance.

SUMMARY

- The young child's eating habits during the 6- to 8-year period are influenced by the school setting, coaches, and teachers.
- Girls will continue into adolescence having a higher proportion of their weight as fat.
- Supplementation with vitamins and minerals is needed only in children at high risk for poor dietary intake.
- No attempt should be made to restrict the young child's intake of a variety of nutrient-dense foods on the basis of fat, sodium, or cholesterol. By age 6, the diet can conform to the Dietary Guidelines for Americans and include no more than 30% of total calories as fat.
- To limit fat to 30%, substitutions should be found for high-fat snacks.
- Fabricated foods are those that generally substitute for high-fat foods. Further evaluation is needed before their use is recommended.
- Parents as well as the school play a critical role in providing opportunities for 6- to 8-year-olds to participate in both structured and unstructured physical fitness activities.

DISCUSSION QUESTIONS

1. What principles from this chapter were followed in developing the guides and food plans?
2. How do the nutrient and energy needs of the school-aged child compare to those of the preschooler?
3. Calculate the energy you need each day and list foods usually eaten. How can your diet be modified using only 30% calories from fat?

4. Can snack foods with more than 30% fat be included in the diet? What snacks in addition to those already mentioned could be recommended to the mother of a young child?
5. Discuss the need to both modify and increase physical education activities.

REFERENCES

1. American Academy of Pediatrics, Committee on Nutrition: Pediatric nutrition handbook, ed. 2, Chicago, 1985, American Academy of Pediatrics.
2. Cook, C. C., and Payne, I. R.: Effect of supplements on the nutritional intake of children, J. Am. Diet. Assoc. 74:130, 1979.
3. Sheridan, M. J., and McPherrin, G.: Fast food and the American diet, Summit, NJ, 1981, American Council on Science and Health.
4. American Heart Association, Nutrition Committee and the Cardiovascular Disease in the Young Council: Diet in the healthy child, Circulation 67:1411, 1983.
5. American Academy of Pediatrics, Committee on Nutrition: Toward a prudent diet for children, Pediatrics 71:78, 1983.
6. Walter, H. J.: Modification of blood cholesterol levels in a school based population in primary prevention of atherosclerosis in childhood: the role of lipids, Proceedings from a videoconference March 28, 1985, NY, Biomedical Information Corporation, 1987.
7. Peck, E. B., and Ullrich, H. D.: Children and weight: a changing perspective, Berkeley, CA, 1985, Nutrition Communications Associates.
8. Summer, S. K.: Obesity in the school age child, School Food Service Review 10(2), 1986.
9. Brownell, K. D., and Kaye, F. S.: A school-based behavior modification, nutrition education and physical activity program for obese children, Am. J. Clin. Nutr. 35:277, 1982.
10. Stitt, K. R.: Weight control and school food service, School Food Serv. Res. Rev. 3:5, 1979.
11. Arnheim, D. D., and Sinclair, W. A.: The clumsy child: a program of motor therapy, St. Louis, 1979, C. V. Mosby Co., p. 21.
12. Fitness: The myths and the facts, American Academy of Pediatrics Fact Sheet, Elk Grove Village, IL, 1987.
13. National Association for the Education of Young Children: Position statement on developmentally appropriate practice in the primary grades, serving 5 through 8-year-olds, Young Children, 43, January 1988, pp. 64-68.
14. Policy statement from American Academy of Pediatrics, Physical fitness and the schools, Pediatrics 80(3):449-450, September 1987.
15. The President's Council on Physical Fitness and Sports, National School Population Fitness Survey, HHS—Office of the Assistant Secretary of Health, Research Project 282-84-0086, University of Michigan Press, 1986, p. 2.

LEARNING OBJECTIVES

Students will be able to

- List the daily food plans for infants, toddlers, and preschoolers
- Define which foods are an acceptable part of the Child Care Food Program
- Describe how food service personnel and teachers may participate in menu planning
- Define cycle menus and plan daily menus that meet the needs of the young child
- State the parents' contributions to the menu
- List the management principles that must be considered in the food service operation
- Define the community dietitian's role in center activities

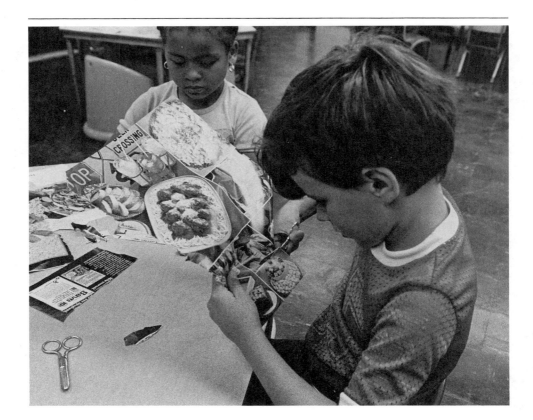

6

The Menu

Food service for the child cared for away from home can occur in a variety of settings. Some of the settings, especially those receiving public funds, must follow regulations outlined by such federal agencies as the U.S. Department of Agriculture and the Department of Health and Human Services, as well as various other state and local agencies.

In addition to providing nourishment, the foods served can be used to teach nutritional practices that will lead to a life of good nutrition. To provide nourishment and nutrition education in the classroom, the principles of food service must first be understood and practiced. The menu can be the tool used to help coordinate the nutrition and food needs of children with learning activities in the various settings.

When teachers and food service personnel work together to select foods and plan the style in which they are served, both professional groups feel committed to making food and nutrition work in the classroom. Although you as a care giver may not take direct responsibility for writing the menus or preparing foods, you are an important component of the process if the menu, food preparation, foods, and food service are to be used in the curriculum or learning activities of the children.

Without center food service there can be no nourishment. Likewise, without curriculum planning involving food service activities there can be few educational activities around mealtime. The food service system described in this chapter is planned jointly by the preschool teacher and food service supervisor or "cook." An outcome of this joint planning may be seen when teachers do not "beg the cook" for a fresh pineapple or have to purchase one themselves for the classroom. Instead, the teacher and food service personnel plan "menus for learning" from which educational experiences naturally evolve.

WHAT TO EAT—FOOD PATTERNS

Before one begins to plan menus or to discuss the planning of the curriculum around the menu, it is necessary to review the basic food patterns for the infant, toddler, and young child. The nutrient and food requirements have been discussed in general terms in earlier chapters. This chapter presents menu or food patterns that meet the Child Care Food Program guidelines [1]. The guidelines are practical for child-care center or home day-care food production. Some centers provide one to three feeding periods. The menus in this chapter provide the minimum amount of nutrients. We have included a cycle menu for those centers that have children for at least one meal and one snack.

Meals served in preschool or school lunch programs are required to provide one third of the child's RDA. If the lunch provides only one third of the recommended amounts of the nutrients, the parents at home must supply an additional two thirds of the recommended allowances through the other meals. In many cases the child must leave home early, possibly without a morning meal, and return late in the evening. Unless the center provides more than the one third of the RDA, children will be consuming fewer nutrients than their recommended allowance.

The Infant

Table 6–1 provides an infant meal pattern that allows for the optional introduction of infant cereals, fruits, and vegetables by 4 months. Children should not take solid foods until after 4 to 6 months of age. In practice, however, many parents are providing their children with solid foods earlier.

Whole milk should not be given until at least 7 months of age and only when the infant is consuming one third of calories from a balanced mixture of foods. The milk should be homogenized, vitamin D–fortified whole milk or diluted evaporated milk. Solid foods rich in carbohydrates are the best choices; when paired with whole milk, which is rich in protein and fat, the diet will contain an acceptable calorie distribution.

Schedule. Depending on the age of the infant, a feeding schedule may be established before the child enters the center. This should be carefully recorded from the interview with the mother or father and discussed with the food service personnel. Taking a dietary history, including a 24-hour recall (Chapter 1), when the infant enters the center is important in determining the child's schedule. A master feeding schedule for infants is advisable (Chapter 9) to help communicate with all staff as well as parents. Centers often set 4-hour feeding schedules, but our experiences show that some babies, both breast- and bottle-fed, demand nourishment every 2 to 3 hours. Food is one of the primary means whereby the very young child can interact with the care giver. This opportunity may be lost if the child is either hungry and irritable or fed too often and disinterested.

Table 6-1
Child-care infant meal pattern

Birth Through 3 Months	4 Through 7 Months	8 Through 11 Months
	Breakfast	
4-6 fl. oz. formula*	4-8 fl. oz. formula* or breast milk	6-8 fl. oz. formula*, breast milk, or whole milk
	0-3 Tbsp infant cereal† (optional)	2-4 tbsp infant cereal† 1-4 tbsp fruit and/or vegetable
	Lunch or Supper	
4-6 fl. oz. formula*	4-8 fl. oz. formula* or breast milk	6-8 fl. oz. formula*, breast milk, or whole milk
	0-3 tbsp infant cereal† (optional)	2-4 tbsp infant cereal† and/or
	0-3 tbsp fruit and/or vegetable (optional)	1-4 tbsp meat, fish, poultry, egg yolk, or cooked dry beans or peas, or ½-2 oz cheese or
		1-4 oz cottage cheese, cheese food, or cheese spread
		1-4 tbsp fruit and/or vegetable
	Supplement	
4-6 fl. oz. formula*	4-6 fl. oz. formula* or breast milk	2-4 fl. oz. formula*, breast milk, whole milk, or juice‡
		0-½ bread slice or 0-2 crackers (optional)§

Source: Data from Federal Register 53(129):25309, July 6, 1988.

*Iron-fortified infant formula.

†Iron-fortified dry infant cereal.

‡Full-strength fruit juice.

§From whole-grain or enriched meal or flour.

Formula Preparation.   It is best for the center to purchase or have parents bring in unopened cans of formula and prepare infant formulas on-site for children who will remain in the center all day (see Chapter 2). The preparation methods and correct sanitation procedures are included in Appendix V. If the formula is prepared in the center, there can be no question as to its freshness or the extent to which proper methods have been used during preparation. The date on the label of the container of formula should be checked by the food service personnel before purchasing and after formula has been stored for some time. Although past-dated formula may not be injurious to the child's health, the taste is often affected by prolonged storage. In most cases powdered formulas are available and can be stored in freezer or refrigerator to retain freshness longer than concentrated or ready-to-feed formulas, which may separate on freezing. A partially used bottle of formula should be discarded at the end of the day. When parents bring formula in bottles to the center, bottles should be refrigerated immediately by care givers, or a policy should be established to allow parents to place bottles in the refrigerator. Each bottle should be clearly labeled with the individual child's name.

Strained or Solid Foods.   The recommended practices for feeding infants were reviewed in Chapter 2. The basic requirements of the infant until 6 months and even longer can be met with iron-fortified formulas. Therefore, there appears to be no advantage in introducing solid foods during the first 6 months of life. In fact the substitution of cow's milk, especially skim milk, causes an excess of protein in the diet and seems to encourage the child to take additional calories from solid foods.

However, social customs favor earlier introduction of solid foods, and each center must establish guidelines and policies that consider these practices. Whenever solid foods are introduced, *do not overfeed.* A 6-month-old's persistent refusal of the spoon with food previously accepted is saying "stop!" to the care giver—discard the last 2 teaspoons of food (Figure 6–1).

Our recommended sequence for introduction of strained foods is

1. Infant cereal—iron-fortified, single-grain
2. Vegetables
3. Meats and fruits

In the past, studies have shown that sodium intakes during infancy rapidly increase when commercially prepared infant foods are added to the diets [2,3]. Most of the companies manufacturing baby foods have eliminated salt from their products. It appears that a taste for salt may be acquired by the preschool years and is not predetermined.

Some infants given home-prepared strained foods or table foods received more sodium than if commercial baby foods would have been used [4]. Care givers who prepare food for infants should add no salt or seasoning with sodium.

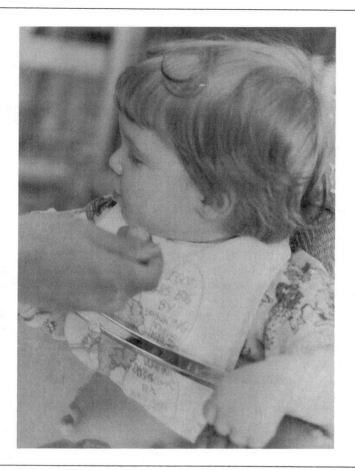

Figure 6-1
Child turns head as a signal to stop feeding.

Commercially Prepared Foods.   Purchasing commercially prepared foods may be advisable for infants at child-care centers with fewer than four to six children. To obtain the best nutrition for the least cost for the infant who is beginning to accept solid foods, the following guidelines should be followed.

Recommended	Not Recommended
Strained vegetables	Creamed vegetables
Strained meats	Vegetable and meat dinners
Single-grain infant cereal	High meat with vegetable
Plain yogurt	dinners

Fruits without added sugar or starch	Custards
	Fruit puddings and desserts
	with tapioca or cornstarch
	Cereal and fruit
	Fruit-flavored yogurt
	(flavored with preserves)
	Fruits with sugar and starch
	Cream cheese, cheese spread

Creamed vegetables include whole-milk solids, modified cornstarch, and in some instances sucrose. Therefore, their caloric density is greater than that of plain strained vegetables. The nutrition content of the combination dinners is lower than if the plain meats and plain vegetables were purchased and given to the child. Sucrose is added to prepared cereal with fruit that is sold in jars, although this product may be fortified with vitamin C and iron. Freeze-dried fruits and sugar are added to some iron-fortified infant cereals.

Approximately one third of some commercially prepared fruits contain modified tapioca starch; however, the name of the food may include this fact (for example, prunes and tapioca). In some cases food may have sugar and food starch added without any indication on the label ("strained bananas"). Puddings and desserts have a low nutrient density compared with milk, plain fruits, and vegetables and are not recommended for center use. Other foods such as yogurt and cottage cheese may be used; however, fruit-flavored yogurt should be avoided because substantial quantities of sugar have been used in the preparation of this product. Instead, use plain yogurt to which pureed or chopped fruit is added.

Center-prepared Foods. If possible, serve fresh or frozen foods that have been properly prepared in the kitchen of the infant center. They can be pureed or ground from fresh or frozen vegetables (no salt added) and fruits that have not been overcooked ("crunchy cooked"). These may be the same as those prepared for the preschool center. A crunchy cooked vegetable or fruit is one that requires chewing and cannot be mashed with the tongue. Leftovers that have been prepared for older children and allowed to stand in cooking water or on the table are not acceptable. Extra portions of freshly cooked food can be prepared (ground or pureed), placed in ice cube trays, and immediately frozen. One or two cubes per feeding will be sufficient for the young infant. Frozen cubes kept in a covered container can be thawed in the refrigerator overnight or cooked in the microwave oven before serving.

Hot spots in microwaved foods can cause serious burns. Foods or beverages heated by microwave may become hot even though the container or bottle feels cool. Stir or shake the fluid and test foods before offering to infants or young children.

By 6 to 7 months the infant will be ready to accept center-prepared foods with a texture other than pureed. The infants are developmentally ready to chew and will do so with their gums, even though teeth have not erupted. Any chopped or mashed bite-sized pieces of table foods, crunchy cooked, are acceptable. These

Dietary Intake

Amount Consumed	Food	Amount Consumed	Food
2 C	*Whole milk (1¼ C served at home)	1 oz	*Cornbread
¼ C	*White beans, cooked	4	Graham crackers
2 oz	Bologna	1 C	Wheat puffs, w/sugar coating
1½ oz	*Frankfurter	2 C	Kool-Aid fortified with vitamin C
½ C	Fried potato	½ C	Sweetened gelatin, plain
1 oz	Potato chips	—	*Carrot/celery strips
1 slice	White bread		

*Denotes foods served during center meal service.

Percent Energy Distribution: Fat 35%
Carbohydrate 53%
Protein 12%

```
TOTAL         NUTRIENT     %RDA   0%   20%   33% 40%   60% 66%   80%   100%
                                   I----I-----I---I-----I---I-----I-----I
1674.5KCAL ENERGY           99%   X X X X X X X X X X X X X X X X X X X X X X X X X
  50.1 GM  PROTEIN         167%   X X X X X X X X X X X X X X X X X X X X X X X X X X X X X X X X X X X X X X X X
2632.3 IU  VITAMIN A       105%   X X X X X X X X X X X X X X X X X X X X X X X X X X X X
 253.7 IU  VITAMIN D        63%   X X X X X X X X X X X X X X X X X
   4.8 IU  VITAMIN E        60%   X X X X X X X X X X X X X X X
  87.1 MG  VITAMIN C       194%   X X X X X X X X X X X X X X X X X X X X X X X X X X X X X X X X X X X X X X X X X X X
 208.3 MCG FOLACIN         104%   X X X X X X X X X X X X X X X X X X X X X X X X X X
  16.0 MG  NIACIN          145%   X X X X X X X X X X X X X X X X X X X X X X X X X X X X X X X X X X X
   1.8 MG  RIBOFLAVIN      183%   X X X X X X X X X X X X X X X X X X X X X X X X X X X X X X X X X X X X X X X X X
   1.4 MG  THIAMIN         154%   X X X X X X X X X X X X X X X X X X X X X X X X X X X X X X X X X X X X X
   1.2 MG  VITAMIN B6       88%   X X X X X X X X X X X X X X X X X X X X X X X
   2.3 MCG VITAMIN B12      90%   X X X X X X X X X X X X X X X X X X X X X X X X
 713.3 MG  CALCIUM          89%   X X X X X X X X X X X X X X X X X X X X X X X
1000.2 MG  PHOSPHORUS      125%   X X X X X X X X X X X X X X X X X X X X X X X X X X X X X X X
   8.3 MG  IRON             83%   X X X X X X X X X X X X X X X X X X X X X X
 126.5 MG  MAGNESIUM        63%   X X X X X X X X X X X X X X X X X
   5.5 MG  ZINC             55%   X X X X X X X X X X X X X X X
```

Figure 6-2
Dietary intake of preschool child with nutrient analysis (Source: NDDA Laboratory, Southern Illinois University at Carbondale.)

Table 6-2
Child Care Food Program required meal pattern

Foods	Ages 1 up to 3*	Ages 3 up to 6	Ages 6 up to 12
Breakfast			
Milk, fluid†	½ C	¾ C	1 C
Juice/vegetable(s) and/or fruits	¼ C	½ C	½ C
Bread/bread alternates‡			
Bread, cornbread, biscuits, rolls or	½ slice	½ slice	1 slice
Cereal:			
Cold, dry, or	¼ C or ⅓ oz	⅓ C or ½ oz	¾ C or 1 oz
Hot, cooked, or	¼ C	¼ C	½ C
Cooked pasta, noodle products, or rice	¼ C	¼ C	½ C
Snack			
(Select 2 out of 4 Components)			
Milk, fluid†	½ C	½ C	1 C
Meat/meat alternates§			
Lean meat, poultry, fish‖ or	½ oz	½ oz	1 oz
Cheese or	½ oz	½ oz	1 oz
Egg, large, or	½ egg	½ egg	1 egg
Cooked dry beans or peas or	⅛ C	⅛ C	¼ C
Peanut butter, soynut butter, other nut or seed butters or	1 tbsp	1 tbsp	2 tbsp
Peanuts, soynuts, tree nuts, or seeds	½ oz	½ oz	1 oz
Juice/vegetable(s) and/or fruit#	½ C	½ C	¾ C

Bread/bread alternates‡			
Bread, cornbread, biscuits, rolls or	½ slice	½ slice	1 slice
Cereal:			
Cold, dry, or	¼ C or ⅓ oz	⅓ C or ½ oz	¾ C or 1 oz
Hot, cooked, or	¼ C	¼ C	½ C
Cooked pasta, noodle products, or rice	¼ C	¼ C	½ C

Lunch/Supper

Milk, fluid, served as beverage	½ C	¾ C	1 C
Meat/meat alternates§			
Meat, poultry, fish‖ or	1 oz	1½ oz	2 oz
Cheese or	1 oz	1½ oz	2 oz
Egg, large, or	1	1	1
Cooked dry beans or peas or	¼ C	⅜ C	½ C
Peanut butter, soynut butter, other nut or seed butters or	2 tbsp	3 tbsp	4 tbsp
Peanuts, soynuts, tree nuts, or seeds**	½ oz = 50%	¾ oz = 50%	1 oz = 50%
Juice/vegetable(s) and/or fruits‡‡	¼ C total	½ C total	¾ C total
Bread/bread alternates‡			
Bread, cornbread, biscuits, rolls or	½ slice	½ slice	1 slice
Cooked pasta, noodle products, or rice	¼ C	¼ C	½ C

*For required serving amounts for infants up to age 1 year, refer to program regulations.

†Fluid milk should be used as a beverage, on cereal, or in part for each purpose.

‡Or an equivalent serving of an acceptable bread, pasta, or noodle product. Cereals must be whole grain, enriched, or fortified.

§Or an equivalent quantity of any combination of foods listed under meat/meat alternates.

‖Cooked lean meat without bone, breading, or skin.

#Juice may not be served when milk is served as the only other component.

**Tree nuts and seeds, except acorns, chestnuts, and coconuts, may be used as meat alternates. Nuts and seeds may supply no more than half of the meat alternate requirement at lunch/supper. Nuts and seeds must be combined with another meat/meat alternate. For purposes of determining combinations, 1 ounce of nuts or seeds is equal to 1 ounce of cooked lean meat, poultry, or fish.

‡‡Serve two or more kinds of vegetable(s) and/or fruit(s) or a combination of both. Full-strength vegetable or fruit juice may be counted to meet not more than one half of this requirement.

foods should not contain seasonings or additional sugar and salt. Foods that are hard and can become lodged in the throat (such as raw celery, nuts, and popcorn) should be avoided.

The Toddler and Preschooler

The methods for feeding the toddler versus the preschooler are different, as discussed in Chapters 3 and 4. Interaction among children is limited at the toddler stage; however, this does not preclude the use of conversation about foods and eating. The amount of foods is generally smaller and served more frequently for the toddler as compared with the preschooler. Young children, 12 to 20 months, may still be fed individually, but shortly after age 2 years, they like and can learn from other children in the center. By 30 months, they can be using tablespoons to take food from serving bowls.

Chapters 3 through 5 include the recommended food patterns to meet children's daily nutritional needs. Frequent use of legumes and green vegetables contributes significantly to specific nutrients often difficult to acquire in the diet. Whole-grain cereals have been included, while "dessert" (something sweet at the end of the meal) is a forgotten word. Children are allowed to take a serving of all the menu items at the start of the meal. No food is withheld at the beginning of a meal.

Figure 6–2 shows the actual foods eaten by a 4-year-old during the day, including foods eaten at the center. The bar graph shows the nutrient composition of the foods for the entire day. The child attended a half-day program, and the menu is like that served in many centers.

Over 80% of the iron allowance was met by serving fortified cereal, bread, meat, and beans. The energy values are not excessive and the caloric distribution is close to that recommended, although fat intake is higher than 30%. Although the child ate a large quantity of food, no fresh vegetables or fruits were eaten. The vitamin C came primarily from gelatin and Kool-Aid, which were fortified.

The preschool center often serves lunch and a snack or breakfast. The food pattern requirements established by the USDA for the Child Care Food Program for children 1 to 12 years old are included in Table 6–2. Programs that qualify can receive reimbursement for serving meals that follow the approved USDA patterns. See Appendix VII for instructions on how to apply for the USDA Child Care Food Program.

PLANNING MENUS WITH STAFF

Menus are often planned to include foods that children like and will eat. This process seems logical because it reduces food waste and appears to be most cost-effective. However, this approach is based on the fact that food service personnel are in charge of planning as well as serving foods, and the teacher or care

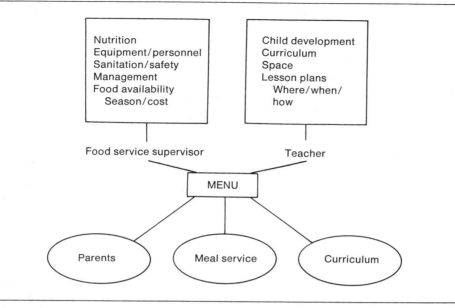

Figure 6-3
Components for the successful implementation of a menu

giver has little, if any, responsibility for these activities. This concept has its roots in hotel and restaurant food service, where pleasing the palate is cost-effective regardless of nutrient content.* Children eat the foods they know, but new or less familiar foods may be viewed with suspicion or rejected. Therefore, a fast food restaurant moving into an elementary school cafeteria is a success in decreasing plate waste but may provide few food choices.

The appearance of fast food establishments with limited variety in schools hinders the objective of helping children consume a wide variety of foods. As stressed throughout, childhood is the best time to develop food habits and favorable attitudes toward many different foods. The menu-planning system that involves teachers and food service personnel can accomplish this goal.

Menus are usually viewed as the foundation of food service operation. The *process* of using an educational approach to develop a center's menu requires the food service personnel and the teacher to coordinate activities. The menus still must contain the basic foods and consider the constraints of the food service facility, but, in addition, the menu will be used as a tool for learning (Figure 6-3). The day's menu, *the product,* is a written translation of the general nutrient requirements discussed previously into a description of specific foods (chicken,

*There is currently an effort to encourage all restaurants and fast food establishments to display the nutrient content of food served along with menu items.

greens, and so on). The proper menu has foods with the appropriate combinations of taste, texture, and color. Producing a menu that meets the child's requirements and the constraints of the food service facility takes management skills.

Food Service Supervisor's Contribution

As indicated in Figure 6–3 the nutrition consultant and food service personnel come to the menu-planning session with a set of nutritional guidelines or needs of children. In addition, there are generally accepted patterns of foods to be included in the menu, such as the meat or alternate, vegetable, bread, fruit, and milk.

Other considerations also affect which foods are prepared and served and how. The equipment and personnel may limit the number and kinds of food items. Baked potatoes and meat loaf may not be served together, since the oven may not be large enough to prepare both at the same time. Likewise, the number of products to be prepared in the preschool kitchen may be limited by personnel. Some foods may need to be prepared from mixes. Most food service personnel can solve these problems if freezer and refrigerator space is available. For example, freshly baked hot rolls, meat loaf, fresh green beans, and salad may be prepared by first selecting a recipe for refrigerator rolls and preparing the rolls for storage in the freezer or refrigerator or by using a basic mix. Ingredients for meat loaf can be combined and frozen early in the week or refrigerated the night before. If fresh green beans are available, they must be prepared on the day of service but could be washed, stemmed, and placed in plastic bags the day before. The salad could then be prepared while other foods are cooking.

Preparing mashed potatoes for 30 to 50 children requires special equipment, and instant potatoes may be the only solution. Baked ham, baked sweet potatoes, and hot rolls require excessive oven space. Fruited gelatin (unsweetened gelatin prepared with fruit juice), tossed salad, and cold meat and cheese platters may require too much refrigerator space. Fruited gelatin is impractical to serve on Monday in a Monday-to-Friday center, since it must be prepared on Friday and allowed to stand over the 2-day weekend.

Availability of foods may change the menu. Availability depends on locality, season, budget, and inventory (which foods are on hand). Most of these factors are interrelated. The foods in season are usually available in your locality and fit within the budgetary constraints. However, in some areas many fresh foods, especially fruits and vegetables, are available all year. Table 6–3 shows the monthly availability of fresh vegetables and fruits.

Some programs receive commodity foods under the USDA Commodity Food Program, and these foods must be taken into consideration in planning menus. The foods on hand should be rotated regularly to ensure that foods served are fresh and of the highest quality.

Some programs serve food prepared in one site and transported to another. Some foods cannot maintain their quality with this treatment, no matter how they are handled. It is best if some preparation can be done on-site. Microwave ovens have become popular for child-care centers that have foods prepared in locations other than the centers.

The use of various types of meal services may also be limited by equipment and personnel. Large numbers of bag lunches may be difficult to prepare. If the center has not purchased serving equipment for family-style meal service, this service may be impossible. However, to use the concepts discussed in this text and to ensure the child's participation, family-style meal service is recommended.

Teacher's Contribution

The teacher brings to the menu-planning session knowledge of the educational needs of children. Available space, equipment, and location will limit some activities; for example, inner-city schools find it difficult to pick apples from nearby orchards, whereas rural preschoolers cannot walk to the grocery or nearby parks.

The food service personnel can suggest various options for involving children in food preparation, service, and cleanup, but the teacher or care giver is the director of the learning activities. Without the teacher's cooperation the food service will not be used effectively to help children learn about food.

The teacher may use the menu as a tool to learning through a specific food service style, for example, family (formal, informal), buffet, cafeteria, bag lunch, and picnic. A particular food item may also be used in conjunction with a learning resource center in the classroom. A new food or preparation method with which the child is becoming familiar may be used along with a science activity (see Chapter 8).

When food service personnel are planning menus, a list of foods and preparation methods can be made available to the teacher. The teachers can circle or indicate which food items or preparation methods are new for the child and should be introduced. Several lists of foods can easily be made available for individual centers. A checklist of various foods and preparation methods is included in Table 6–4.

STYLES OF FOOD SERVICE

Children love variety. Therefore, weather permitting, teachers may plan some meals outside, picnic style. Inside, a variety of settings are available (for instance, a Christmas buffet for older preschoolers). Food service styles include family, buffet, cafeteria, picnic, and bag lunch.

In *family style* food service, all children sit at a table, which has been prepared with individual plates and flatware. Food is placed on the table in serving bowls and is passed. Children help themselves from serving bowls with the assistance of the teacher. A *modified family style* may be used with a group of children new to the center. Only one or two items would be placed in serving

Table 6-3
Monthly availability of fresh vegetables and fruits

Commodity	Jan	Feb	March	April	May	June	July	Aug	Sept	Oct	Nov	Dec
Apples	|*												
Apricots							†		‡				
Asparagus													
Avocados													
Bananas													
Beans, green or wax													
Beets													
Berries, miscellaneous§													
Blueberries													
Broccoli													
Brussels sprouts													
Cabbage													
Cantaloupe													
Carrots													
Cauliflower													
Celery													
Cherries													
Chinese cabbage													
Corn													
Cranberries													
Cucumber													
Eggplant													
Escarole-endive-chicory													
Grapefruit													
Grapes													
Greens													
Honeydew melon													
Lemons													
Lettuce, head, leaf, romaine													
Limes													

Mangoes
Mushrooms
Nectarines
Okra
Onions, green
Onions, mature
Oranges
Parsley and herbs
Parsnips
Peaches
Pears
Peas, green
Peppers, green
Pineapples
Plums
Potatoes, white
Pumpkins
Radishes
Rhubarb
Spinach
Squash, summer, winter
Strawberries
Sweet potatoes
Tangerines
Tomatoes
Turnips (rutabagas)
Watermelons

Source: Modified from U.S. Department of Agriculture Food and Nutrition Service: Food purchasing pointer for school food service, Program Aid No. 1160, Washington, DC, Aug. 1977, U.S. Government Printing Office.

* ——— 6% to 23% of the total annual supply.

† over 43% of the total annual supply.

‡ 24% to 42% of the total annual supply.

§ Berries, miscellaneous, refers mostly to blackberries, dewberries, and raspberries.

Table 6-4
Checklist of foods and preparation methods for menu planning

Vegetables

Beans
  Fresh lima beans
    Raw
    Buttered
    Cooked with bacon or ham
    With tomatoes
  Snap beans
    Raw
    With bacon or salt pork
    With crisp bacon chips
    With cream sauce
    With new potatoes
    With tomatoes
    With carrot circles
    Salad
Beets
  Buttered
  Harvard
  Cold sliced
  And lettuce salad
Broccoli
  Raw
  Buttered
  With lemon sauce
  With cheese sauce
  With cream sauce
Cabbage*
  With carrots, cooked
  Buttered
  Cole slaw
  Creamed
  In gelatin
  Raw wedge
  Salad with fruit or other
    vegetables
  With corned beef
  Sauerkraut
Carrots
  Raw sticks, curls, wheels
  Baked
  Cooked with celery
  Cooked with peas
  Creamed
  Glazed
  In gelatin (with fruit juice)
  Mashed
  Scalloped

And cabbage slaw
And raisin salad
Cauliflower
  Raw
  With cheese sauce
  Buttered
  Cream sauce
  With peas
Celery
  Raw sticks
  Braised
  Buttered
  With carrots, cooked
Corn
  On ear
  Buttered
  Creamed
  With lima beans
  Popped
Cucumber
  Raw slices
  In salads
Eggplant
  Baked
  Scalloped
  With tomatoes
Green peas
  Buttered
  Creamed
  Scalloped
  With onion
  With bacon or ham
  Raw
Green pea pods (snow peas)
  Raw
  Sauteed
  Buttered
Lettuce
  Raw
  Shredded
  Wilted
  Combination salad
  Wedges
  Cooked
  Fried
  Creamed

Okra
  Raw
  Boiled
  Buttered
  Stewed with tomato
Onions, green, yellow, white dry
  Fried
  Raw
  Boiled with peas
  Salad
Parsnips
  Buttered
  Browned
  Raw strips
Potato (white)
  Raw
  With cheese sauce
  Baked
  Boiled and sprinkled with
    parsley and butter
  Browned in oven
  Creamed
  Pancakes
  Mashed
  Salad
  Scalloped
  Peeled baked
  Hash browns
  French fries
Pumpkin
  Baked
  Mashed
  Cooked whole—cut lid and
    remove seeds and roast
Rutabagas
  Raw
  Cubes
  Mashed
  Raw strips
Spinach/other greens
  Buttered
  Creamed
  Raw leaf
  With celery
  With hard-cooked eggs
  With cheese sauce
  With onions and bacon

*Strong-flavored vegetables taste best when cooked in milk.

Table 6-4
continued

Squash (summer)†
  Raw
  Buttered
  With tomato
  Seasoned with bacon and/
    or onion
  Baked
Squash (winter)†
  Raw sticks, curls, wheels
  Baked
  Mashed
  Cooked in shell
  Roast seeds

Apple
  Applesauce
  Applesauce with cinnamon
    hearts or raisins
  Baked
  Brown Betty
  Fresh wedge
  Pudding
  Snow
  Tapioca
  And raisin salad
  Fried
Apricot
  In fruit cup
  Plain
  Stewed dry fruit
  Whip
  With cheese
Banana
  Baked
  In fruit cup
  In gelatin
  In orange juice
  Pudding
  Sliced
  Snow
  Whole or half
  With milk
  Fried
Berries
  Plain

Sweet potato
  Baked
  Mashed
  Scalloped with apple
  With marshmallows (rarely)
  Fried
  Buttered
Tomato
  Baked
  Broiled
  Raw wedge
  Juice
  Scalloped

Fruits

  With milk
Cantaloupe
  Balls
  In fruit cup
  Sliced
Cherries
  Plain
  Pudding
Grapefruit
  Juice
  Salad
  Sections
Grapes (seedless)
  In gelatin
  Plain
Melons
  Balls
  Cubes
  Fruit cup
  Sliced
Orange
  Betty
  Custard
  Juice
  Sections
  Wedges
  Wheel
Peach
  In gelatin
  Plain—sliced, half
  Salad

Stewed
Cold canned
Sliced
And okra
And cucumber salad
And lettuce salad
Aspic
Turnips
  Buttered
  Mashed
  Scalloped
  Raw strips

  Sauce
  Snow
  Stewed dry fruit
  Tapioca
Pear
  Plain
  Stewed dry fruit
  Whip
  With cheese
  Sauce
  With other fruit
  Fried
Pineapple
  Crushed
  Cubes, plain
  In gelatin (cooked)‡
  With cabbage or carrot
Plum
  Plain
Prunes
  Custard
  Snow
  Stewed
  Whipped
  With applesauce
Pumpkin
  See vegetables
Raisins
  In bread or rice pudding
  Plain
  Stewed
  In salad

---

†Summer squash is white or very light yellow inside; winter squash is dark yellow inside.   *(continued)*

‡Gelatin will not become firm if fresh rather than cooked pineapple is used.

Table 6-4
continued

Meat

Beef
  American chop suey
  Beef-noodle casserole
  Beef and liver loaf
  Ground beef patty
  Roast
  Hot beef sandwich with
    gravy
  Beef stew with vegetables
  Cold sliced beef
  Meat balls and spaghetti
  Meat balls and vegetable
    casserole
  Beef hash

Ground beef and macaroni
  casserole
Cold sliced beef sandwich
Meat sauce and spaghetti
Corned beef with cabbage
Beef stew with brown gravy
  over rice
Beef stew with red gravy
  over noodles
Sloppy Joe
Meat loaf with tomato gravy
Pork
  Chop suey
  Creamed ham and peas on
    toast

Ham salad
Ham and sweet potato
  casserole
Lean pork steak
Scalloped ham and potato
Sliced baked ham
Ham sandwich
Pork roast
Lamb
  Lamb patty
  Lamb meat loaf
  Lamb stew
  Roast leg of lamb
  Scalloped lamb

Poultry and Fish

Poultry
  Stewed chicken with rice
  Chicken and dumplings
  Chicken with noodles
  Chicken with vegetables
  Creamed chicken
  Smothered chicken
  Baked chicken
  Fried chicken

Chicken salad
Baked turkey
Turkey hash
Hot turkey sandwich with
  gravy
Cold sliced turkey sandwich
Turkey salad
Turkey supreme
Fish
  Baked fish fillet with creole

Creamed fish with celery
  and peas
Salmon loaf
Tuna fish salad
Tuna-noodle casserole
Tuna boats
Salmon patty
Baked fish sticks
Fish flake balls

Other Meats

Liver
  Baked
  Braised, plain
  Braised, tomato sauce
  Loaf

Strips
With gravy
Smothered with onions
Rice dressing with giblets

Kidney
  Baked
  Chopped
  Sauteed with onions

Meat Alternates

Cheese
  American cheese cubes or
    wedges
  Cheese and noodle or
    macaroni
  Cheese, tomato, and
    macaroni
  Cheeseburger
  Cheese toast
  Cheese and vegetable
    casserole

Cottage cheese with fruit
American cheese sandwich
Grilled cheese sandwich
Dried beans, peas, and
  peanut butter
Baked beans with ham
  seasoning
Bean, rice, tomato, and
  cheese casserole
Bean soup with ham

Red beans with ham
Lima beans with ham
Lima beans and cheese
  casserole
Lima beans with tomato,
  celery, and wieners
Pinto beans and wiener
  rings
Black-eyed peas with
  ham

Table 6-4

continued

Egg
  Baked egg and cheese
  Baked egg and vegetable
  Creamed egg and spinach

Egg à la king
Goldenrod eggs
Hard-cooked eggs in tomato
  sauce

Scrambled eggs
Scrambled eggs with cheese
Stuffed deviled eggs
Tofu§

Breads, Sandwiches, and Cereals

Bread
  Plain
    Whole wheat
    Raisin
    Rye
    Biscuit
    Corn bread (pan or sticks)
    Corn spoon bread
  Hot
    Biscuits
    Corn bread
    Muffins
    Rolls
  Shapes
    Strips
    Squares
    Triangles
    Circles
    Animals
  Sandwiches
    Butter

Cheese
Meat
Peanut butter
Vegetable
  Grated carrots and
    cabbage
  Sliced tomato/green
    pepper
Cream cheese

Macaroni
  Buttered
  Bouillon
  Plain
  Salad
  With cheese
  With tomato sauce
  See beef list

Noodles
  Buttered
  Plain

With sauce
See meats
Rice (brown)
  Buttered
  Bouillon
  Pudding
  With raisins
  With cheese
  With chicken
Grits
  Buttered
  With ham
  With cheese
  Baked
Crackers
  Graham
  Whole grain
  With peanut butter
  With cheese
  With cream cheese

Other Foods (Use Occasionally)

Cake (using whole-grain flour)
  Gingerbread
  Plain cake with fruits
Cookie (with whole-grain
    cereal)
  Gingersnap
  Oatmeal/raisin
  Peanut butter

Plain vanilla
Molasses
Gelatin (unsweetened)
  Plain, add fruit juice
  Whipped, add fruit juice
  With fruit
Pudding
  Cornstarch

Vanilla with fruit
Squash or pumpkin
Custard
  Bread pudding with raisins
  Egg
  Rice
Tapioca
  With raisins

§Not a replacement for protein source in the Child Care Food Program.

bowls, and the teacher would place other foods on the plates. This method is used only until the children are familiar with this style of meal service.

Food, flatware, and plates are placed on the serving table in a *buffet style* presentation. The child takes a plate, flatware, and food from the table with or without assistance from adults, but foods are not "dished up" for the child. This style may be used with an experienced group of preschoolers to add variety.

The younger children's flatware may be placed at the table, and the child takes only a plate on which food is placed from the buffet table.

In cafeteria style service food, flatware, and plates are placed on a serving tray. An adult places foods on the child's plate or tray. One or more items may be selected by the child. Portion sizes are usually set by the server. However, children may be asked how much they can eat. This service is not recommended for preschoolers.

No formal definition exists for *picnic style* meal service, except that the meal is usually eaten at a picnic table or on the ground out-of-doors. This style has been used indoors where playgrounds or parks have not been available or where the weather has not cooperated. Children love picnics! Foods should be easy to prepare and carry. One or more of the foods may be prepared outside over an open fire; however, outdoor cooking is not necessary for a successful picnic. Paper plates, cups, and plastic utensils may be used. Remember, infants as well as preschoolers like to eat outside.

For the *bag lunch*, easy-to-prepare foods are packed in a bag. A spoon may be added for eating some foods but most foods should be finger foods. This meal service is therefore limited to children who can eat finger foods. Bag lunches can be used for field trips. All the nutrients in a regular lunch can be supplied through the bag lunch—candy bars, potato chips, and sweet cakes do not have to be included. A menu may include peanut butter or cheese sandwich on whole-wheat bread, raw vegetables and fruit, and milk. Remember, providing liquids for children in hot weather is important.

PLANNING PROCEDURE

The menu should include the foods that

1. Provide the recommended nutritional components
2. Satisfy the curriculum needs
3. Are prepared and served successfully with the available resources
4. Are eaten by the children

Cycle Menus

Planning menus well in advance is a key to good management. *Cycle menus* are a series of carefully planned menus, used for a definite period of time and then repeated. They are planned for an odd number of days not divisible by five, such as 11, 13, 21, or 29 days, to ensure that a menu is not repeated on the same day in consecutive weeks.

Using cycle menus reduces the time required for menu planning. After the initial cycle has been completed, the menu can be changed to account for special occasions such as holidays and vacations. To make a cycle menu successful, at least three to four new menus should be added in the subsequent cycle. This ensures that meals do not become monotonous or boring. In addition, with a cy-

SAMPLE FORMAT:
For Child Care Center
Discretionary Use

Date _____

FOOD PRODUCTION RECORD

Day (Circle)   M   T   W   Th   F

Food Item	Recipe Source	Number of Units Used	Unit Size	Portions Served				Leftovers/Notes
				1-3 years	3-6 years	6-12 years	Adults	
LUNCH								

_____
Signature of Designated Person

Figure 6–4 Food production record
(Source: Illinois State Board of Education, Department of Child Nutrition, Springfield, IL, 1987, The Board.)

WEEKLY MENU PLANNING WORK SHEET

Week of _____

Requirements					
BREAKFAST Milk, fluid Juice or fruit or vegetable Bread or bread alternate (including cereal)					
A.M. SNACK *(Select two of these four components)* Milk, fluid Juice or fruit or vegetable Bread or bread alternate (including cereal) Meat or meat alternate					
LUNCH Milk, fluid Meat or meat alternate Vegetables and/or fruits (two or more) Bread or bread alternate					
P.M. SNACK *(Select two of these four components)* Milk, fluid Juice or fruit or vegetable Bread or bread alternate (including cereal) Meat or meat alternate					
SUPPER Milk, fluid Meat or meat alternate Vegetables and/or fruits (two or more) Bread or bread alternate					

Figure 6-5

Menu planning worksheet [Source: Illinois State Board of Education, Department of Child Nutrition: Child Care Food Program—a guide to crediting foods, Springfield, IL, 1987, The Board.)

cle menu, food preparation procedures can be standardized and costs can be identified and controlled.

Teacher activities can be easily varied from the first 3- or 4-week cycle to the second time the cycle is used. A menu can be thought of as a road map, always allowing opportunities to change direction. The menu should be flexible for side trips, but the food service supervisor and teacher should be conscientious enough not to get seriously sidetracked into a poor nutritional program.

Menu Plans

Several forms will assist the food service manager and the teacher in the preparation of menus. Figures 6–4 and 6–5 can assist you in daily and weekly menu planning. The work sheet (Figure 6–5) is for three meals and two snacks, which, together, should provide foods meeting 100% of the RDA. This form is useful if the center serves more than one meal. The production record (Figure 6–4) serves to help make sure all foods can be produced with the staff and provides a record for the next time the menu is served.

Try preparing a menu using the forms in this book. Referring once more to the requirements in Table 6–2 for the young child, begin to fill out at least one weekly menu planning work sheet. Although no rule dictates how the menu should be planned, food service planners usually start with the meat, meat alternate, or protein foods and add other components in order to get a wide variety. You could begin with any food component. Table 6–4 gives a variety of foods and preparation methods to assist in planning.

At least two fruits and/or vegetables for lunch and dinner (main meals) should be chosen. One fruit or vegetable should be raw if possible. Table 6–5 lists many fruits and vegetables high in vitamins A and C. Remember that these foods are nutrient-dense sources of many vitamins and minerals.

CHILD CARE FOOD PROGRAM GUIDELINES—1 YEAR AND OLDER

There is often confusion about which foods are included under the Child Care Food Program guidelines. Table 6–6 presents specific foods for the older child that do not meet the Child Care Food Program requirements. Frequent, if not daily, use of whole-grain cereals and meat alternates are recommended to meet the RDA for the child. Preparation with limited quantities of sugar and fat helps to control excessive calories in the diet while encouraging the young child to eat other more nutrient-dense foods.

Child Nutrition Labeling

To assist in purchasing foods that meet meal pattern requirements, some foods are identified with a Child Nutrition (CN) label. Child Nutrition labeling is a voluntary federal labeling program that provides a warranty for CN-labeled products.

Table 6-5
Fruit and vegetable list

Rich in Carotene (vitamin A value)	Rich in Vitamin C (ascorbic acid) (serve every day)	Other Fruits and Vegetables
Good Sources	*Good Sources*	Fruits
Fruits	Fruits	Apples
Apricots	Grapefruit and juice	Applesauce
Cantaloupe*	Grapefruit-orange juice	Avocados
Mangoes*	Guavas	Bananas
Papayas*	Kumquats	Berries
Purple plums (canned)	Mangoes†	Cranberries
Vegetables	Oranges and juice	Cranberry sauce
Beet greens	Papayas†	Dates
Broccoli*	Strawberries	Figs
Carrots	Tangerines and juice	Fruit cocktail
Chard, Swiss	Vegetables	Grapes
Chicory greens	Broccoli†	Olives
Collards*	Brussels sprouts	Peaches (canned)
Cress, garden*	Cauliflower	Pears
Dandelion greens*	Collards†	Persimmons
Kale*	Cress, garden†	Pineapple
Mixed vegetables (frozen)	Kale†	Plums
Mustard greens*	Kohlrabi	Raisins
Peas and carrots (frozen)	Mustard greens†	Rhubarb
Peppers, sweet, red*	Peppers, sweet, red and green†	Watermelon
Pumpkin		Vegetables
Spinach*	*Fair Sources*	Bean sprouts
Squash, winter	Fruits	Beans, green or wax
Sweet potatoes*	Cantaloupe†	Beans, lima, green
Turnip greens*	Honeydew melon	Beets
Fair Sources	Raspberries, red	Celery
Fruits	Tangelos and juice	Chinese cabbage
Cherries, red, sour	Vegetables	Corn
Nectarines	Asparagus†	Cucumbers
Peaches (except canned)	Cabbage	Eggplant
Prunes	Dandelion greens†	Lettuce
Vegetables	Okra	Mushrooms
Asparagus, green*	Potatoes (cooked in skins)	Onions
Endive, curly	Rutabagas	Parsley
Escarole, curly	Sauerkraut	Parsnips
Tomatoes*	Spinach†	Peas, green, immature
Tomato juice, paste, or puree*	Sweet potatoes†	Pimientos
Vegetable juice cocktail	Tomatoes, tomato juice, paste, or puree†	Potatoes (not cooked in skins)
	Turnip greens†	Radishes
	Turnips	Squash, summer
		Watercress

*Also valuable for vitamin C.

†Also valuable for carotene.

Table 6-6
Foods that do not meet Child Care Food Program requirements

Milk Components	*Jams*	*Imitation cheese*
Evaporated milk	Jellies	Nut or seed meal or flour
Nonfat dry milk	Dried vegetables for seasoning	Commercial packaged
Cocoa mix (added to water)	Fruit breads (pumpkin,	macaroni and cheese*
Pudding, custard	banana, carrot, and	Pot pies (store bought)*
Ice cream, sherbet	zucchini)	Canned ravioli*
Yogurt	Cranberry juice cocktail	Canned spaghetti*
Half and half	Coconut	
Sour cream		*Miscellaneous Foods*
Whipping cream	*Bread Component*	Soda pop
Cream cheese	Hominy	Tea
Eggnog	Popcorn, caramel corn	Marshmallows
Powdered drinks	Cake, snack cakes	Catsup
	Dessert pie crust	Pickle relish
Fruit/Vegetable Component	Hard pretzels	Mustard
Fruit nectar	Shaped snack chips	Gelatin
Fruit drinks or punch	Brownies	Candy
Garnishes, e.g., pickles,	Shoestring potatoes	Honey
parsley, that amount to less		Sour cream
than ⅛ C	*Meat/Meat Alternate Component*	Syrup
Potato chips, corn chips, and	Bacon	Butter
similar packaged snacks	Cream cheese	Margarine
Pickle relish	Tofu	Salad dressing
Lemonade	Parmesan cheese, if used as	Yeast
	garnish	

*These foods cannot be used unless the label obtained by the center indicates Child Nutrition (CN) or it includes a manufacturer's statement of composition.

A CN label allows manufacturers to clearly state the contribution of a product toward the meal pattern requirements while protecting the consumer from exaggerated claims about a product. However, it does not provide any assurance of product quality.

Products eligible for CN labels include main dish products that contribute significantly to the meat/meat alternate component of the meal pattern requirements and juice and juice drink products that contain at least 50 percent full-strength juice by volume.

A facsimile of a CN label is presented in Figure 6–6. Note the distinct border of the CN logo, the meal pattern contribution statement, the 6-digit product identification number, the USDA/FNS authorization, and the month and year of approval.

Questions Frequently Asked

The answers to the following questions were supplied by the Illinois State Board of Education, Department of Child Nutrition.

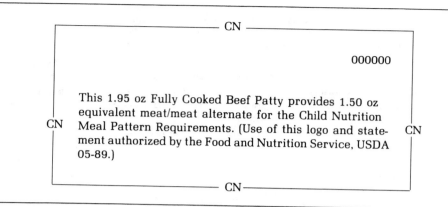

Figure 6–6
Facsimile Child Nutrition Label

Milk Component

1. Which types of milk can be served to meet the Child Care Food Program regulations?
   The milk must be a pasteurized fresh fluid product that is served as a beverage, poured over cereal, or used partly for each purpose. Reconstituted milk from a dry powder or canned milk cannot be used to meet the milk requirement. Likewise, a cocoa mix made from dried milk powder or canned milk products will not count toward the milk requirement. At breakfast milk may be used on cereal, as a beverage, or as a beverage and on cereal. At lunch and supper you must serve milk as a beverage.

2. Can the milk used in preparation of custards, puddings, and ice cream be counted toward the milk requirement?
   No. The milk must be served as a beverage, poured over cereal, or used partly for each purpose.

3. Can yogurt be used to meet the milk or meat requirement?
   Under current Child Care Food Program regulations, yogurt is an extra food and cannot be used to meet basic meal pattern requirements, but it can be used as a meat alternate for a supplement only.

4. Can imitation milk products be used to meet the milk requirement?
   No. Imitation milk products do not meet the definition of fluid milk and cannot receive credit toward the meal pattern requirement. The imitation milk products are made from the following ingredients: whey, corn syrup solids, coconut oil, sodium caseinate, and nonfat milk. In addition, there may be added artificial colors, sugar, and gum.

5. Can a milkshake be served to meet the milk requirement?
   Yes. If it contains 8 fluid ounces of milk for 6- to 12-year-old; 6 fluid ounces for 3- to 6-year-old and 4 fluid ounces for 1- to 3-year-old.

6. Is fluid milk mixed with grape juice, orange juice, and other juices creditable?

   Yes. The milk-juice mixture is creditable in both the milk and fruit/vegetable categories when served for breakfast, lunch, or supper if the required amount of milk plus the required amount of fruit juice is served.

7. If I use fluid milk, can hot chocolate or cocoa be served to meet the milk requirement?

   Yes. When made with fluid milk, this beverage is creditable. Flavored hot chocolate mixes reconstituted with water are not creditable.

Bread and Bread Alternate Component

The following criteria must be met for food items to be creditable as bread or bread alternates, whether purchased or prepared in the home or center:

- The item must contain whole-grain and/or enriched flour and/or meal as the primary ingredient(s) by weight as specified on the label or according to the recipe, or must be enriched in preparation or processing and labeled "enriched." If a cereal is fortified, the label must indicate it is fortified.
- The item must be provided in quantities specified in the Child Care Food Program regulations.
- The item must serve the customary function of bread in a meal. For lunch or supper, the item must be served as an accompaniment to, or a recognizable integral part of, the main dish (and not merely as an ingredient).
- The item must meet minimum weight standards. (See the bread and bread alternates weight table at the end of this section.)

1. Can cake, cookies, and snack-type foods be used at lunch?

   No. Desserts or snack-type foods such as cakes, cookies, and pie cannot be used for the bread requirement at lunch and supper.

2. If spaghetti with meat sauce is served, must bread be served in addition?

   If sufficient quantities of enriched spaghetti are served, an additional slice of bread is not needed. Rice, pasta, or other cereal products can be served in combination with bread or other bread alternates to meet the minimum bread requirement (for example, ¼ cup rice and ½ slice bread).

3. Can glorified rice and bread or rice pudding be credited as a bread or bread alternate?

   At lunch or supper, bread or rice pudding cannot be used to meet the bread requirements, because it is not served as an accompaniment or integral part of the main dish. However, for supplements, bread or rice pudding can be used to meet the bread component if there is at least ¼ cup cooked rice or approximately ½ slice of bread per serving.

4. Can Rice Krispies bars or similar cereal bar products be credited toward the bread or bread alternate at supplement?

   Rice Krispies bars or similar bars made from a cereal product may be credited as an acceptable bread/bread alternate for breakfast and snacks if the cereal is whole grain or enriched and if the amount of cereal can be measured to ⅓ cup (volume) or ½ ounce (weight), whichever is less per one half serving. Because these have a high sugar content, they should be served no more than twice per week.

5. Can cinnamon rolls and quick breads be credited as a bread alternate?
Yes. Center-made or homemade cinnamon rolls made with whole-grain or enriched flour as the predominant ingredient by weight can meet the requirements for breakfast, snack, lunch, and supper, since these rolls are traditionally served as bread.

6. Can Danish pastries, Long Johns, and rich sweet rolls be used at breakfast or at supplements?
No. Because the predominant ingredient by weight is generally not enriched flour, they cannot be used as a bread item.

7. Can the breading in corn dogs be counted as part of the bread requirement?
Yes. The breading can be counted if it contains enriched or whole-grain cornmeal and flour. The breading can be credited in the following manner:
   a. Multiply the weight of the corn dog (meat plus breading) by 28.35 g to determine the weight of the product in grams.
   b. Multiply by 35% to determine the weight of breading.
   c. Divide by 25 g to determine the number of bread equivalents. For example:

   3-ounce corn dog
   $3 \times 28.35 \text{ g} = 85.05 \text{ g}$ for total weight of product
   $85.05 \text{ g} \times 0.35 = 29.77 \text{ g}$ of breading
   29.77 divided by 25 g = 1.19 bread servings

Or remove the cooked batter from a serving and weigh. If the weight is in ounces, multiply by 28.35 to convert to grams. Divide this number by 25 g to determine the number of bread credits.

   2-ounce corn dog will provide approximately ¾ bread serving
   3-ounce corn dog will provide approximately 1 bread serving
   4-ounce corn dog will provide approximately 1½ bread servings

8. Can cookies and animal crackers be used as a snack to meet the bread alternate?
Yes. Cookies may be used as an acceptable bread alternate when the following criteria have been met:
   a. Whole-grain or enriched meal or flour must be the predominant ingredient(s) as specified on the label or according to the recipe.
   b. The total weight of a serving must be a minimum of 35 g. This quantity represents a serving equivalent to one slice of bread.
Cookies should not be served more than twice a week. Cookies can only be used as the bread alternate for supplements.

9. Can items such as potato sticks, popcorn, corn chips, potato chips, hard thin pretzels, and so on, be used to meet the bread requirement?
   No. Extruded grain products and snack-type foods such as these cannot be used for the bread requirement. These foods are counted as extras.
10. Can corn tortillas and other corn products be credited as a bread alternate?
    Corn tortillas and other corn products can be credited if the main ingredient is one of the following: whole-grain corn, whole-ground corn, whole-germed corn, cornmeal, corn flour, enriched cornmeal, enriched corn flour, or enriched corn grits. However, if the main ingredient is listed as corn grits, degerminated corn flour, or degerminated cornmeal, the corn products cannot be credited.
11. Can graham crackers be used as a bread alternate?
    Yes. The main ingredient is whole-grain or enriched flour.
12. Can pie crust be credited as a bread alternate?
    Yes. If the crust is being served as an accompaniment to, or as an integral part of, the main dish (the main dish contains the meat/meat alternate). Also, the primary ingredient by weight must be whole-grain or enriched flour or meal. Pie crust served as part of a dessert is not creditable because it is not served as an integral part of the main dish.
13. Can cereals be mixed and served as a "party mix"?
    Yes. Cereals that are whole-grain, enriched, or fortified may be mixed and served for a supplement only. However, ingredients such as hard pretzels, nuts, and seeds are not creditable as bread alternates and their weights must be subtracted from the cereal portion of the mix. Nuts and seeds could be counted toward the meat alternate.
14. Are rice cakes a creditable bread alternate?
    Yes. Rice cakes are creditable as a bread alternate and part of the crackers and low-moisture bread group. Three rice cakes are required for one bread serving. The portion size per child may be too large to be practical. Rice cakes must contain whole-grain or enriched meal or flour as the primary ingredient by weight. The brown rice contained in rice cakes is a whole grain.

Partial List of Bread Equivalents

Group A: Breads, Rolls, and Quick Bread (1 serving)

Bagel	57 g or 2 oz
Cloverleaf roll	30 g or 1.1 oz
Frankfurter bun	40 g or 1.4 oz
Hamburger bun, medium	50 g or 1.8 oz
Hamburger bun, small	40 g or 1.4 oz
Hard roll (kaiser)	57 g or 2 oz
Hoagie or submarine	68 g or 2.4 oz
Parkerhouse roll	30 g or 1.1 oz
Pretzel, soft	57 g or 2 oz

Group B: Crackers and Low-Moisture Breads; 1 Serving = 20 g (0.7 oz)

Graham	21 g or 0.7 oz
Saltines	23 g or 0.8 oz
Melba toast	20 g or 0.7 oz
Rye wafers	25 g or 0.9 oz
Taco shells	20 g or 0.8 oz
Zwieback	21 g or 0.7 oz
Bread sticks (7¾ inches long, ¾-inch diameter)	20 g or 0.7 oz

Group C: Miscellaneous Items; ½ Serving = 15 g (0.5 oz); 1 Serving = 30 g (1 oz)

Dumplings
Hush puppies
Meat/meat alternate pie crust
Meat/meat alternate turnover crust
Pancakes
Pizza crust
Sopapillas
Spoonbread
Tortillas (6-inch)
Waffles
Cookies and granola bars for snacks only; 1 serving = 35 g

Note that because weights of these bread products differ, it is impossible to list how many crackers, pieces of bread, taco shells, and so on it takes to equal one bread serving. To accurately determine serving size, these products must be weighed individually.

Fruit/Vegetable Component

1. What foods cannot be counted toward the fruit/vegetable component? The following food items do not qualify as vegetable or fruit and may not be credited toward meeting the fruit/vegetable requirement in any meal served:
   a. Snack-type foods made from vegetables or fruits, such as potato chips, corn curls, and banana chips
   b. Pickle relish
   c. Tomato catsup and chili sauce
   d. Dry vegetables for seasoning
   e. Garnishes such as parsley, pickle slices, pimentos, and olives that amount to less than ⅛ cup per serving
   f. Coconut
2. Can a chef's salad be counted toward meeting two servings of fruit and vegetable?

The fruit/vegetable component must be two different servings. Menu items such as fruit cocktail and mixed vegetables are considered as only one item. Large combination vegetable or fruit salad entrees, containing at least ½ cup (for 3- to 6-year-olds) of two or more vegetables and/or fruits in combination with meat or meat alternates (such as chef's salad or fruit plate with cottage cheese), are considered two or more servings and will meet the full requirement.

3. Which types of juice can be used?

   Any product, either liquid or frozen, that is labeled "juice," "full-strength juice," "single-strength juice," or "reconstituted juice" is considered full-strength juice. Examples of full-strength juice are apple, grape, grapefruit, grapefruit-orange, lemon, lime, orange, pear-apple, pineapple, prune, tomato, and vegetable juice.

   "Juice drinks" and other combination products such as a frozen juice bar may contain only a small amount of full-strength juice. The product label may indicate percentage of full-strength juice in the product. To be used in meeting a part of the fruit/vegetable requirement, the product must contain a minimum of 50% full-strength juice. Only the full-strength juice portion may be counted to meet the fruit/vegetable requirement.

   Products labeled as "ade," "juice cocktail drink," or "drink" cannot be used. Nectars, lemonade, and cranberry juice cocktail contain less than 50% full-strength juice and cannot be used to meet the fruit/vegetable requirement.

4. How do you determine if sweet apple cider is full-strength juice?

   There are no USDA grade standards or FDA standards of identity for sweet apple cider; thus, the cider may be diluted and sweetened. If a brand of sweet apple cider is prepared without the addition of sweetened ingredients and without dilution, then it is full-strength fruit juice. If this information is not indicated on the label, contact the manufacturer.

5. Can pickles be counted as part of the fruit/vegetable component?

   Pickles can be served and counted as part of the fruit/vegetable component if at least ⅛ cup is served. Pickle slices served with a sandwich usually cannot be counted because ⅛ cup is not normally served. If products such as gherkins, whole dill pickles, or lengthwise-sliced pickles are served in sufficient quantities, they can be counted. However, good menu planning practices suggest that pickles are not used frequently to meet the fruit/vegetable requirement.

6. Can the fruit or vegetable contained in banana bread, zucchini bread, applesauce cake, and raisin cookies be counted toward the fruit/vegetable requirement?

   There are not sufficient amounts of fruits or vegetables in these products to credit toward fruit/vegetable components.

7. Can the fruit in pie filling count?

   Yes. The fruit contained in canned pie filling can be counted based on ½ credit. For example, ½ cup canned pie filling will count as ¼ cup of fruit.

In a homemade or center-made pie, the amount of fruit can be credited based on the amount of fruit placed in the product divided by the number of servings received.

8. Which soups can be used to meet the fruit/vegetable component?
Canned condensed soups (1 part water and 1 part soup) that contain vegetables such as clam chowder, minestrone, tomato, tomato with rice and/or vegetable, and vegetable with other basic components such as meat and poultry can be counted (1 cup reconstituted soup counts as ¼ cup vegetable). One-half cup bean, lentil, or split pea soup can be counted as ¼ cup vegetable. French onion, cream of celery, and cream of mushroom soup do not contain sufficient amounts of vegetable to count toward the fruit/vegetable requirement. Chicken noodle soup and beef and noodle that do not contain vegetable products cannot be counted toward fruit/vegetable components.

Dehydrated soups that contain vegetables can be used if the volume of vegetables is measured. The soup must be reconstituted according to package directions and the vegetable products separated from rice and noodles to determine the amount of vegetables contained in the product.

Homemade and center-made soups that contain vegetable products can be counted based on the amount of vegetables contained per serving.

Meat/Meat Alternate Component

1. Must all the protein foods be in the main dish?
The meat/meat alternate must be served in the main dish or the main dish and one other menu item. This means that two menu items are the maximum number that may be used to meet the meat/meat alternate requirement.

2. Can items such as Parmesan cheese be counted?
Small amounts of meat or meat alternate used as garnishes, seasonings, or in breadings do not count toward meeting the meat/meat alternate requirement of the meal. Examples are grated Parmesan cheese used as a garnish over spaghetti or egg in breading.

3. Do cooked beans count as meat or vegetable?
Cooked dry beans or peas may be used to meet the meat/meat alternate requirement or the fruit/vegetable requirement but not both in the same meal.

4. Do nuts count as a meat alternate?
Yes. Peanuts, soynuts, and tree nuts such as walnuts and seeds, which are nutritionally comparable to meat or other meat alternates, may be used. Due to their extremely low protein content and iron values nuts that cannot be used as a meat alternate are acorns, chestnuts, and coconuts. Nuts and seeds may fulfill all the meat alternate requirements for snacks, but not more than one half of the meat/meat alternate requirement for lunch/supper.

Table 6-7
Foods common to most ethnic food patterns

Meat and Alternates	Milk and Milk Products	Grain Products	Vegetables	Fruits	Others
Pork*	Milk, fluid	Rice	Carrots	Apples	Fruit juices
Beef	Ice cream	White bread	Cabbage	Bananas	
Chicken		Noodles, macaroni,	Green beans	Oranges	
Eggs		spaghetti	Greens (especially spinach)	Peaches	
		Dry cereal	Sweet potatoes or yams	Pears	
			Tomatoes	Tangerines	

*May be restricted because of religious custom.

5. Can vegetable-protein products be used?
   Hydrated vegetable-protein products (such as those made from soy) may be used to meet no more than 30% of the meat/meat alternate requirement or a maximum ratio of 30 parts hydrated vegetable protein to 70 parts uncooked meat, poultry, or fish. A vegetable-protein product must be hydrated to a 60% to 65% moisture level or ratio of 1 part dehydrated textured vegetable protein to 1½ parts water.

CULTURAL FOOD PATTERNS

Knowledge of cultural food patterns helps the care giver establish rapport with the child and family. Serving foods that represent different cultural food patterns can be a nourishing and educational experience for children. What people eat depends on ethnic, social, and economic factors. Children who were born in this country generally like and will eat foods that are readily available. Table 6-7 illustrates the similarities among traditional foods of six ethnic groups—black, Hispanic-American, Japanese, Chinese, Vietnamese, and American Indian. Using these common foods, menu planners will find it relatively easy to accommodate diverse tastes. However, preparation methods vary greatly from one ethnic group to another.

Although there are many similarities, the teacher should capitalize on the diverse ethnic cuisines found in this country and make an effort to incorporate as many of the foods as possible into the child-care menu and curriculum. Calling on parents from a variety of backgrounds to help plan menus is an excellent way to provide cultural experiences.

MENU CHECKLIST

The following questions will serve as a convenient checklist in your menu planning. If you are now participating in a preschool center and have access to the menus, use that center as a guide.

Table 6-8
Winter cycle menus for preschooler

Day 1	Day 2	Day 3	Day 4
Beef and vegetable stew 1½ oz beef ¼ C carrots and potatoes Molded salad (orange sections, ¼ C) Whole wheat bread, ½ slice Margarine, 1 tsp 2% milk, ¾ C SNACKS: Deviled egg, ½ 2% milk, ½ C	Chicken livers, 1½ oz Green beans, ¼ C Cooked tomatoes or tomato wedges, ¼ C Whole wheat bread, ½ slice Margarine, 1 tsp 2% milk, ¾ C SNACKS: Pineapple chunks, ½ C 2% milk, ½ C	Fish, baked, 1½ oz Seasoned brown rice, ¼ C Asparagus spears, ¼ C Plums, 2 Margarine, 1 tsp Whole wheat muffin, 1 2% milk, ¾ C SNACKS: Mandarin oranges, ½ C 2% milk, ½ C	Roast pork, 1½ oz Sweet potato, ¼ C Baby lima beans, ¼ C Carrot sticks, 4 (6 in. long) Whole wheat bread, ½ slice Margarine, 1 tsp 2% milk, ¾ C SNACKS: Grapefruit sections, ½ C 2% milk, ½ C

Day 5	Day 6	Day 7	Day 8
Baked chicken, 1½ oz Cooked zucchini, ½ C Tossed salad, ½ C Whole wheat bread, ½ slice Margarine, 1 tsp 2% milk, ¾ C SNACKS: Dried fruits—peach slice, apricot slice, dates, approximately 8 slices 2% milk, ½ C	White beans and ham ½ C beans 1 oz ham Coleslaw, ¼ C Tomato, ¼ C Corn bread, 1 to 2 in. square Margarine, 1 tsp 2% milk, ¾ C SNACKS: Grapes (green), 18 2% milk, ½ C	Beef cubes, 1½ oz Brown rice, ¼ C Broccoli, ¼ C Applesauce, ¼ C Whole wheat bread, ½ slice Margarine, 1 tsp 2% milk, ¾ C SNACKS: Floating banana (½ banana and ¼ C orange juice) 2% milk, ½ C	Fried chicken, 1½ oz Mashed potatoes, ¼ C Cranberry sauce, ⅛ C Brussels sprouts, ¼ C Whole wheat bread, ½ slice Margarine, 1 tsp 2% milk, ¾ C SNACKS: Pineapple, ½ C 2% milk, ½ C

Day 9	Day 10	Day 11	Day 12
Broiled fish, 1½ oz Scalloped corn, ½ C Cooked greens, ¼ C Whole wheat bread, ½ slice Margarine, 1 tsp 2% milk, ¾ C	Chili, ½ C 1 oz. hamburger ¼ C beans 2 tbsp tomato sauce Vegetable salad, ½ C Grapefruit, ¼ C Whole wheat crackers, 3	Omelet 1 large egg ½ oz cheddar cheese Oven browned potato, ¼ C Broccoli, ¼ C Whole wheat bread, ½ slice Margarine, 1 tsp	Meat loaf (1½ oz hamburger) Mashed potatoes, ¼ C Cooked cabbage with carrots, ¼ C Whole wheat bread, ½ slice Margarine, 1 tsp 2% milk, ¾ C

SNACKS:
Cooked prunes, ½ C
2% milk, ½ C

Margarine, 1 tsp
2% milk, ¾ C
SNACKS:
Sliced peaches, ½ C
2% milk, ½ C

2% milk, ¾ C
SNACKS:
Bread sticks, 2
Peanut butter, 1 tbsp
Tomato juice, ½ C

SNACKS:
Pear halves, 2, with raisins and sunflower seeds
2% milk, ½ C

Day 13	Day 14	Day 15	Day 16
Roast turkey, 1½ oz Sweet potatoes, ¼ C Cranberry salad, ¼ C Whole wheat bread, ½ slice Margarine, 1 tsp 2% milk, ¾ C SNACKS: Citrus cup, ½ C Toasted wheat germ, 1 tsp 2% milk, ½ C	Beef liver, 1½ oz Beets, ¼ C Buttered noodles, ¼ C Lettuce salad, ½ C Whole wheat bread, ¼ slice Margarine, 1 tsp 2% milk, ¾ C SNACKS: Waldorf salad: ½ C apple, 1 tsp raisins, ½ tsp walnuts, 1 tsp mayonnaise 2% milk, ½ C	Pizza 5⅛ in. arc whole wheat crust with 1 oz beef Carrot sticks, 2 Green pepper rings, 2 Sweet cherries, ¼ C 2% milk, ¾ C SNACKS: Orange sections, ¼ C Banana chunks, ¼ banana 2% milk, ½ C	Baked breaded fish sticks, 3 (1½ oz fish) Au gratin potatoes, ¼ C Spinach salad ¼ C spinach 2 tbsp chopped egg 1½ tsp salad dressing Pineapple slice 2% milk, ¾ C SNACKS: Bread pudding (bread, ½ slice) Orange juice, ½ C

Day 17	Day 18	Day 19
Ham and cheese sandwich 1 oz ham ½ oz cheese Baked beans in tomato sauce, ¼ C Apricots, ¼ C Whole wheat bread, 1 slice Margarine, 1 tsp 2% milk, ¾ C SNACKS: Apple and peanut butter snacks 2 crosscut slices apple, ¼ in. 1 tbsp peanut butter 2% milk, ½ C	Spaghetti dinner ¼ C spaghetti 2 tbsp sauce 1½ oz meat Tossed salad ¼ C lettuce ¼ C greens ¼ tomato Whole wheat roll, ½ Margarine, 1 tsp 2% milk, ¾ C SNACKS: Whole wheat crackers, 4 Tomato juice, ½ C	Seafood or chicken chop suey 1½ oz meat Bean sprouts, bamboo shoots, water chestnuts, and green pepper, ½ C Brown rice, ¼ C Whole wheat bread, ½ slice Margarine, ½ tsp 2% milk, ¾ C SNACKS: Strawberries, ½ C 2% milk, ½ C

Note: Menus provide 33% of RDA for 4-year-old per week and meet Child Care Food Program Regulations, 1983. Appreciation is extended to Maureen Conley, R.D., Supervisor, Food and Nutrition Programs, Illinois State Board of Education.

1. Do the lunches meet the minimum requirements for the group served? (See Tables 6-1 and 6-2.)
2. Is a raw vegetable or fruit included daily for preschoolers and finger foods for toddlers?
3. Is a carotene-rich fruit or vegetable included at least twice a week? Is a dark green vegetable included almost every day?
4. Is a vitamin C-rich fruit or vegetable included each day?
5. Are foods that are good sources of iron included daily (5 mg)?
6. Are sugar and salt used in limited quantities (for example, potato chips not served with ham or lunch meats, no sweet desserts)?
7. Do the lunches include a good balance of color, texture, shape, flavor, and temperature?
8. Are the foods varied from day to day and week to week from cycle to cycle?
9. Is at least one new food or preparation method introduced each week?
10. Are new foods introduced in combination with popular foods?
11. Are the instructor's objectives integrated into the menus?

```
PERCENT ENERGY DISTRIBUTION


                  PROTEIN     21%          FAT     32%       CARBOHYDRATE    47%

NUTRIENT    %RDA 0%              20%     33%  40%          60%  66%      80%          100%
----------------I----------------I---------I-----I----------------I-----I---------I----------------I
ENERGY       33%  X X X X X X X X X X X X X X X X
PROTEIN      93%  X X X X X X X X X X X X X X X X X X X X X X X X X X X X X X X X X X X X X X X X X X X X X X
VITAMIN A   156%  X X X X X X X X X X X X X X X X X X X X X X X X X X X X X X X X X X X X X X X X X X X X X X X X X X X X X
VITAMIN D    33%  X X X X X X X X X X X X X X X X
VITAMIN E    48%  X X X X X X X X X X X X X X X X X X X X X X X X
VITAMIN C    84%  X X X X X X X X X X X X X X X X X X X X X X X X X X X X X X X X X X X X X X X X X X X
FOLACIN      33%  X X X X X X X X X X X X X X X X
NIACIN       42%  X X X X X X X X X X X X X X X X X X X X X
RIBOFLAVIN   81%  X X X X X X X X X X X X X X X X X X X X X X X X X X X X X X X X X X X X X X X X
THIAMIN      47%  X X X X X X X X X X X X X X X X X X X X X X X
VITAMIN B6   35%  X X X X X X X X X X X X X X X X X X
VITAMIN B12  72%  X X X X X X X X X X X X X X X X X X X X X X X X X X X X X X X X X X X X X
CALCIUM      60%  X X X X X X X X X X X X X X X X X X X X X X X X X X X X X X
PHOSPHORUS   68%  X X X X X X X X X X X X X X X X X X X X X X X X X X X X X X X X X X X X
IRON         34%  X X X X X X X X X X X X X X X X X
MAGNESIUM    52%  X X X X X X X X X X X X X X X X X X X X X X X X X X
ZINC         33%  X X X X X X X X X X X X X X X X
----------------I----------------I---------I-----I----------------I-----I---------I----------------I


TOTAL NUTRIENTS

     4-5 GM DIETARY FIBER        78.5 MG CHOLESTEROL      553.3 MG SODIUM      1170.3 MG POTASSIUM
```

Figure 6-7
Nutrient analysis of cycle menus from Table 6-8 (*Source:* NDDA Laboratory, Southern Illinois University at Carbondale.)

12. Can the lunches be prepared successfully within the time available?
13. Can the lunches be prepared with the staff, facilities, and equipment available?
14. Can food be purchased with money budgeted?
15. Do cycle menus reflect both the children's own culture and that of unfamiliar cultures?
16. Do the menus give opportunities for the child to develop motor skills (foods for spoon, knife, and fork for the preschooler; finger foods and foods for the spoon for the toddler)?

Table 6–8 is a set of menus for 19 days. These menus have been planned for one meal and a snack, meeting approximately the required one third of the RDA for all nutrients for the 4-year-old (see Figure 6–7). With carefully chosen additional snack items, these menus will meet 50% of the RDA, providing an additional 1 mg of iron. The energy allotment has been set at 1500 kcal for the 4- to 5-year-old.

GOOD MANAGEMENT PRINCIPLES

The teacher or care giver and food service personnel must work jointly to decide on the foods purchased, prepared, stored, and eaten. Menu planning is not the same as that carried out by the family at home. Not only is the number of persons to be served larger, but also certain controls must be established on ordering and purchasing foods, scheduling, preparation, and recording costs. Whim, fancies, or food idiosyncrasies of personnel have no place in the well-operated center.

Many preschool day-care facilities can receive some food assistance if they are nonprofit centers (see Appendix VII, Child Care Food Program), but with this assistance comes the need for controlling cost and for keeping accurate records. This does not mean that food and the eating experience are lost to the cost-control expert. On the contrary, it encourages advance planning and allows an ideal opportunity to have teacher, administrator, and food service personnel plan menus together.

Quantity food service principles and procedures are applied through planning the menu, ordering and purchasing food, controlling supplies, preparing food, and analyzing costs. The following highlights each area:

Planning the Menu

1. Plan preferably a month or more in advance.
2. Maintain up-to-the-minute inventories on which menus can be based.
3. Use locally abundant foods.
4. Order and use donated commodities, if available.
5. Evaluate menus for adequacy, appearance, acceptance, and workload.

Ordering and Purchasing Food

1. Develop purchase orders or grocery lists in advance.
2. Order by the case or in quantities that are least expensive. (Small centers may purchase with other nearby child-care centers, senior citizen programs, or schools.)
3. Obtain competitive quotations each time purchases are authorized.
4. Check deliveries for quantity, quality, weight, and conformity to all specifications.

Controlling Supplies

1. Record correctly all merchandise issued from storage.
2. Refrigerate food that needs to be kept cold, and keep frozen foods in a freezer.
3. Prevent loss from the kitchen and warehouse by keeping records and making regular checks. (Keep freezers locked.)
4. Allow no leftover food to be taken from the kitchen.

Preparing Food

1. Follow tested recipes. This assures a uniform product, prevents waste, and makes it easier to provide portions of the correct size. (Recipes for child-care services are available from USDA [5].)
2. Avoid providing too much or too little food by keeping accurate records of participation. If all the food is used, the extra handling and storage of leftover food is avoided. If there is too little food, nutrition and educational programs will suffer.
3. In estimating the number to be served, consider the weather, center activities, and other factors.
4. Simplify preparation and serving.
5. Maintain food production records (Figure 6-4).

Analyzing Costs

1. Keep accurate daily cost records.
2. Do not repeat expensive menu items unless they can be balanced by inexpensive items or unless funds are available.

Food service personnel should be encouraged to attend School Food Service Certification Workshops as well as to receive the Certification for Food Service Managers in states where such services are available. Contact the regional or state agency that administers the USDA Child Care Food Program for more information and the specific requirements of each state.

SANITARY PRACTICES

The topic of sanitation deserves special attention, especially in preparation of foods for vulnerable, "high-risk" groups such as infants and young children. Some states now require a food handler's certificate. Food service textbooks can provide additional information on sanitary practices and other aspects of quantity food production [6–8].

Organisms

Bacteria, which cause food-borne illnesses, are so tiny they can only be seen with a microscope. They are found everywhere on everything, in the air we breathe, on the things we touch—we even carry them on our skin, hair, and clothing. Food, moisture, and moderate temperatures promote life and growth of these organisms. When all these conditions are present, they grow and multiply at a rapid rate. About every 20 minutes the organism may split, grow, and divide again and again. In 24 hours one may grow and divide into 281 trillion organisms.

Three common types of organisms are *Staphylococcus*, *Salmonella*, and *Clostridium*. Knowing their sources and how they are spread, the food service worker can protect food from these organisms. *Staphylococcus* or "staph" organisms come in contact with food through someone who has an infected sore, cut, or burn. Coughing and sneezing can also bring *Staphylococcus* organisms in contact with dirty equipment. They grow most rapidly in custards, cream fillings, egg, tuna and potato salads, and most of the high-protein foods. As the *Staphylococcus* organisms quickly multiply, they produce a poisonous substance called a *toxin*. The toxin is the cause of sickness. If food is left at room temperature, these organisms grow and produce toxin, but if food is kept refrigerated or hot—above 140° F—after preparation, *Staphylococcus* organisms will not grow and produce toxin. Once a food is exposed to *Staphylococcus*, cooking will kill the organism, but the poisonous toxin will remain.

It is possible that food may enter the kitchen with the *Salmonella* organism already in it; these organisms may be spread by someone who has handled the infected food and then handled other foods. *Salmonella* organisms may also be spread by someone who has been ill and still carries the organism. The foods that are most often involved in this type of food poisoning are eggs, poultry, meat pies, and unpasteurized milk products.

Salmonella organisms from uncooked meats may get onto your cutting board and be spread to any cooked meats prepared on the same board. To prevent this you should use separate boards for uncooked and cooked meats and wash the cutting boards frequently. Proper refrigeration, 40° F and under, will stop the growth of *Salmonella* organisms. Thorough cooking will kill this organism and prevent foodborne illness.

Two types of *Clostridium* organisms can affect food. The first of these is *Clostridium perfringens*. Its major source is meat. This organism originally comes from soil. It infects animals that are used for meat products, so it is possible that freshly delivered meat may be infected. *Clostridium perfringens* multiplies rapidly, not only in meat products, but in broths and gravies as well. These bacteria are heat resistant, so they cannot be destroyed by cooking. To prevent further bacteria growth, broths, gravies, and meats that are not to be served immediately should be placed in shallow pans and refrigerated promptly.

The second *Clostridium* organism *(Clostridium botulinum)* causes botulism, which is a rare but deadly form of food poisoning. It occurs mainly in foods that are canned, perhaps developing when a can is damaged. Therefore, cans that are dented, bulging, or leaking or have contents that foam, smell bad, or have an off color or milky appearance should not be used. Also, botulism may occur in home canning when foods that have a low acid content—green beans and beets—are canned either in an "open kettle" or "water bath." It may also occur when some low-acid fruits are home canned without the use of a pressure cooker. Therefore, child-care centers should not accept home-canned foods from well-meaning parents. You, the care giver or administrator, could be held responsible for a child who becomes ill from contaminated food.

Dangerous organisms may get into your kitchen through several ways:

1. Food service personnel may bring in disease-causing organisms and, because of careless personal hygiene, pass these on to food. Therefore, it is important that those in food service maintain a high degree of personal hygiene.
2. Disease-ridden insects and rodents will carry organisms in with them. It is the responsibility of the kitchen employee to be on the lookout for signs of pest infestation, such as droppings and food damage, and report any findings to the supervisor so that proper steps for extermination may be taken.
3. The organisms may be carried into the child-care center already on the food.

Remember, living organisms need food, moisture, and moderate temperature to grow. *After preparation, keep foods in a cold refrigerator, 40° F and under, or hot, over 140° F.* Do not leave food out in warm kitchen temperatures. All refrigerators and freezers should contain thermometers (Figure 6–8).

Personal Sanitation

Personal hygiene means more than just a clean face and hands. It means a clean body, clean clothes, and clean habits. Everyone's skin harbors organisms.

Food service personnel should wear clean uniforms or aprons each day. An apron should be changed when it gets soiled. It is necessary that a kitchen cap, chef's cap, or hairnet be worn, since organisms are on hair. Also, caps or nets prevent hair from falling onto the food. The hands of a food service worker should be kept clean, with short, clean nails and no jewelry other than a watch or wedding ring.

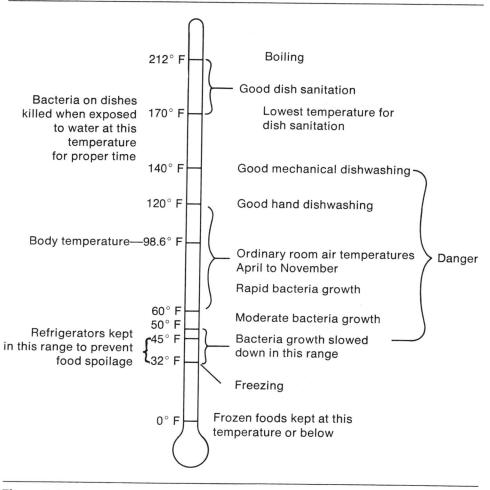

Figure 6-8
Temperature and food sanitation

Hands frequently harbor organisms that can be transferred to food. Because of this, it is essential that hands be washed before working, each time they become dirty, after smoking (organisms from your mouth get onto cigarettes and then onto fingers), and after using the toilet. To effectively wash hands use soap and hot water. The mechanical scrub of hand against hand gets the trapped dirt and grime out. Take time to do a thorough job. Do not lean against the basin; organisms outside the basin will get on your uniform and then onto the work counter and work area. Rinse and dry hands thoroughly with a fresh paper towel. Do not use your clean hands to turn off water. Use a paper towel. This will keep the clean hands from touching the unsanitary water faucet. Food service personnel should not handle the food if they have boils, running sores, skin eruptions, or infected cuts, since these conditions may be sources of infection. It is possible to work in a non-food-handling part of the kitchen until the skin condition has disappeared.

Food should not be handled by anyone with an illness. Turn away from food to sneeze or cough, and cover mouth and nose with a disposable tissue. (A sneeze alone will explode millions of organisms into the air and contaminate not only food but also work areas, equipment, and coworkers.) Because organisms from a sneeze or cough can penetrate the tissue used and get onto the hands, dispose of the tissue after use and wash hands.

The warmth of a kitchen often causes one to perspire. When wiping perspiration from the face, use a paper towel, not a kitchen towel. After using, dispose of the paper towel and wash hands. Always comb hair in the lavatory, not in the kitchen. Try not to touch hair or skin while working, for the hand could then serve as a carrier of organisms to the food.

Food Handling

The following guidelines for food handling must be followed:

1. Select food from clean, wholesome sources.
2. Examine food when it is delivered to make sure it is not spoiled or dirty and that no insects are present.
3. Sort, wash, and store foods in tightly covered, labeled containers at proper temperatures at all times.
4. Keep perishable foods refrigerated between processing operations and before serving.
5. Use only fluid pasteurized milk.
6. Always check food supplies before using—when in doubt, throw it out!
7. Always wipe all can tops before opening.
8. Maintain all potentially hazardous foods at safe temperatures, below 40° F or above 140° F.
   a. Take food temperatures in the *center* of the food mass.
   b. Make sure all hot food reaches an internal temperature of 165° to 170° F.
   c. Serve hot food immediately, or refrigerate immediately in shallow pans. Refrigerating a hot food will not spoil it. Foods should *never* be left out at room temperature to cool.
   d. When chilling food, the center of the food mass must reach 40° F within 4 hours.
   e. Bake casserole-type foods in shallow pans to ensure adequate heating in the center of food.
   f. Do not stack foods such as cooked meat in deep pans. It should be put in shallow layers in shallow pans for refrigeration and for heating.

    g. Do not stack food containers on refrigerator shelves, but place covered containers individually on shelves to allow maximum heat removal.

    h. Do not line refrigerator shelves or oven shelves, because this practice prevents air movement.

9. Place thermometers in the center of the refrigerator and oven, facing toward the front. Ensure that they are clean and easy to read.

10. Use two spoons when tasting foods. Dip into food with one spoon. Transfer food from spoon 1 to spoon 2 without touching the two spoons together. Taste food from spoon 2. Never put spoon 1 into mouth. Never put spoon 2 into food.

11. Always use clean utensils instead of fingers to pick up food. If you must use fingers to guide food into serving dishes, always wear sanitary plastic gloves.

12. Take hold of drinking glasses at the bottom and cups and utensils by the handles.

13. Do not let fingers touch the contents of dishes, bowls, or glasses. Keep fingers under the rim of bowls, plates, and dishes.

14. Use tongs or forks to pick up rolls, butter squares, and bread.

15. Pick up silverware and knives by the handles.

Care Givers and Food Service

In many cases it is necessary and even advantageous for child-care workers to assist the food service personnel. In some centers unions may forbid this activity. However, where permitted, the care giver should follow the same procedures to ensure maintenance of sanitary conditions in the food service facility.

Personal hygiene principles should be followed. (Hands should be washed before personnel come into the kitchen area.) Likewise, providing a clean apron and wearing a hairnet or cap are essential during food preparation and cleanup.

Eating and drinking of food by staff should be permitted only outside the kitchen or food preparation area. Taking "tastes" from the container of food by care givers while food service personnel are preparing and serving food is disruptive and should not be permitted.

PARENT PARTICIPATION

Most centers assume the large task of educating parents as well as children about nutrition. Menus and basic nutrition education programs are shared with parents. Because food idiosyncrasies and poor eating habits may be a result of relatively few foods being served or offered in the home, preventing possible nutritional deficiencies and maintaining the child in the best possible nutritional status involves the parents' continuation of sound principles at home. Parents can be participants in the food programs by helping plan menus and by participating in food preparation and service.

Many preschool centers require parents to serve on advisory or policy boards, which approve cycle menus before they are used. However, too often this means "rubber stamping" a menu or set of menus without being provided with proper information on which to judge the quality of the menus. If possible, a parent should serve along with teacher and food service personnel in the total planning process. At minimum, the parents should receive a copy of the menus, which should explain how foods will be used in the center to help the child learn about new foods and accept a wide variety. In some states the licensing regulations require that menus be posted at least 2 weeks in advance and must be kept on file for up to 6 months.

Many centers arrange group sessions conducted by a nutritionist on the food and nutrition needs of children. These sessions include the nutritional needs of children as related to the specific menus of the center. The nutritionist, along with the food service personnel and care giver, must be accountable to parents for the food served, how foods are used in the child-care center, and for the education of the child's parents so that the efforts begun in the center will be continued at home.

COMMUNITY DIETITIAN

Both child-care workers and food service personnel find it helpful to consult with a community dietitian or public health nutritionist. The public health nutritionist has had courses in public health and community nutrition from an accredited college or university and an approved dietetic internship or equivalent training and experience in a health care program that meets requirements for the registered dietitian (R.D.). The community dietitian, also an R.D., is experienced in working with food and nutrition programs for mothers and children in a variety of settings such as day care, supplemental feeding programs, and institutions. The community dietitian's education includes not just the study of foods and nutrition but also the social and psychological aspects of food and eating for the child and family as a unit.

Nutrition consultation can be located by contacting universities with a public health nutrition or dietetics program, the state or local health departments, local or regional health systems agencies, home extension programs, child and family or welfare agencies, and local hospital dietary departments. Most state health agencies, a large number of city and county health agencies, and many community health projects employ nutrition personnel to plan, direct, and carry out nutrition services. Nutritionists, professionally trained in the science of nutrition, are involved in the delivery of nutrition services in these health care programs and are available to child-care centers.

Qualified nutritionists may also be found in special projects or programs, such as the maternal and infant care projects; rural health projects; Women, Infants, and Children Supplemental Food Program; and Head Start, that may be operated independently of other community health and welfare agencies. The local

American Dietetic Association, Home Economics Association, or National Dairy Council may be contacted to help your center locate professionals with experience in the areas of child feeding.

The dietitian should have available a means of verifying the nutrient content of the menus for you and the ability to evaluate the menus according to the established state and federal guidelines. The availability of a computerized system can ensure that a substantial portion of the nutrient recommendation (RDA) has been included; this subject is discussed in Chapter 1. Many dietitians and nutritionists have access to such systems through state health departments or universities. Without access to such a system, hand calculations serve as well. Simple comparison to the established food guides does not always ensure meeting the RDA.

The nutritionist should be available when representatives from regulatory agencies visit the program. This person, knowledgeable in food service, can ensure that food service personnel are properly trained, sanitary requirements met, and safe practices followed and can verify through nutrient data that the foods provide the nutrients recommended for young children in the right amounts.

The menu-planning session with teacher representative and food service director is the best time to communicate the planning and implementation process of the entire food and nutrition program. The nutritionist should be expected to elaborate in greater detail the applications of principles discussed in this text. With knowledge of local, state, and federal agencies' guidelines, child and family nutrition programs, and resources and materials, the nutritionist can serve as an excellent resource person for centers and the families served.

Training

Some training for the food service personnel is required. In no other facility where food is prepared do we expect the extent of involvement of the teacher and food service personnel. The Child Care Food Program often provides workshops (usually free or at a small cost) on food service and nutrition for food service personnel as well as teachers. The School Lunch Program, usually operated by the state educational agency, conducts workshops for food service personnel that the center staff may attend. These are generally geared to specific aspects of food service. In addition, in-service training should be requested of nutritionists consulting for the program.

SUMMARY

- The daily food plans for toddlers and preschoolers may differ in texture and amounts served; however, table foods can be used for all groups.
- If the menu is to become a tool for the educational curriculum, the food service personnel and teachers must participate together in menu planning.

- Cycle menus, which are flexible enough to be changed frequently, not only help meet the nutritional needs of the individual child but also assist the food service personnel and teacher in planning food service and the curriculum.
- Without the use of good management principles, foods will not provide the quality necessary to encourage children to actively participate in the educational process.
- The Child Care Food Program provides reimbursement for meals that meet USDA specifications. These guidelines can be followed in helping provide infants, toddlers, and preschoolers with the RDA.

DISCUSSION QUESTIONS

1. How are the food patterns for the various age groups different?
2. How might the teacher and food service personnel participate in planning?
3. Are there foods or combinations of foods that meet the Child Care Food Program requirements but might be questioned for the preschool child given the principles outlined in Chapters 3 and 4?
4. Have you observed the good management principles outlined in this chapter in preschool or day-care facilities?
5. List possible constraints from the food service management viewpoint of preparing the following menu: meat loaf, baked potato, cooked broccoli, tossed salad, freshly baked whole wheat rolls, baked apple, and milk.
6. Which factors must be considered in food storage, preparation, and cleanup in order to follow good sanitary practices?

REFERENCES

1. Illinois State Board of Education, Department of Child Nutrition: Child Care Food Program—a guide to crediting foods, Springfield, IL, 1987, The Board.
2. Payaw, F. A., and Hampton, L. P.: Infant feeding practices, 1966, Salt content of the modern diet, Am. J. Dis. Child. 111:370, 1966.
3. Guthrie, H. A.: Infant feeding practices—a predisposing factor in hypertension, Am. J. Clin. Nutr. 21:863, 1968.
4. Endres, J., Poon, S. W., Welch, P., et al.: Dietary sodium intake of infants fed commercially prepared baby food and table food, J. Am. Diet. Assoc. 87:750–753, 1987.
5. U.S. Department of Agriculture, Food and Nutrition Services: Quantity recipes for child care centers, FNS-86, Washington, DC, 1986, U.S. Government Printing Office.
6. Morgan, W. J.: Supervision and management of quantity food preparation, ed. 2, Berkeley, CA, 1981, McCutchan Publishing Corp.
7. Kinder, F., Green, N. R., and Harris, N.: Meal management, ed. 6, New York, 1984, MacMillan Publishing Co.
8. Knight, J., and Kotscheyar, L.: Quantity food production, Boston, 1979, CBI Publishing Co.

LEARNING OBJECTIVES

Students will be able to

- List and describe the four major curriculum approaches used in early childhood education programs
- List the characteristics of the cognitive-interactionist approach
- List six programmatic insights to be gained in using any approach to learning
- State the goals and objectives for teaching nutrition directly to young children (3 to 5 years)
- Using one food from each of the food groups, describe how the food can be used according to Blank's model [1]
- Write nutrition education objectives and list activities to teach the young child (birth to 3 years) good nutrition principles

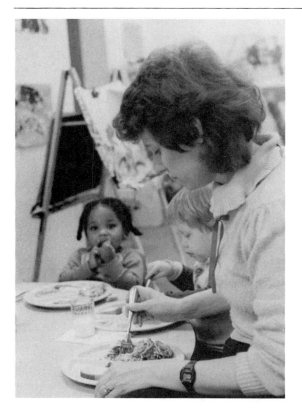

Curriculum Approaches and Teaching Basic Nutrient Concepts

In compiling information for this chapter, we considered the following questions: How do children develop intellectually? Which concepts do they acquire? At which age do they begin to develop these concepts? How can we as teachers of young children teach concepts using foods as one of the primary teaching tools? We have attempted to answer these questions through the use of one approach or model, while presenting additional common teaching approaches that are practical in early childhood settings. All these approaches can be adapted to the nutrition curriculum.

PROGRAMMATIC APPROACHES TO LEARNING

As we examine the development of thought and the many implications it has for teaching, it becomes evident that the environment and the kind of stimulation and interaction with adults to which a child is exposed in the early years will have a significant impact on the child's capabilities.

The child learns through interaction and encounters with objects and persons in the environment. Food, the eating situation, and those persons who provide the food and food service are components of the environment. Thus, the child learns through observing and interacting with foods and the eating situation, manipulating foods, and modeling or imitating those significant adults who participate with the child in the eating situation. The child's perception of the world becomes stabilized, and concepts about the world develop into usable entities.

How much and how well this is learned and the kinds of things learned depend on the child's exposure to examples of foods and the eating experiences. The nutrition education curriculum in early childhood settings should provide the appropriate kinds of experiences, materials, and opportunities to explore and interact for each child's complete development.

It is generally agreed that the early years in a child's life are critical to development and that appropriate early childhood programs can have a positive influence [2]. There is less agreement on which kind of educational program is appropriate, and this, too, has a significant relationship to nutrition education for the young child. The Head Start planned variation studies [3] and numerous educational laboratories and universities have been and are involved in trying to answer that question.

There are at least four major types of approaches to early childhood education: the cognitive-interactionist, traditional nursery school, perceptual motor, and the academic skills [3]. We have chosen the cognitive-interactionist approach to express ways of teaching nutrition education concepts to children. This does not mean that the other approaches are not appropriate for helping children select the proper foods. Any of the methods can be used with success.

Cognitive-interactionist Approach

Cognition refers to mental growth and activity. It defines most of the processes of thinking and knowing that children employ daily—planning what to do in the morning, learning the rules of a game, or making up an excuse for not going to bed early. Cognition includes thinking, remembering, problem solving, understanding, planning, imagining, judging, and deciding. These processes develop in a predictable way according to Piaget [4]. Cognitive ability, which makes understanding possible, develops in two major stages—sensorimotor (birth to 24 months) and preoperational (24 months to 6 years).

Sensorimotor Stage.   This stage covers the period of growth from birth through 24 months. During this period the child depends on inborn sensorimotor reflexes for interaction with the environment. The environment does not just turn on and off those tools provided by heredity. The infant profits from experience and actively modifies the reflex schemes. For example, the child learns to recognize the nipple and to search for it [4]. The smell or sight of food can cause the older infant to crawl to the kitchen in pursuit of it.

Preoperational Stage.   This stage of development extends from 2 to 6 years of age. During this period the child starts to play symbolically and to explore the world in a more able way than the random exploration of an infant. The child has gained more control over the body and thus has freer movement within the environment. Socializing and interacting with others has started. The child's powers of thought are still at a primitive stage, and the sense organs, which have further developed from the sensorimotor period, are still the primary tools for learning. The child needs to look, feel, taste, smell, and even listen to food before, during, and after preparation and to experience this involvement over and over until different experiences (that is, eating a variety of foods) make sense and are internalized.

Concepts. Concepts play an important role in cognitive development. Understanding is based on concepts, which in turn determine what one knows and believes and, to a large extent, what one does. Flavell [5] states that "once a concept develops, it serves as an experimental filter through which impinging events are screened, gauged, and evaluated, a process that determines in large part what responses can and will occur."

As you work with children, you will find that they frequently possess a number of misconceptions. These misconceptions are often caused by incorrect information, limited experience, gullibility, faulty reasoning, vivid imagination, unrealistic thinking, and misunderstanding of words. For example, a child might say, "Milk comes from the grocery store, not from cows." Once a misconception is formed, it is difficult to change. This is where the care giver plays an important role, since it is the care giver's responsibility to provide experiences that teach children about food, thus minimizing the development of nutritional misconceptions.

The cognitive development approach, also referred to as *verbal cognitive* or *interactionist,* includes a variety of diverse types of programs. These approaches share a common emphasis on the development of cognitive skills and abilities such as understanding and using language; concept formation, association, and discrimination; problem solving; and memory. The amount of structure and teaching vis-à-vis child-directed activity varies among programs.

The Perry Preschool Project is a program that exemplifies the cognitive-interactionist approach [6]. This program follows the Piagetian sequence of content areas with respect to motor and verbal levels of operation. Mayer [3] describes the daily routine as one in which teachers carry out their goals and objectives. When teaching nutrition to children, the care giver takes on a directing role. The routine involving food, food service, and nutrition principles is made as tangible and concrete for the child as possible. The approach is similar to the traditional nursery school, or child development model (discussed later), in the number and kinds of materials used and in the prearranged activity areas.

Lay and Dopyera summarized conditions that interactionists believe should be found in programs for young children:

1. All kinds of experiences would be available, not merely those labeled academic. Learners are provided with many possibilities for active "hands on" involvement, which is the basis for later abstract thought processes.
2. Long unstructured activity periods should be provided so that children can engage in the independent planning and execution of projects.
3. A variety of peers should be available for social interaction so that personal views can be validated or modified.

4. Adult input is largely provided on a one-to-one basis or through small groups formed for a specific purpose (for example, to compose a group story or learn to set up a terrarium) and disbanded immediately thereafter (in contrast to being maintained over a period of time).

5. Adults frequently request input from children that requires recall, synthesis, conjecture, estimation, demonstration, and experimentation.*

Other Approaches

Three additional approaches to early childhood education described by Mayer [3] are the academic skills, traditional nursery school, and perceptual-motor approaches. The *academic skills approach* teaches the preschool child the academic skills usually learned in the first years of elementary school through a program of planned, sequenced, highly structured activities. The best known example is the Bereiter-Englemann academically oriented preschool program. Children receive direct instruction in language, arithmetic, and reading, with some time for music and semistructured play. Each teacher takes responsibility for one of the subject areas, and the children in small ability groups rotate from one subject area and teacher to the next. The method of instruction is intense oral drill. Sentence patterns are taught as didactic repetitive formulas, and they increase in complexity as children master them. Concepts such as number and volume, for example, are presented as rules and learned by rote memorization. Children may be expected to memorize examples of the concepts "fruit" or "vegetable."

Another common approach is often termed the *traditional nursery school*. This type stresses the social and emotional development of the child through free play and organized group activities, such as making placemats for mealtime table settings, reading stories about food, and singing songs about food. Also referred to as the *child development model* [3], this curricular approach has been the pattern for most preschools serving middle-class populations. It is based on the physiological belief that effective development fosters cognitive development. This approach ranks highest in child-child interaction, providing opportunities for children to participate together without teacher intervention. The care giver's role is subtle. By planning and arranging the eating environment, children learn about foods. Observations of each child's readiness to profit from a food experience determine the use of that experience.

The *perceptual-motor approach*, or sensory-cognitive model, is best illustrated in the Montessori preschool program. This type of program emphasizes self-corrective sensorimotor activities with specially designed materials. The approach ranks high in child-material interaction but lowest of the four approaches in teacher-child interaction [3]. Learning occurs through "doing," with emphasis on concrete nonverbal experiences. The child is free to choose the activity and to move from task to task, and the teaching materials are planned in a carefully

*From *Becoming a Teacher of Young Children*, second edition, by Margaret Lay-Dopyera and John Dopyera. Copyright © 1982 by D. C. Health & Co. Reprinted by permission of the publisher.

prescribed sequence. The importance of the child's having contact with the natural environment is stressed. Specific experiences with food are planned and encouraged.

Programmatic Insights

Much is yet to be learned from educational philosophies and practices inherent in various early child development curriculum approaches. Each has been carefully and meticulously thought through, tested over a considerable period, and critically evaluated in terms of later school achievement and the personal adequacies of the children involved. From the many models and approaches we can glean important information about children and their learning. Important programmatic insights can be summarized as follows [7]:

1. There is no absolute or preferred approach to learning for all children.
2. Educational goals are determined by an emphasis on child growth or child learning. Where growth objectives dominate, curricular items are introduced when the child can integrate them. Where learning is emphasized, a systematic planned sequence of events is in order.
3. The recognition of individual differences is vital in effective preschool training.
4. A child should experience a continuity in education with curriculum introduced at the developmentally appropriate time and reinforced until the behavior indicates the desired achievement.
5. The teacher's commitment to imparting new social and intellectual skills is necessary for a positive educational experience.
6. Stimulating child-centered environments that provide numerous opportunities for exploration and experimentation are crucial for normal personality and intellectual development.

Early childhood problems cannot be homogeneous in a pluralistic society [8]. There is no single "best" approach or system. Each program should reflect the particular orientation, background, and aspirations of the children's community in the educational setting. This provides us the opportunity to maximize the development of each group rather than attempting to equalize the development of all groups in our society.

GOALS AND OBJECTIVES FOR NUTRITION EDUCATION

The goal of the nutrition education program, whether using a direct or indirect method, may be stated as follows:

Children will eat a well-balanced diet daily to establish and protect their nutritional health for life.

Ideally, after a sound and effective nutrition education program, it should be expected of preschool children that the following would occur:

Given a choice of foods, the child will select those foods with a high nutrient density (quality) as frequently or more frequently than those with a low nutrient density.

The implication of this objective can be far-reaching. If the nutrition education program is successful, children when confronted with candy or soda should be willing to choose vegetables, fruit, fruit juices, or foods high in nutrient density. Because it is perhaps not practical to expect to change the total environment of the child and the eating habits of all persons coming in contact with the child at home, in the community, and at the marketplace, an alternate overall objective would be the following:

Given a variety of foods through a well-planned, prepared, and served menu, the child will accept (taste) all foods provided.

This objective is based on the belief that young children with a sufficient number of positive experiences with many high-quality foods will learn to eat a wide variety of foods.

At the close of their preschool experiences children should be able to

1. State names of all foods served.
2. Identify foods by taste, odor, or touch.
3. Classify foods into food groups, such as vegetables, fruits, meats/meat alternates (nuts, legumes, lentils), cereals/grains, milk and milk products, fats (butter, margarine, oil), and other foods (low nutrient density foods or "empty calories").
4. Match foods served at mealtime with the basic food groups.
5. Match foods served at home with the basic food groups.
6. State number of times each day a child should eat foods from each food group (optional).
7. Name major nutrients in each food group (optional).

Although it is our belief that the last two objectives are too advanced for the preschooler, some centers find that their children can progress to this stage. Objectives 1 through 5 should be accomplished before progressing to objectives 6 and 7.

TEACHING CHILDREN TO EAT NOURISHING FOOD

The basic food groups provide the basis for teaching children to eat a wide variety of nourishing foods. The menu provides the substance for the nutrition education activities that ultimately lead to the child's acceptance of these foods.

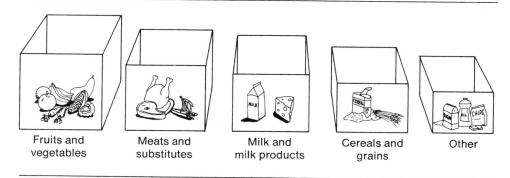

Figure 7–1
Boxes representing basic food groups

Basic Food Group Reference

A visual aid provides a concrete reference point to help young children (3 to 5 years) understand the food groups. One such aid can be constructed with five or more boxes. The boxes can be large enough to hold empty food containers brought from home, or they can be used as a receptacle for food models and pictures of foods. Children can help prepare each box as you progress through the food groups, teaching them the concepts of vegetables, fruits, meats and meat alternates (nuts, legumes, lentils), grains/cereals, milk and milk products, fats, and "other" group (Figure 7–1).

You may choose to combine the food groups into only five categories:

Group 1:   fruits and vegetables
Group 2:   meats and meat alternates
Group 3:   milk and milk products
Group 4:   cereals/grains
Group 5:   other (fat, sugars, low nutrient density foods)

The preparation can include gathering boxes of various sizes. Because the vegetable and fruit group should contain the most variety, these boxes may be largest, followed by those for the meat, nuts, legumes, and lentils group. The fat group would be the smallest. The boxes can be sprayed white or color coded, and children can cut out pictures of food from magazines to paste onto the boxes. The meat and meat alternates box may need to be divided to emphasize the importance of including nuts, legumes, and lentils in the diet (Figure 7–2).

Each food box should be prepared separately, and the foods should be matched with foods served on the menu (objective 4).

The tasting of food items before, during, and after preparation is exciting and educational for children. For example, select a day when white beans appear on the menu. Although children cannot chew a hard dry bean, they can identify it by touch (objective 2). Materials for this activity include:

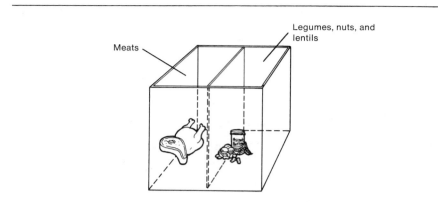

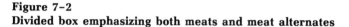

Figure 7–2
Divided box emphasizing both meats and meat alternates

Menu with beans
Food boxes
Uncooked beans
Partially cooked beans
Pictures of beans in food boxes
Pictures or models of other meats and meat alternates
Covered can

Let the child feel beans placed in a covered can. Pictures of beans can then be placed in the meat and meat alternates food group box (objective 3), and children can note other pictures in the meat alternates box that look similar and that look different. Pinto beans and red beans are similar to white beans, but hamburger and eggs are much different from beans, although they all fall into the meat and meat alternate group.

When planning this event with the cook or food service personnel, you will ask for some partially cooked beans, still crunchy, to taste (objective 1), to feel, to smell, and to note how they have become soft. (In addition, beans may be soaked overnight to allow the children an opportunity to see how they have expanded and become softer.) It is best to teach nutrition education concepts before a meal or snack, since the interest in food and food-related activities will be stronger. At mealtime children can compare the fully cooked beans with the uncooked and partially cooked product as well as to the basic food group "meat and meat alternates" (objective 4).

We have presented the nutrition concept of beans informally. However, if lesson plans were to be written and one needed a model to follow, the following is another illustration using a six-stage model.

Teaching a Nutrition Concept

Objectives 1 through 5 can be taught directly to the child, and each involves teaching a concept. The food and nutrition concepts may be taught through a modified hierarchical sequence of six steps. This is especially true for the 2- through 4-year-old. The six stages as described by Blank [1] are (1) a clear instance, (2) a clear definition of the function or attribute of the instance, (3) extension of the concept to similar instances, (4) extension of the concept to less obvious positive instances, (5) consideration of negative instances, and (6) extension of category.

In giving a preschooler a clear instance, we are in fact giving an example. We associate a word with an object. The following presents a modified version of the hierarchical sequence and examples of the use of this scheme. Whenever possible, let the child taste the example presented—regardless of how small the portion is.

MATERIALS: The food group boxes; menu with apples; red and yellow apple, preferably with stem; fresh samples or pictures of dissimilar fruits; other red fruits and vegetables (e.g., onion, red grape); pictures or models of apples and apple pie; covered can (Figure 7–3).

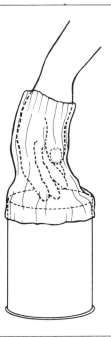

Figure 7–3
Identifying item in covered can by touch

Steps	*Example—The Red Apple*
1. Give an example.	"This is an apple; watch the apple roll; this is a big apple."
2. Give a clear definition of the function or attribute of the instance characteristic of the concept. Actions must accompany the verbal dialogue to make the concept clear to the child.	"This apple is round; it has a stem; its skin is smooth. Apples are from the fruit group." ACTIONS: Have the child feel, taste, smell, and listen to the crunchy sound of the apple. Use covered can (Figure 7–3).
3. To extend the concept to similar instances, use contrast. Choose items that are definitely dissimilar.	Use nonfood items or dissimilar food items. An apple may be compared with all the food groups other than fruit. Once again, review the characteristics of the apple.
4. To extend the concept to less obvious instances, present foods with confusing characteristics. These most often will be within food groups but may also be across groups.	Given bananas, grapes, pineapples, lemons, and a yellow apple, ask the child to find another apple. Let the child taste as many fruits as possible.
5. Consider subtle negative instances meaning that the characteristics of the food are primarily present, yet the food is different.	"Let's find something that is red and round and not an apple." Display red grapes, a red plum, red onion, or a red-orange nectarine. Let child taste even the onion.
6. Extend the category to relate to activities using the apple either at mealtime or during a special activity.	When baked or fried apples are served, the children can be asked, "How can we prepare (cook) apples?" Note that the question "What can we make with apples?" will be answered undoubtedly with "apple pie." When this happens, be prepared. Pictures of low density foods are readily available. Have children place the picture of apple pie in the "other" food group box, thus emphasizing the low nutrient quality.

Because we have provided an example of a meat alternate (beans) and a fruit (apple), vegetables cannot be forgotten. Choose a vegetable high in nutrient quality to provide the child not only with a learning experience but also with a chance to become more familiar with a food that has a high nutrient density. Beans were chosen over other meat products because they have many nutrients that the American diet appears to need in greater quantity. In addition, dietary intake studies show that consumption of meat protein generally is adequate to high. Most homes provide children with meat products (See preceding chapters for discussion of nutrition and foods.)

Because greens and broccoli have a high vitamin C (ascorbic acid), vitamin A, and iron content, they should be included in the educational curriculum of the preschool center. Because greens are usually less expensive than broccoli, this food has been chosen for illustration.

MATERIALS: The food group boxes; menu with greens; facilities to stir-fry greens in center*; fresh (if possible) or frozen greens; fresh broccoli, lettuce, cabbage, and celery leaves, or pictures of these foods.

Steps	*Example—Greens*
1. Give a clear example.	Each child is given a fresh leaf of spinach, turnip, beet, or mustard. "This food is called greens—beet greens, mustard greens, turnip greens, spinach greens."
2. Give a clear definition of the function or attribute.	"Greens are colored green; they are crisp to taste; greens are from the vegetable food group." ACTIONS: Have the children feel, taste, smell, and listen to the crispy sound of the green when they taste it raw.
3. Extend the concept to similar instances.	Use food items from other food groups (e.g., breads, milk, or meat). Compare the greens to at least one item from each of the other food group boxes. Children may select the picture from the boxes of meat, cereals, milk, and fruit. Using the vegetable box with pictures of greens and other vegetables, find a picture of greens.
4. Extend the concept to less obvious positive instances.	In a group of items having the same color and texture (e.g., lettuce, celery leaves), have the child notice the difference between beet greens, spinach greens, and turnip greens.
5. Consider negative instances.	Using broccoli, lettuce, and cabbage leaves (or models or pictures), discuss the differences between these green vegetables.
6. Extend the category.	"Let's eat these greens, raw, cooked with salad dressing, cream sauce, or margarine." Be sure greens are on the menu. Do not be concerned if the cooked (remember, crunchy cooked) greens are not hot; children prefer foods that are not hot and will eat many cooked vegetables cold.

*The stir-fry method can be used with a frying pan in the classroom. Just use ½ tablespoon of margarine for a pound of greens, and stir in frying pan to the "crunchy cooked" stage (takes less than 5 minutes).

Teaching About Nutrients

Those care givers who wish to stress nutrient content of specific foods (such as protein in meats, iron in meats, vitamins A and C in fruits and vegetables) can follow the same format. Appendix I provides the nutrient composition of most foods. A discussion of protein, fat, and carbohydrate can be found in Chapter 1 and in basic nutrition textbooks.

The Very Young Child. With a child of 4 to 6 months (when food is first introduced) or one of 12 to 16 months (when language becomes useful), the preceding objectives are inappropriate. The child is not expected to indicate wants by pointing until approximately 15 to 18 months. Many children can, however, indicate desire for food before this time and can identify the foods they are eating by repeating or imitating care givers and the names given to the food. Therefore, with the 1-year-old child, begin with objective 1, "State names of all foods served." The child at 12 months can look at pictures of foods and hear the sound of their names, can begin to imitate words, and can and generally will follow simple instructions such as "Please eat the carrots."

Children may first need to become familiar with the food and like it before they actually eat it. With foods high in nutritive value we may have to allow the child practice getting acquainted with the texture and flavors by frequently serving and having the child taste the food item. Infants will refuse some new foods, but given continual exposure they will accept them. This is perhaps best illustrated in breast-fed infants. When breast-fed infants are suddenly switched to infant formula, they often do not like the formula and refuse to drink it. Likewise, infants who are milk intolerant dislike being switched to soy formulas, but parents and care givers persist, since the health and well-being of the child are at stake. Eventually they "learn" to like the new formula, as older infants and toddlers learn to like a variety of foods.

Specific activities for the very young child from birth to 12 months include the following:

1. Hold the very young infant while bottle-feeding. Occasionally when two infants must be bottle-fed at the same time, this is not possible. Although schedules may have to be negotiated with parents, we believe it is important to hold the young infant who is being bottle-fed, just as infants who are breast-fed are held. This is especially true if the infant is in the center for more than 3 to 4 hours.
2. Talk to the infant and young toddler about the food in a pleasant voice while looking at the child, although the child cannot respond with verbal communication.
3. State the names of all foods and eating utensils you are using or that you let the child use; for example, "Would you like a drink of milk? Here is your blue cup. Can you take the handle of the cup? See the milk in the cup. You're drinking the milk by yourself. Good! I only put a small amount of milk into the cup, but I will give you more milk. Would you like more milk? I'll give you just a little more milk from this carton to see if you would like

more milk. See, I'm pouring the milk from the carton into the blue cup. Now, I'll give you the blue cup. Can you take the blue cup? (Baby does not take cup.) Okay, I think you've had enough milk and you don't seem to want any more milk. Perhaps later you'd like some more milk." The child needs to hear your voice and the names of food and eating utensils. Note that after the child has taken at least a taste of the food, any signal from the nonverbal child that additional food or drink is not desired should cause you to stop feeding at once.

When the toddler or older infant is accepting table foods and is fed individually, the care giver must provide a model for the child to imitate by eating the same foods.

1. Make the eating experience pleasant by allowing the child to eat the quantity of a variety of foods desired. Praise the child for trying new, less favorite foods, but expect the child to taste all foods. Refusing a food one day should signal that this food must be reintroduced in small quantities on another day.
2. Give the child finger foods as soon as the child can manipulate the foods in the hand. It is important for the child to experience the touch of the food as well as the taste. This also encourages hand-to-mouth coordination and strengthens finger manipulation. Ideas for finger-feeding have been given in previous chapters. Be sure food is appropriate (for example, cubes of cheese, crunchy cooked vegetables, dry whole-grain toast).
3. Encourage the child to share finger foods with you.
4. Be sure infant seats are fastened to table when feeding small infants, or strap the infant into the high chair securely.
5. Use dishes with sides that facilitate filling by spoon. Use spoons and forks sized for the young child.
6. Tolerate spills and learn to plan for them. Have equipment for spilled milk ready for the cleanup job. As soon as children are capable, have them participate in the cleanup activity.

The Young Toddler (12 to 24 Months)

1. Initiate objective 1. Name all foods served.
2. Let the child begin to put cup, plate, spoon, and fork on table setting.
3. Allow the child to develop self-help skills at mealtime.
4. Allow the child to help you prepare food. Children this age can mix several ingredients with spoons, and they like to taste as they explore.
5. Introduce all foods by this period, except those that may become lodged in the throat (popcorn, nuts).

The Older Toddler (24 to 36 Months)

1. Continue with objective 1. Name all foods served.
2. Begin with objectives 2 and 3. Classify and match foods eaten with basic food groups.

3. The child should be able to set the table with minimal assistance.
4. The child should be able to use spoon and fork and begin using knife for spreading.
5. Provide a low cabinet drawer or shelf for unbreakable cooking utensils to use in play to imitate food preparation activities.
6. Provide a table and table-setting equipment—cups, plates, flatware—to practice table setting.
7. The child should be able to serve self from serving bowls.
8. Provide opportunity to prepare food and practice objectives 1 to 3. Prepare fresh green beans, make tossed salad, mix ingredients for fruit breads, etc.

SUMMARY

- The development of thought and the process of learning are significantly influenced by a child's interactions with objects and persons in the environment. Nutrition may be learned through a curriculum that provides enriching experiences and materials and encourages interaction and exploration for the developing child.
- Four major approaches to early childhood education are cognitive-interactionist, academic skills, traditional nursery school, and perceptual-motor. Any of the methods can be used to successfully teach nutrition education concepts to children.
- The cognitive-interactionist method approaches cognitive ability as a process that develops in a predictable way. This process is separated into two major categories, according to Piaget. The sensorimotor stage ranges from birth to 24 months, and the preoperational stage ranges from 2 to 6 years.
- Concepts play an important role in cognitive development. The care giver is extremely important in guiding and forming sound concepts.
- The cognitive development approach incorporates a variety of diverse types of programs. Common to all the approaches is the emphasis on the development of cognitive skills and abilities such as understanding and using language; concept formation, association, and discrimination; problem solving; and memory.
- There is no one best approach to learning for all children. Six important programmatic insights are presented as applicable to any approach to learning. The child-care worker is encouraged to choose and develop a program that will maximize the development of the group under consideration.
- The basic goal of the nutrition education program is to establish a lifetime pattern of eating a well-balanced daily diet.
- Teaching based on the basic food groups and the menu can help lead the child to accepting and eventually eating a wide variety of nourishing foods.

- The optimal time for teaching nutrition concepts directly to young children is just before a meal or snack, since the interest in food-related activities will be stronger.
- A hierarchical six-stage sequence for teaching a concept to young children was developed by Blank. The food and nutrition concepts may be taught through a modified version of this hierarchy. The six stages consist of giving a clear instance, giving a clear definition of the function or attribute of the instance, extending the concept to similar instances, extending the concept to less positive instances, considering negative instances, and extending the category.
- The very young child (birth to 18 months) can benefit from verbal stimulation provided by the care giver. Hearing the voice describe foods and eating utensils during mealtime enriches the eating experience of the young child. The older infant or toddler learns through observation of the care giver, who provides a model of appropriate nutrition and eating practices.

DISCUSSION QUESTIONS

1. Discuss the similarities and differences of the four programmatic approaches used in early childhood programs.
2. Define cognition as it applies to mental growth and activity of children.
3. Children frequently possess a number of misconceptions. How are these misconceptions formed? Can they be changed?
4. Name the program characteristics of the cognitive-interactionist approach.
5. List six programmatic insights to be gained in using any approach to learning.
6. What is the basic goal of the nutrition education program? Name an objective that would be representative of this goal.
7. Describe how the basic food groups can be used to present nutrition education activities in early childhood centers.
8. Using Blank's hierarchical stages, select and describe a nutrition concept as you would present it to a group of preschoolers.
9. List the activities that would be appropriate to teach good nutrition principles to the very young child (6 months to 2 years).

REFERENCES

1. Blank, M.: Teaching learning in the preschool—dialogue approach, Columbus, OH, 1983, Bell & Howell Co.
2. Leeper, S., et al.: Good schools for young children, ed. 5, New York, 1984, Macmillan Publishing Co.
3. Mayer, R. S.: A comparative analysis of preschool curriculum models. In Anderson, R. H., and Shane, H. G., editors: As the twig is bent, Boston, 1971, Houghton Mifflin Co.

4. Ginsburg, H., and Opper, S.: Piaget's theory of intellectual development, Englewood Cliffs, NJ, 1979, Prentice-Hall, Inc.
5. Flavell, J. H.: Concept development. In Mussen, P. H., editor: Carmichael's manual of child psychology, ed. 3, vol. 1, New York, 1970, John Wiley & Sons, Inc.
6. Weikart, D. P.: Curriculum vs. staff model in preschool education, IRCD Bull. Three:52–53, 1971.
7. MacFadden, D. N., editor: Early childhood development programs and services: planning for action, Washington, DC, 1972, Publications Department, National Association for the Education of Young Children.
8. Lasser, G.: The need for diversity in day care. In Grotberg, E., editor: Day care: resources for decisions, Washington, DC, 1971, Office of Planning, Research, and Evaluation.

SUGGESTED READINGS

Margarey, A., Worsley, A., and Boulton, J.: Children's thinking about food: 1. Knowledge of nutrients, J. Nutr. 43:1, 2–8, 1986.

Margarey, A., Worsley, A., and Boulton, J.: Children's thinking about food: 2. Concept development and beliefs, J. Nutr. 43:1, 9–16, 1986.

LEARNING OBJECTIVES

Students will be able to

- Discuss the use of the menu as a key resource for nutrition education in early childhood programs
- Write a lesson plan for at least one curriculum area incorporating food or nutrition in the activities
- List the four developmental areas used to integrate food and nutrition activities in the learning environment
- Justify the need for clearly defined objectives in the development of an effective early childhood curriculum
- List the 10 elements that may be used to construct an operational curriculum using behavioral objectives
- Develop written lesson plans using nutrition activities related to the four developmental skills
- Convert a written recipe into a nonreader recipe
- List some precautions to be observed when cooking in the classroom

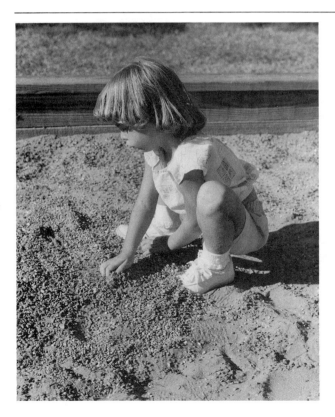

Making It Work in Early Childhood Education

Chapter 7 presented curriculum approaches for teaching nutrition and food concepts directly to the child. This chapter centers on integrating food and nutrition concepts into various curriculum areas as an indirect means of teaching children about food. Activities make use of foods served as part of the menu or those prepared from a recipe in the classroom.

Although feeding or eating times are excellent settings for nutrition education, the staff must be cautious not to make them the only setting, since nutrition education can be incorporated in the *total early childhood curriculum*. Careful consideration should be given to a method of curriculum construction, and a plan should be developed for implementation.

It is not unusual to see children as young as 2 years old serving themselves at mealtime in early childhood centers across the nation. They set the table and pass dishes filled with fresh vegetables and meat. They butter bread that they have baked themselves. They pour their own milk (Figure 8–1). They are joined at the table by their teachers and other staff members who engage in conversation. The children eat, giggle, and talk about their favorite foods, often discussing important nutrition concepts in the process.

Through this process, positive attitudes toward food can be developed in early childhood settings. However, only through planning based on assessment of needs of individual children and calculations of future status can you be sure that you are helping the child.

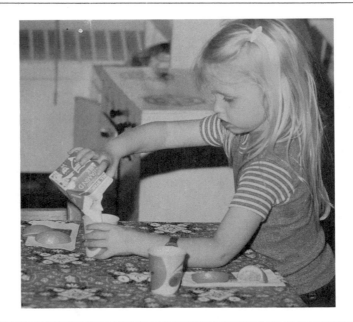

Figure 8–1
A toddler pours milk.

THE MENU

The menu can be considered the major raw material in planning and implementing nutrition learning activities in early childhood education. Chapter 6 discussed use of the menu as a process for planning with the food service personnel. Chapter 7 emphasized using menu items to teach basic nutrition concepts. Figure 8–2 shows the menu at the hub of many of the curriculum areas, including nutrition education.

Care givers may integrate the menu into the early childhood curriculum in a variety of ways; two approaches are presented in this chapter. In the first approach, the care giver uses a single food (in our example, a raisin) to develop instruction in various curriculum areas—language, science, art, math, social studies, music, and physical education (motor coordination). Next, the behavioral-objective approach is used to teach skills related to personal-social, sensorimotor, language, and perceptual-cognitive areas.

Use of Food from the Menu

When you are selecting a food for use in the curriculum, the first consideration should be its nutritional quality. To encourage the intake of nourishing foods, exposure to these foods is important. Raisins are used as the first example [1].

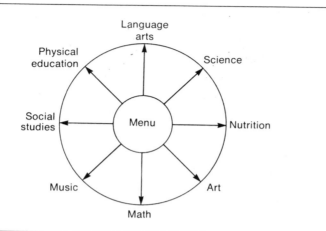

Figure 8-2
The menu as source for activities in all curriculum areas

Class Introduction to Raisin

Nutrition
½ cup approximate measure
230 kcal energy (15% of energy allowance, based on 1500 kcal)
2 g protein
Trace fat
60 g carbohydrate
45 g calcium
3 mg iron (30% of iron allowance)

General Introduction. Raisins can be introduced in the following way:

ACTIVITY: Let's solve a mystery
MATERIALS: Menu with raisins, opaque container with holes, raisins, clear glass or plastic container with water, and clear glass or plastic container (empty).
PROCEDURE: Have each member of the class smell raisins that have been placed in an opaque container with holes in the lid. Ask them not to guess what is in the container until everyone has smelled the raisins. Then ask those who think they know to raise their hands but not to name the mystery item. (About half of some 4-year-old groups will have no idea what they have smelled.) Then have the class members close their eyes. Hand each child a few raisins and have them describe the mystery item. Such observations may be "small," "squishy," "soft," "round," and even "square"—one child squished the raisin into a perfect cube after hearing classmates agree that raisins were round. After much discussion, ask the children to open their eyes to check their identification. Discuss such additional questions as: What color is a raisin? How big is it? Is it smooth? What do you do with it? Finally, ask, what does it taste like? Following the discussion, the children again can close their eyes and count as several raisins are dropped into water ("plop") and then into an empty cup, noting the difference in sound. Talk about how the raisins look in the water; they do not float, but they fall more slowly than when dropped into an empty cup. At the end of the day, compare

the raisins in the two cups. What happened? Are they the same color? Are they the same size? Do they float? How do they taste? Note that the raisins in water have absorbed liquid, diluting the concentration of natural sugar and making them taste less sweet than the dried product. At mealtime be sure to review and ask the children to identify raisins in other foods such as salads (menu) or raisin bread or cereal. Discuss how to prepare grapes to make raisins. Grapes may be covered with cheesecloth and set to dry in the sun. Let the children observe the changes in the grapes and try to guess what will happen next. A warm oven turned off, door ajar, may be used for drying overnight (see Science Activity).

Language Arts. Let children discuss a variety of sensory experiences with raisins. How do they smell? (Put in opaque container with holes in lid.) How do they feel? Squishy, small, round, soft. How do they look? Black, little, bumpy, sort of shaped like an egg. How do they sound? Drop raisins in water, empty cups, on paper, and so on. How do they taste? Do different kinds have different tastes?

ACTIVITY: Mr. Raisin pictures
PROCEDURE: Have each child draw a picture of Mr. Raisin and tell you what he is doing. Write dialogue on the picture: "He's going to punch a hole through the raisin box so he can get out!" Have them make other pictures and combine these into their own Mr. Raisin book. A class may talk about iron helping to keep them strong and healthy. Mr. Raisin may be endowed with bionic powers. Ask each child to draw a series of pictures showing how a grape turns into a raisin. Let them cut these out, back them with flannel (or Velcro), and use them for their own flannel board story. How does Mr. Grape feel? What does Mr. Raisin think about when he's sitting out in the sun? For the older preschooler, you may use the letters in the word *raisin*. Find the same letters in the children's names on the name chart or in signs around the room. See how many words, silly or real, you can rhyme with raisin. Then write a poem or song using those words. Find words that start with the same sound and other foods, animals, and things in school that start with the same sound.

Science. What is a raisin? A raisin is a dehydrated grape. What does dehydrated mean? It means "dried." How do you remove the water? Most commercially processed raisins are dried in the vineyard in bunches on wooden or paper trays.

ACTIVITY: Making raisins
MATERIALS: Fresh, ripe, firm seedless Thompson grapes; scales; large pan or bowl of water; plastic-coated trays or paper plates; pieces of clean cheesecloth, mosquito netting, or wire screen, large enough to cover the trays; and glass container with tight-fitting lid.
PROCEDURE: Weigh the grapes and record the weight. (Measuring weight of grapes will only be meaningful for older preschooler.) Handle carefully, as grapes bruise easily. Save a few for comparison later or be prepared to purchase grapes 4 to 5 days later for children to compare to dried grapes. Place grapes in a container of water, and wash them thoroughly. Lift the grapes from the water, and blot with a towel. Remove the grapes from the stem, and spread one layer of grapes evenly on the tray. Cover the tray with the cloth or screen to keep insects and dust from getting on the grapes. Fasten the cloth so it will not blow off. Place the tray in direct sunlight to dry, away from dirt and dust and where air can circulate freely over and under the tray. Temperatures under 80° F are not recommended. Rotate the grapes daily to help in

the drying process. After 4 days test the grapes for dryness by squeezing them in your hand. If there is no moisture left in your hand and the grape springs apart when the hand is opened, they are dry enough. They should be pliable and leathery to touch. If they are not dry enough, test them again the next day. When the grapes are dry, remove them from the tray and weigh. Record the weight and compare with the first weight. Compare raisins' qualities to those of the grapes you set aside (or a fresh bunch of grapes).

Comparisons

Color	Green to brown
Form	Sphere to flat
Texture	Smooth to wrinkled
Taste	Sweet and mild to sweeter and rich

Put several raisins in a cup of water. Do they sink or float? What happens after they soak for an hour or two? Are they the same color? Size? Texture?

How long will raisins keep? In tight containers in a cool, dry place they will keep for 6 months. How long will grapes keep? In the refrigerator they will keep for 3 to 5 days.

Experiment! Try observing the effect of different locations on raisins: What happens to them in the sun, the dark, the refrigerator, the oven, and so on?

If you have pets in the classroom, find out which ones can eat raisins. One teacher reported, "For several days we had a young guinea pig in the class. The children fed him raisins and other bits of fresh fruit and vegetables. Then one day the baby went home, and papa was brought in for a day. The children were very excited and decided the raisins, with all that iron, had made him grow fast."

Art. Raisins can be used for art projects.

ACTIVITY: Edible artwork

MATERIALS: Give the children graham crackers or large cookies, softened peanut butter or cream cheese as paste, and light and dark raisins, and let them make their own pictures—for example, funny faces. You might add nuts, cereal, coconut, or other small edibles for interest.

PROCEDURE: Use raisins for features on gingerbread men or as faces on peanut butter sandwiches. Put them on a table with a bunch of toothpicks, and let the children make raisin critters. Children can make a grapevine by drawing green scribbles and pasting on leaves and raisins (for the grapes). Or they can draw pictures of Mr. Raisin in various moods. (See suggestions in Language Arts.)

Math. Let the children pass out and divide the completed food. Passing out the food is an excellent one-to-one math activity for very young children, and older children can work out how to share a loaf of raisin bread or 31 raisin cookies with 11 children.

Some of the best math work done with foods is in actual cooking. To follow a recipe, you must practice numeral recognition, one-to-one counting, adding and subtracting, measuring, fractions, weights and volume, and time intervals. As the children are cooking, ask them questions that will help them work out how to follow the recipe accurately. How many cups of flour have we used? How many more do we need? Of course, the answers will depend on age level.

Give the children a small cup filled with raisins and nuts. Let them sort and count. How many nuts? How many raisins? Which do you have more of? How can you make them the same? What can you do so you will have more raisins? Children enjoy eating their way through these math problems.

Give each child several raisins. Have the child find and eat the smallest and the largest. Sort the rest by size, and eat the middle one. You may have to use grapes and raisins for comparison, since often young children cannot determine small differences in size.

Have the child close his eyes and count as you drop raisins into a cup of water.

Social Studies. The following are questions from which to develop your plans:

Which kinds of grapes are used to make raisins? Thompson seedless, Muscat, and Black Corinth are used. (Unless you are an expert on grape varieties, buy several kinds, if available, or cut out pictures of grapes.)
What growing conditions do they require? Hot, dry summer climate at harvest time is needed. Could we grow them here?
How are grapes grown? Who grows them?
Are machines used to pick grapes?
How are grapes prepared to be dried? How are they dried? How long does it take?
Who packages them? Do they use a machine?
How are they stored?
What can they be used for?
What are the advantages of drying fruit? Where might we use dried fruit? They may be eaten during camping trips, eaten as snacks, cooked in bread, mixed in salads.

Music. After a number of experiences with raisins, a care giver asked her preschool children to make up a song about raisins, as follows:

Kelly: Five little raisins sitting on a bench. Along came a witch and ate them.
Sarah: Started setting it to music to the tune of "Five Little Ducks Went Out to Play."

Three little raisins sitting on a bench,
Sitting there as quiet as could be
Along came a witch and ate one,
Two little raisins sitting on a bench.

Along came a witch and ate one
One little raisin sitting on a bench.

He jumped off so the witch couldn't get him.
Zero little raisins sitting on a bench.

If you are a 4-year-old, and you made it up yourself, that's a great song! You may write the music for the song using raisins as the musical notes.

Physical Education
Fine motor development. Any of the math or art activities requiring the picking up of individual raisins aids in fine motor development. Stabbing raisins with toothpicks for construction materials or stick people requires a good deal of coordination.
Gross motor development (raisin treasure hunt). Make a treasure map leading to a treasure of individual boxes or containers of raisins. Children can be required to crawl

under tables, hop around chairs, and climb over gross motor equipment or appropriate furniture to find the treasure. You can substitute raisins for the "candy" associated with Easter, along with hard-cooked eggs.

Developmental Areas

The cognitive-interactionist approach and most other approaches to learning feature commonly emphasized areas or skills around which the objectives for a curriculum can be constructed. These areas are personal and social, sensorimotor, language, and perceptual-cognitive.

It is crucial to remember that some children are able to demonstrate all or most of the following behaviors as measured by teacher observation or objective-referenced instruments. Some children attain even higher levels of achievement, whereas others continue to progress toward mastery of some of these objectives during their primary school experience.

Personal and Social Development. Personal and social development involves becoming aware of the environment. Children identify themselves in relation to peers and others in their surroundings. Young children depend on adults to meet their needs, and this dependence motivates children to obey parents' rules and demands. Between the ages of about 2 and 3½ years children go through a transitional period where they are seeking independence and resisting adults. This is a time when the young child attempts to make independent decisions. Personal growth is evidenced by the child's ability to be independent.

In the next stage of development, from ages 3½ to 5 years, the child tries to win the approval and acceptance of peers and is becoming more sensitive to the opinions of adults. Children in this age group are friendly and cooperative. They begin to express emotions and seek solutions to problems. By seeking solutions children learn to control their behavior.

Children need to be loved, enjoyed, and needed. Preparing food helps children to feel both useful and needed and allows direct interaction with adults. Being able to complete a task and having others enjoy the finished product contribute to the child's self-worth and provide convenient avenues for meeting basic ego needs.

Sensorimotor Skill Development. Everything a child learns is dependent on sensorimotor skills. *Sensorimotor* refers to a combination of the input of sensations and the output of motor activity. It reflects the development of the central nervous system. To discover the functions of the body and its parts, the child will try all the possible muscular reactions, large muscle groups, and small muscle groups. Beginning at the head, muscle control moves to the foot in a systematic fashion. In addition, development takes place from the axis of the body outward to the periphery, the outer surfaces of the body.

The body can be used in a variety of ways during food preparation, thereby fostering the development of sensorimotor skills. Stirring, beating, slicing, rolling,

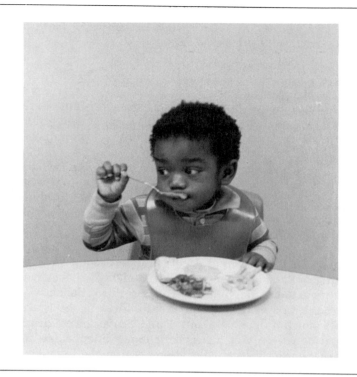

Figure 8-3
Sensorimotor skills are gradually mastered as the child develops.

breaking eggs, peeling, scrubbing, holding, spreading, and shaking are but a few of the movements that, with repetition, evidence gradual mastery and increased coordination (Figure 8-3).

Language Development—Receptive and Expressive. Language development depends on past sensorimotor experiences and exposure to a variety of people, places, and things. Language is learned through imitation and reinforcement. *Receptive language* is language that is spoken or written by others and received by the individual. The receptive language skills are listening and reading. *Expressive language* is language that is used in communicating with other individuals. Speaking and writing are expressive language skills.

Between the ages of 3 and 4, children acquire the ability to comprehend most of the language they will use in conversation throughout their lives. At 3 years of age most children use 900 words; by 4 years they use about 1550.

Expressing emotions and ideas is also vital to language development. Provide stimulating situations in which the child has ample time to give opinions and to express creatively without being interrupted. Language skills will affect all endeavors in learning. Having acquired these abilities, the child will be ready to attempt other learning skills.

Food preparation and serving are heavily supported by communication. The beginnings of communication are between parent and child during feeding. Mealtime can be a prime time for language stimulation as children become older. As children become involved in such situations as planning and preparing snacks and meals, receptive and expressive language are facilitated (Figure 8–4).

Perceptual-Cognitive Skill Development. Cognitive learning prospers when a child is socially competent, emotionally stable, and physically healthy. Cognitive objectives represent an intertwining of creative arts, mathematics, and science skills. A young child is a natural explorer, with a built-in curiosity mechanism that wants to find out how and why. Using real situations, an adult will be able to teach mathematical and scientific concepts. The child will learn to reason and analyze, developing processes for ordering, sorting, spatial relationships, sequencing, and becoming aware of the physical environment.

Providing meaningful experiences in the three areas of *creative arts—music, art, and drama—*develops a child's creativeness and improves self-concept. The

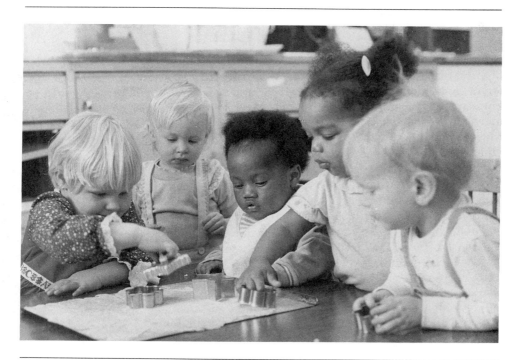

Figure 8–4
Expressive and receptive language development is facilitated while preparing snacks.

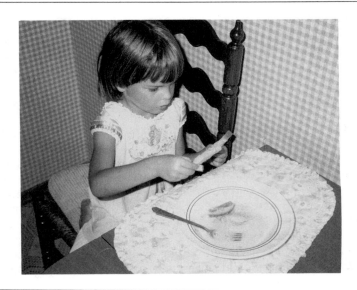

Figure 8–5
Cognitive learning develops through play.

creative arts can also be used to develop and improve personal and social, sensori-motor, and language skills. A social skill that could be taught is distinguishing between happy and sad music; a sensorimotor skill would be clapping and marching to the beat of a song or kneading or patting bread to the sound of music. Music education should encourage all types of movements and sounds. Art allows children to exhibit their view of the world. Because children love to role-play at this stage, drama activities should be an integral part of the curriculum. Children should be allowed to express themselves by acting out a nursery rhyme or a fairy tale or putting on dress-up clothes. Food puppets can help children express feelings about food and what food contributes to their well-being.

Taking part in food preparation is a good way to help create an environment rich in perceptual stimulation and to encourage use of all sensory receptors. The smells, tastes, sounds, textures, and sights of food are varied. As children arrange raw vegetables and fruits on a plate, they are exposed to a variety of textures, shapes, colors, and odors, with unlimited opportunities to discriminate perceptually (Figure 8–5).

OBJECTIVES AND NUTRITION EDUCATION

A curriculum plan serves as a framework through which the staff can implement various approaches to achieving nutrition education goals.

Before writing any curriculum, the teacher must first possess basic knowledge and concepts of the chosen field. In this case, before attempting to write a nutrition curriculum, the care giver should know basic food and nutrition concepts (Chapters 1 to 6) and should have developed a basic educational approach.

When writing a curriculum, the teacher must take the lead in developing a plan or procedure to reach defined goals. This procedure is similar to the development of plays for a football game. In each instance, someone must do the planning, which includes identifying elements and recognizing the inter-relationships that exist so that goals and objectives can be obtained at a specified time. A comprehensive system of steps in which all the elements are interrelated is vital. Steps in the system contribute to a common goal of improved nutrient intake through nutrition education.

Ten Steps

The following steps, essential in any curriculum, provide a systematic approach to instruction:

1. Developing objectives
2. Developing activities
3. Assessing entering skills
4. Choosing a teaching strategy
5. Organizing the group
6. Allocating time
7. Allocating space
8. Choosing teaching resources
9. Evaluating performance
10. Analyzing feedback

Developing Objectives.   The care giver first states in behavioral objectives what the learners should be able to do on completion of the curriculum. Learning objectives vary according to children's chronological age and developmental level. As was mentioned earlier, learning objectives are crucial to the development of an effective curriculum. The teacher must clearly define objectives for children not only to plan the curriculum but also to assess individual progress and to evaluate program effectiveness.

Early childhood programs must acknowledge developmental variability in children but be cognizant of objectives appropriate to their age level and toward which they should be progressing.

Developing Activities.   The care giver selects and develops activities that will help children attain the stated objectives. Content selection should include a variety of activities that are developmentally suitable for preschoolers.

Assessing Entering Skills.   The child's entering behavior must be evaluated. The teacher can make use of the previously developed behavioral objectives with a checklist to record the child's progress. Another approach is to develop an informal inventory to assess the child's existing knowledge of or skill in a particular area. This screening device might indicate a child's ability to define basic terms related to nutrition and the ability to describe basic concepts. For example, if all 3-year-olds can identify all the food items present, the care giver should progress to the next objective.

The essential question to be asked by the pretest is, To what extent has the child previously acquired the terms, concepts, and skills that are a part of this curriculum?

Choosing a Teaching Strategy. An approach should be chosen that will provide the teacher with a method to most effectively present learning activities. We have chosen the cognitive-interactionist approach previously discussed.

Organizing the Group. Group organization is determined by the objectives. Which objectives can be reached by the learner individually? Which objectives can be achieved only through interaction among the learners themselves? Which objectives can be achieved through a presentation by the teacher and interaction between the learners and the teacher?

Allocating Time. The teacher must estimate the time necessary to accomplish defined objectives, teaching strategies, and use of resources, considering the abilities and interest of the children. The teaching plan should take into account the estimated time for each type of activity. Yet no teacher should feel bound by any formula allocating time; rather, analyze the learning objectives and space availability and make the best use of each.

Allocating Space. Space allocation involves the decision to use or have available large spaces, small spaces, and independent learning spaces. Space should be allocated on the basis of meeting the objectives taught by the lesson.

Choosing Teaching Resources. While the teacher is the most important resource for the child, a variety of instructional materials also enable the learner to obtain knowledge.

Gerlach and Ely [2] classify resources into five general categories:

1. Real materials and people (care givers, cooks, parents, food, real things)
2. Visual materials for projection (videotapes, filmstrips, movie projectors, television, opaque projectors)
3. Audio materials (radio, recordings, tapes)
4. Printed materials (books, pictures, duplicating masters)
5. Display materials (food boxes, bulletin boards, flannel boards, chalk boards)

A good curriculum will make use of all these resource categories to provide a rich variety of learning experiences for the child.

Evaluating Performance.   A vital component of the curriculum, performance evaluation asks the question, Did the child meet the objective? When evaluating a preschool curriculum, the teacher observes the child's behavior and actions. Evaluation by child observation is naturally enhanced by properly stated behavioral objectives.

Analyzing Feedback.   The care giver asks, Is this approach to teaching effective? Are all the elements working together as a unit to do what was originally proposed? The care giver self-evaluates performance by continually analyzing the interaction of the children with the activities and by noting their performance evaluations. The teacher can observe not only the strong points the curriculum presents but also those areas that call for improvement. The teacher must be flexible enough to change activities or any step if the objectives are not being met.

Lesson Plans for Preschoolers

Now that you are familiar with a format for curriculum construction, you should be ready to begin the development of nutritional experiences that can be incorporated into the total early childhood program. The following plans follow the objective-oriented format. This formula can be adapted easily to any of the educational approaches (Chapter 7). The activities are used with the interactionist approach, where routines are as tangible and concrete for the children as possible. An activity may be listed under one particular skill but could be applied to several.

Personal and Social Skills

Gross Motor Skills

ACTIVITY: Tacos
OBJECTIVE: Child is able to take turns and share.
MATERIALS: Taco shells, ground beef, taco seasoning and sauce, head of lettuce, cheddar cheese, onions, tomatoes.
PROCEDURE: Divide the children into five small groups. Each is responsible for a particular task in preparing the tacos. Group One—cook ground beef, adding sauce and seasoning. Group Two—heat taco shells for 10 minutes and shred the head of lettuce. Group Three—chop onions. Use a manual chopper, not a sharp knife. Group Four—shred cheese. Group Five—chop tomatoes. All children will then take turns filling the taco shells halfway with ground beef and adding toppings.
EVALUATION: Children are observed meeting the stated objectives.

Sensorimotor Development

Gross Motor Skills

ACTIVITY: Making butter
OBJECTIVE: Child moves body to rhythm of music while making butter from whipped cream.

MATERIALS: Record "Alice's Restaurant"*, small jars with lids (baby food jars), whipping cream (at room temperature), salt (optional).
PROCEDURE:

1. Child or care giver pours 3 tablespoons of whipping cream into the small jars.
2. Child places lid on the jar.
3. The jar is shaken to the tune of "Alice's Restaurant" until whipping cream turns to butter (5 to 10 minutes).
4. Liquid is poured off butter into container. Butter is put into bowl (stirring will take out additional liquid).
5. A pinch of salt is added to butter for taste.
6. Butter can be spread on crackers or bread for eating, and liquid can be drunk.

EVALUATION: Child can keep beat of music until butter is made.

Fine Motor Skills

ACTIVITY: No-bake cookies
OBJECTIVE: The child rolls, pounds, squeezes, and pulls dough.
MATERIALS: Bowl, large spoon, measuring cups, drawing-type recipe that children can read, ½ cup wheat germ, 1½ cups peanut butter, 1½ cups brown sugar, 3 cups dried milk, ¾ cup graham cracker crumbs.
PROCEDURE:

1. Measure ingredients into bowl.
2. Mix ingredients with large spoon.
3. Take small amount of dough in hands and roll into small ball.
4. Roll balls in powdered sugar.

EVALUATION: Child is observed meeting the stated objective.

Kinesthetic Tactile Discrimination

ACTIVITY: Which food is missing?
OBJECTIVE: Child identifies food by touch.
MATERIALS: Ear of sweet corn, cauliflower, carrot (use items on menu), paper or cloth bag or covered can.
PROCEDURE:

1. Show children three types of food, and let them examine each by sight and touch.
2. Place the three foods in a bag or covered can.
3. Have the children remove the food you call for by touch identification only.
4. Replace the food and pass on to another group member.
5. Repeat the process.

EVALUATION: Child is observed meeting the stated objectives.

*Learning basic skills through music, Health and Safety, Vol. 3, AR526, Freeport, NY, 1970, Educational Activities, Inc.

Taste—Olfactory Discrimination

ACTIVITY: Taste and touch

OBJECTIVE: Child discriminates between the following taste qualities: sweet, sour, and salty.

MATERIALS: Variety of foods to taste, including three tastes distinguishable by a preschooler (sweet—fruit, salty—apple slice with salt, and sour—pickle or lemon); pictures of food items; blindfold.

PROCEDURE:

1. Blindfold child.
2. Have child taste item.
3. Remove blindfold.
4. Have child describe what was tasted.
5. Have child find picture of what was tasted.

EVALUATION: Child is observed meeting the stated objectives.

Auditory Discrimination and Memory

ACTIVITY: Rotten potato

OBJECTIVE: The child carries out a series of three or more directions.

MATERIALS: One sheet of poster board, lined and cut into 64 equal pieces; 16 foods from each of the food groups on the cards to facilitate pairing.

PROCEDURE: Play "Rotten Potato" using the same pairing format used when playing "Go Fish."

EVALUATION: Children observed meeting the stated objective.

Visual Discrimination and Memory

ACTIVITY: Tell a story with pictures

OBJECTIVE: The child describes objects or experiences from memory.

MATERIALS: Sequence cards depicting nutritional activity.

PROCEDURE:

1. Give the child cards depicting a previous food activity.
2. Have the child arrange the cards in the proper sequence (Figure 8-6).
3. Have the child relate the story to other children.

EVALUATION: Child is observed meeting the stated objective.

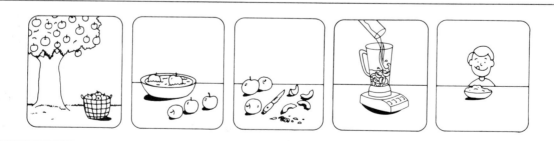

Figure 8-6
Sequence cards depicting the making of applesauce

Language Development (Receptive and Expressive)

ACTIVITY: Relating an experience

OBJECTIVE: Children dictate ideas in an organized, sequential pattern. This activity is to follow a field trip to an apple orchard.

MATERIALS: Newsprint, Magic Markers.

PROCEDURE: Following a trip to an apple orchard, the children dictate to the care giver their interpretation of the trip from its beginning until its end. The care giver records what the children say. This activity also helps children to listen and appreciate the contributions of others as well as enlarging their vocabulary. If the written material can be reproduced, parents enjoy seeing what the child has contributed.

EVALUATION: Children observed meeting the stated objectives.

Cognitive Development

Mathematics and Science Skills

ACTIVITY: Outline matching

OBJECTIVE: The child matches, recognizes, and identifies a variety of shapes. The child also establishes a one-on-one correspondence through matching.

MATERIALS: Two 12 × 18 inch pieces of poster board, outlines of food items to match shapes outlined on poster board (e.g., apple, lemon, banana, grape, peanut, lettuce).

PROCEDURE: Child takes food items out of box one at a time, names the item, and then attempts to place the object on its outline form. Teacher might say, "Can you find which shape this banana is on the answer board?"

EVALUATION: Child is observed meeting the stated objective.

Sets and Subsets

ACTIVITY: Choose a set

OBJECTIVE: The child identifies and constructs sets and subsets from 1 to 10.

MATERIALS: Pocket chart; numerals 1 through 5 written on top line of chart; index cards; pictures of basic food groups in 10 sets of 1, 10 sets of 2, 10 sets of 3, 10 sets of 4, and 10 sets of 5 glued on index cards.

PROCEDURE: The child counts the set on each card and matches the card with the appropriate numeral (i.e., child picks a card). Count five lemons and then place the card with five lemons on it in the pocket chart under the numeral 5.

EVALUATION: The child is observed using the number concepts.

Numeration and Place Value

ACTIVITY: Cans

OBJECTIVE: The child recognizes numerals 1 to 10.

MATERIALS: Ten tin cans, numerals 1 through 10 painted on cans, 55 peanuts in the shell.

PROCEDURE: Child puts the appropriate number of peanuts in the cans. Child then can arrange the cans in order 1 through 10.

EVALUATION: The child recognizes numerals.

Addition and Subtraction

ACTIVITY: Dry fruit mix
OBJECTIVE: The child adds by joining sets.
MATERIALS: Small paper plates for each child, dried fruit (e.g., banana slices, apricots, raisins, and apples).
PROCEDURE: Place small amounts of dried fruit mix on table in front of each child. Direct the child to put two apple slices on his plate. Now ask, "How many pieces of fruit are on your plate?" Next direct the child to add one banana slice. Then ask, "How many pieces of fruit do you have now?" or "How many pieces do you have all together?" Continue process by adding various sets according to the child's ability. When finished, let the child eat the fruit mix.
EVALUATION: Child is able to add or join sets.

Measurement

ACTIVITY: Cups
OBJECTIVE: Child identifies concepts of volume: full, half full, and empty.
MATERIALS: Clear plastic cups of various sizes, container for pouring material, pouring material (water, rice, navy beans, or cornmeal).
PROCEDURE: The teacher discusses and demonstrates the concepts of full, half full, and empty. The children are then given time to take a container and then pour the material following the teacher's or child's directions, "Give me a full cup," "Give me an empty cup," or "Give me a half-full cup." This activity can be reinforced at mealtime or snacktime.
EVALUATION: Child is observed meeting the stated objectives.

Fractions

ACTIVITY: Tangerines
OBJECTIVE: Child determines one half of the whole or small group.
MATERIALS: Tangerines (one per child); graph with children's names, one per column, with a different color for each child's area to aid in their visualization of the graph (Figure 8–7).
PROCEDURE:

1. Have the children peel their tangerines.
2. Break the tangerines into sections.
3. Let the children count their sections and circle the corresponding number on the graph.
4. Teacher-child interaction includes comparisons: "How many in Tim's tangerine?" "How many in Mary's tangerine?" "How many pieces make a whole tangerine?" "How many pieces in half of a tangerine?"

EVALUATION: Child is observed meeting the stated objective.

Geometry

ACTIVITY: Straight and curved
OBJECTIVE: The child recognizes straight and curved lines.

7	7	7	7	7
6	6	6	6	6
5	5	5	5	5
4	4	4	4	4
3	3	3	3	3
2	2	2	2	2
1	1	1	1	1

Sue Tim John Jack Mary Teri

Figure 8–7
Graph for visualizing number concepts

MATERIALS: An assortment of food-packaging materials (e.g., boxes, jars, cans, and bottles).
PROCEDURE:

1. The child examines the food packages.
2. The child separates the packages into two classifications—those with straight planes and those with curved planes.

EVALUATION: Child is observed meeting the stated objective.

Problem Solving

ACTIVITY: Use of a recipe
OBJECTIVE: Child uses the five senses to gather information and then communicates observations to others.
MATERIALS: Illustrated recipe, ingredients for recipe.
PROCEDURE: Give the child an illustrated recipe; see whether the child can "cook" from the recipe.
EVALUATION: Child is observed meeting the stated objective.

Creative Arts

ACTIVITY (ART): Drawing
OBJECTIVE: Child expresses a mental image, design, or happening from actual experience or verbal motivations. This activity follows a field trip to an apple orchard.
MATERIALS: Crayons (primary colors), newsprint.
PROCEDURE: Children are to draw and color their interpretations of the field trip highlights.

ADDITIONAL ACTIVITY: Children can make applesauce, then use the stems, seeds, and peelings to make a collage.

EVALUATION: Children are observed meeting the stated objective.

Sociodramatic Play

ACTIVITY: Fruit stand

OBJECTIVE: The child interprets realistic roles played by family and community members.

MATERIALS: Variety of fruits, shopping bags, a stand made from a refrigerator packing box or cardboard box of similar size, a scale.

PROCEDURE: Set up a fruit stand. Have some small boxes filled with a variety of fruits and set up a cash register, shopping bags, and a scale. After the children have purchased the fruit, they can use it as a snack.

EVALUATION: Children are observed meeting the stated objective.

As stated earlier, the curriculum serves as a guide for the teacher. Often curriculums are placed in folders, filed away, and used only when programs are evaluated or scrutinized by outside consultants. This should not be allowed to happen. A curriculum should always be open-ended. One should keep it updated with new activities and approaches.

RECIPES FOR NONREADERS

The menu, if planned with cooperation between food service personnel and care giver, is perhaps the best tool with which to teach nutrition education; creating a food product in the classroom is also exciting and fun for care giver and student. Often the first task in deciding what to cook is selecting a recipe. There are many cookbooks for children with illustrated recipes for nonreaders. However, any standard cookbook recipe may be used for cooking in the preschool center.

Use of a Recipe for Nonreaders

One of the most important lessons in reading readiness for the preschool student is that words have value. They tell us something. In a recipe, they tell us how to make something that we want to eat. The preschooler discovers that reading is something that can be personally exciting and useful.

By reorganizing, simplifying, and using illustrations, a recipe can be written so that a preschooler can read it nearly independently. A properly organized recipe gives the child such prereading skills as top-to-bottom and left-to-right sequencing. Most recipes as they appear in cookbooks do not do this. Usually the ingredients are listed, followed by a series of instructions. The teacher can rewrite the recipe on a large poster so that cooking can progress from the first to the last step in sequence. (These posters should be saved and used again and again.) After a few cooking experiences, the child will be able to help you to

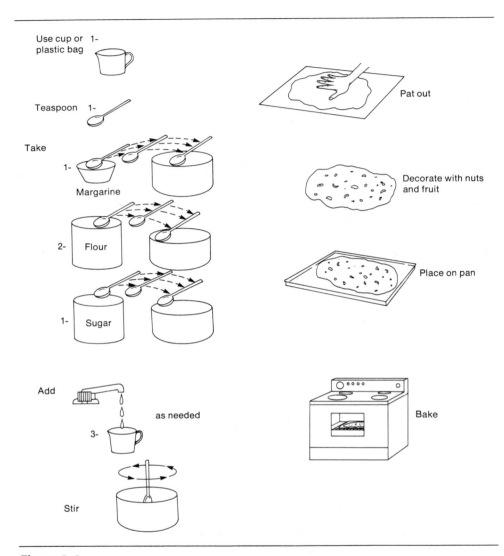

Use cup or 1-
plastic bag

Teaspoon 1-

Take

1-
Margarine

2- Flour

1- Sugar

Add

as needed

3-

Stir

Pat out

Decorate with nuts
and fruit

Place on pan

Bake

Figure 8-8
A recipe poster for nonreaders for "Never-Fail Cookies"

read the next step in sequence and will recognize the words that appear frequently on recipe posters.

The large recipe poster also teaches a variety of math concepts: numeral
recognition, counting, measurement, and so on. Following the steps of a recipe
gives an added dimension to the actual measuring the child is doing and gives
the children who are waiting their turn something to refer to as they help count
the ingredients being added. Figure 8-8 is a recipe for nonreaders for "Never-
Fail Cookies," which can be made as follows:

EQUIPMENT: Cookie sheet; oven (preheat to 350° to 375° F); old newspapers for floor; waxed paper—approximately 12 × 12 inch pieces, one piece per child—or plastic bags; washcloth and water or hand-washing facilities nearby; deep cup and spoon; napkins or paper towels for eating cookies; at least 3 large bowls; 3 serving tablespoons; and 3 serving teaspoons.

INGREDIENTS: Margarine (shortening or fat); sugar (granulated or brown); flour (whole wheat) with 1 teaspoon baking powder per cup of flour; water or milk; decorative items such as raisins, coconut flakes, fruit, and nuts (chopped). Allow approximately 1½ tablespoons of the ingredient per child (e.g., 10 children = 1 cup fat, 1 cup sugar, and 1¼ cups flour).

PROCEDURE: The child takes a spoon of each of the ingredients from the bowls and places it on waxed paper. The child then makes one cookie and puts it on the cookie sheet. The teacher observes and adds more liquid or flour as needed. The cookies may be marked with a slip of paper. Have children help put cookies into oven. After cookies are cool, children can remove them to a plate. Sit at a table or in a circle to review activities for children, and let children explain what they have accomplished.

NOTE: A "never-fail muffin" can be made using the same principles. The child should add eggs (one or two), milk, and raisins, nuts, or fruit to the batter. The batter must be thinner, and the child uses bowl and spoon. Personal experiences with 3-year-olds indicate that they can accomplish this task! (No matter what the product looks like they eat it!)

Reading, math, and science skills have much more value if the child actually experiences them. Cooking affords this opportunity. A recipe allows you to expose the child to a number of specific academic skills without formal instruction.

In using a recipe with preschoolers, do not belabor each step or insist that they understand each concept (Figure 8–9). Treat the recipe as a tool. For example, say, "Let's see what we do first." Ask occasional questions about what

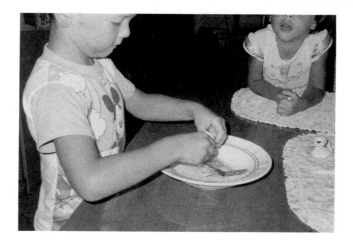

Figure 8–9
A child learns from experience.

you are doing, and let the children's comments and questions guide the discussion. Let the equipment and ingredients be the tools to stimulate the discussion.

COOKING IN THE CLASSROOM

Relatively few early childhood programs have child-sized cooking facilities; therefore, electrical appliances are frequently used. When using electrical appliances, be sure that the equipment is in proper working order. It is dangerous to allow children to stand on stools and chairs to do stove-top cooking in the kitchen. No matter where cooking is done or how, safety precautions must be emphasized, and supervision is imperative. Children can be taught the precautions to use around cooking equipment. There will undoubtedly be some burns and cuts, but it is hoped that with adequate supervision these will not be serious.

If a child should get burned or cut, administer first aid immediately. Sharp knives should be kept by the teacher. The children can be taught how to use them properly for slicing, cutting, or chopping but only under close supervision. Of course, along with food preparation comes cleanup. Children can and should be involved in the various cleanup chores, which vary from wiping counter tops and tables to washing, rinsing, and drying dishes. The degree of involvement in cleanup will depend on the facilities and legal requirements.

Classroom Recipes

Dried Fruit Treats

MATERIALS: Food grinder, crackers (to clean grinder), measuring cup, large mixing bowl and spoon, shallow bowl for sugar, platter for finished candy.

1 C raisins	1 C dried apricots
1 C dried prunes	Powdered sugar or coconut
(pitted)	flakes

Put the raisins, prunes, and apricots through a grinder. Run a few crackers through the grinder after the fruit. They will clean the grinder so any fruit sticking to it will not be wasted, and the crackers can be added to the candy. Mix the ground dried fruit together. Make small balls of it with your hands. Roll the balls in powdered sugar so they will not be sticky. Lay them on waxed paper to get firm.

NOTE: You can also roll this candy in coconut flakes.

ACTIVITIES: This cooking activity is especially useful in teaching the following:

1. *Social studies.* This recipe comes from a book prepared for use by cooks in Alaska, including Eskimo women. Lead the children through a discussion of why raisins and other dried fruits might be especially important in Alaska.
   a. How are these foods prepared?
   b. How long can they be stored?
   c. How long can fresh grapes be stored?

d. Which other methods of food preparation and storage might people in a cold climate use?

2. *Motor development.* The grinding, mixing, and rolling of the fruit into balls give great opportunity for physical involvement.

3. *Math*
   a. Compare the volume of fruit before and after grinding.
   b. Compare weight before and after.
   c. How many candy balls can be made?
   d. Are they all the same size?

4. *Safety.* Teach proper use of food grinder and discuss cleanliness.

Polka-Dot Bread

MATERIALS: Measuring cups, measuring spoons, saucepan, large mixing bowl and spoon, portable mixer, flour sifter, loaf pan (8½ × 4½ × 2½ inches), shortening to grease pan, knife to level measure, timer.

1½ C seedless raisins	1 tbsp grated orange peel
1½ C water	2½ C sifted whole-wheat flour
1 slightly beaten egg	1 tsp salt
1 C dark brown sugar	2 tsp baking powder
2 tbsp salad oil	½ tsp soda

Combine raisins and water; let soak. Mix next four ingredients. Stir in raisin mixture. Sift together dry ingredients; beat well. Pour into greased loaf pan. Bake at 325° F for about 60 minutes or until done.

ACTIVITIES: This classroom cooking activity is useful in teaching the following:

1. *Socioemotional development.* Send a child home with a slice of warm bread to share with parents. Few mothers can resist asking questions about bread still hot from the oven. The children also feel a sense of accomplishment because they have completed a complicated job. Let the children help decide how to share the work of completing the recipe. Let them decide how to share the finished product equally.

2. *Math.* Using a large poster recipe, let the children "read" how many cups or teaspoons of each ingredient should be added. Have them keep track of how many cups of flour or teaspoons of baking powder have been added and how many more are needed. Discuss baking time—units, measurement, and importance. Discuss oven temperature—units and importance of the numbers on the dial.

3. *Science.* Talk about the various ingredients used—liquids, powders, and so on. Discuss changes in texture and color, from the mixing of liquid and flour, to completed batter, and finally to baked bread. How does the oven stay at one temperature? Discuss preheating. What would happen if we changed oven temperatures or timing? Use a toothpick to test for doneness. Start testing 10 minutes or more before it should be done, or lower the temperature and see whether the bread is done in the length of time stated in the recipe.

4. *Safety.*
   a. Why can we not put our finger in the batter for a taste?

b. Give each child a Popsicle stick for a "lick."
c. Why can we not use the stick more than once?
d. Why do we have hot pads as cooking equipment today?
e. Encourage children to set safety rules for use of the stove.

Banana Krunchies

MATERIALS: Waxed paper, plastic knife.

Bananas
Wheat germ

Give each child half of a banana. Let the children slice the bananas into small pieces. Place approximately 2 tbsp of wheat germ on the waxed paper. Let the children roll the banana slices in the wheat germ until completely covered.

ACTIVITIES: This classroom cooking activity is especially useful in teaching the following:

1. *Motor development.* Fine motor skills can be developed by peeling, slicing, and rolling the bananas.
2. *Language development*
   a. Descriptive terms can be learned or reinforced: smooth, ripe, firm, crunchy, hard, soft.
   b. Verb tense can be expressed (past, present, and future): "We *had* a whole banana; we *have* half a banana now; we *will* slice the banana."
3. *Reading and writing*
   a. After completing the recipe, help the children record their "cooking" experience. A large classroom chart can be constructed by illustrating the recipe with simple pictures or drawings of the steps involved.
   b. Individual recipes can be sent home with the children to share with their parents. Repeating the recipe at home reinforces the experience and gives meaning to the written words on the recipe.

Yogofroosicle

MATERIALS: Small paper cups, Popsicle sticks, mixing bowl and spoon.

1 6 oz can frozen juice concentrate (any flavor)
1 pint yogurt
1 tsp vanilla

Mix the ingredients until well blended. Pour mixture into paper cups. Place cups in the freezer. Add Popsicle stick to each when the mixture is thick and slushy. Continue freezing until the yogofroosicles are completely hard.

ACTIVITIES: This classroom cooking activity is especially useful in teaching the following:

1. *Science*
   a. Simple concepts can be learned, including changes in states of matter and cause-and-effect relationships (freezing, melting).
   b. Concentration (juice) can be explained.

2. *Social studies*
    a. Where did yogurt originate?
    b. How is it used in different countries and cultures?
3. *Nutrition*
    a. What nutritional value is there in yogurt? In juice?
    b. Which other ways can we use yogurt in cooking?
    c. Introduce the many varieties of juices and their nutritional value.
4. *Math*
    a. One-to-one correspondence can be learned: one paper cup for each child, one popsicle stick for each cup.
    b. Children can learn measuring concepts. In this recipe we used ounces to measure the juice, a teaspoon to measure the vanilla, and a pint to measure the yogurt.

Fruit Kabob

MATERIALS: Toothpicks, plastic knives, cutting board.

Bananas
Strawberries

Cut a banana into three sections. Give each child one section and two or three whole strawberries. Help the children cut the strawberries and bananas into slices. Give each child three toothpicks. Have them alternately place a strawberry, then a banana on a toothpick until it is full.

ACTIVITIES: This classroom cooking activity is especially useful in teaching the following:

1. *Language development*
    a. The children can learn the names of equipment they are using (toothpicks, cutting board).
    b. The teacher can present new words by presenting them in a demonstrative manner. "We will slice the banana into three sections—just about this thick."
2. *Fine motor skills.* This activity uses both hands to push the fruit onto the toothpick. This is a complex activity that also promotes eye-hand coordination.
3. *Math.* The division of the banana provides an excellent opportunity for counting and for discussion of concepts such as quantity and equivalents.

Purple Cow

MATERIALS: Measuring cups, blender, cups for serving

½ C plain yogurt
½ C milk
½ C unsweetened grape juice

Mix ingredients in blender and serve.

ACTIVITIES: This classroom cooking activity is especially useful in teaching the following:

1. *Math*
   a. Explain the concept of equal parts. All ingredients in this recipe are of the same amount—½ cup.
   b. Discuss the difference between a half and a whole. (Explain that a whole is twice as much as a half.)
2. *Science*
   a. Discuss the color change when all ingredients are mixed together.
   b. Explain the transformation from milk to yogurt.
3. *Safety.* Instruct the children on the proper use of the blender and discuss the importance of safety when using any electrical appliance.
4. *Motor and perceptual skills.* Allow the children to pour the "purple" milk into serving cups. This develops manipulation skills and eye-hand control.

Popcorn

MATERIALS: Corn popper (with transparent top, if possible), paper cups for individual servings.

½ C popcorn
2 tbsp oil

Soak the popcorn in oil; pour into the corn popper and pop!
ACTIVITIES: This classroom cooking activity is especially useful in teaching the following:

1. *Sensory development.* All the senses can be tapped through this experience:
   a. *Sight.* The children observe the color differences between the popped and unpopped corn.
   b. *Sound.* The children hear and describe the sounds of the oil heating and the wonderful sounds of the corn as it pops.
   c. *Smell.* They notice the aroma of the popcorn as it cooks.
   d. *Taste.* They can eat popcorn that is cooked; they cannot eat popcorn that is not cooked. They can compare the difference in taste of popcorn with and without salt.
2. *Science*
   a. Condensation can be described as the moisture gathers inside the corn popper during the heating stage.
   b. Encourage thought about prediction of future action, "What will happen when this unpopped corn gets hot inside the corn popper?" (It *will* jump; it *will* burst; it *will* pop.)
3. *Social studies.* Unshelled popcorn is available in some areas. This could lead to a discussion as to where popcorn comes from, where it originated, and so on.
4. *Language development.* Children can learn certain grammatical structures:
   a. Is this corn popped or unpopped? Is it cooked or uncooked?
   b. Would you like your popcorn salted or unsalted?
   c. Some people like popcorn buttered; others like it unbuttered.

Kid's Quiche

MATERIALS: Measuring cups, measuring spoons, knife for chopping, grater, large bowl for mixing, a pie plate.

1 C creamed cottage cheese
½ C plain yogurt
1½ C grated cheese (cheddar, Monterey Jack, or Swiss.)
3 eggs
½ tsp dry mustard
½ tsp salt
1 small onion, chopped or grated
½ tsp curry powder

Mix everything together until well blended. Pour mixture into a lightly greased pie plate. Bake for 10 minutes at 425° F and then for 15 minutes at 350° F.

ACTIVITIES: This classroom activity is especially useful in teaching the following:

1. *Nutrition*
   a. Allow children to observe the various ingredients. Explain that cottage cheese, yogurt, and grated cheese are all part of the milk group.
   b. Discuss the nutritional value of milk products.
   c. Identify the seasoning ingredients in the recipe. Why do we use seasonings?
2. *Language development*
   a. How do the tastes, colors, and textures of the ingredients differ? (Allow children to express these differences.)
   b. Some seasonings (salt) are also used to prevent spoilage of foods. (Discuss fresh foods and spoilage.)
3. *Science*
   a. Stress the importance of accurate measurement and timing of the baking process.
   b. Adjustments in temperature are necessary to prevent burning of the quiche.
4. *Social studies.* Where did *quiche* originate?

Munchwich

MATERIALS: Knife for chopping, measuring cups, measuring spoons.

⅓ C chopped peanuts
⅓ C dried apricots
⅓ C chopped, pitted dates
⅓ C raisins
4 oz cream cheese, softened
2 tbsp orange juice

Mix peanuts, apricots, dates, and raisins. Cream together cream cheese and orange juice. Blend everything together and spread on whole-grain bread.

ACTIVITIES: This classroom cooking activity is useful in teaching the following:

1. *Motor development.* Chopping, mixing, and spreading develop manipulation and eye-hand coordination.
2. *Nutrition.* Discuss the value of dried fruit (nutritive value and longer storage).
3. *Language development.* The ingredients in this recipe can stimulate a great deal of discussion:
   a. Discuss differences in color, size, shape, and texture.
   b. Classify the ingredients according to food groups.
   c. Descriptive terms can be emphasized: crunchy, hard, soft, ripe, dried, sweet, salty.

Friendship Salad

MATERIALS: Mixing bowl and spoon, knife for chopping, cutting board, orange juice for dipping fruit, paper cups for serving.

Each child brings a piece of fresh fruit from home. This can be planned the day before preparation.
Wash fruit. Pare and core fruits, if needed. Chop fruit. Slice bananas, apples, and pears into orange juice to prevent darkening. Mix all fruit together. Serve.
ACTIVITIES: This classroom cooking activity is useful in teaching the following:

1. *Socioemotional development*
   a. Children learn a great deal about cooperation. They learn that working together can be fun and beneficial to everyone.
   b. They learn responsibility for planning, bringing food from home, preparing, and sharing in the work experience.
2. *Math*
   a. Children can learn through a counting experience: "We have one apple; how many raisins do we have? Let's count them. Do we have more cherries or more raisins?"
   b. They can learn one-to-one correspondence. "If we have six children, how many different kinds of fruit will we have?"
3. *Language development.* Children can learn to compare and contrast: "The apple is round; what other fruit do we have that is round?" "The banana and cherry are different—how are they different?" (Discuss size, shape, and color.)
4. *Motor development.* The children learn fine coordination skills through peeling, chopping, and slicing.
5. *Science*
   a. They learn the concept of "sink and float" by dropping the various pieces of chopped fruit into the orange juice.
   b. They learn to predict by guessing which fruit will sink or float.
   c. They can speculate as to why these things happen.

Guacamole Dip

MATERIALS: Fork for mashing, mixing bowl, measuring spoons, knife for chopping.

1 large ripe avocado
1 medium onion, minced

1 tbsp lemon juice
1 large tomato, peeled and chopped
Dash of Tabasco sauce
¼ tsp pepper

Mash avocado with a fork. Mix all the ingredients together until well blended. Serve as a dip with a variety of raw vegetables or whole wheat crackers.
ACTIVITIES: This classroom cooking activity is useful in teaching the following:

1. *Social studies*
   a. Avocadoes were originally grown in Mexico. They are also grown in the United States today (California, Florida, and Hawaii).
   b. Some people call avocados "alligator pears" because of the shape, the color, and the rough texture.
2. *Science*
   a. The seed can be removed and allowed to root. The children can plant the seed and watch it grow into a tree.
   b. Discuss the shape of the seed.
   c. Discuss what seeds and plants need in order to grow.
3. *Motor development.* Mashing, mixing, and dipping enhance motor development.

Energy Marbles

MATERIALS: Measuring cups, knife for leveling, large mixing bowl and spoon, tray for chilling the finished product.

1 C sugar-free peanut butter
⅓ C instant nonfat dry milk
¼ C sesame seeds
¼ C raisins
½ C unsweetened coconut

Mix all ingredients and roll into small balls. Chill and eat.
ACTIVITIES: This classroom cooking activity is useful in teaching the following:

1. *Health*
   a. Why do we need energy?
   b. Which foods in this recipe provide us with energy?
   c. Why is it important to have clean hands before rolling the dough into balls?
2. *Math*
   a. Discuss the differences between the portion sizes of the ingredients (e.g., "Is the ¼-cup measuring cup smaller or larger than the ½-cup?").
   b. Allow the children to count the number of balls as they are rolling them and also count the total number at the conclusion of the recipe.
   c. Do we have more dough now that it is in little balls? Do we have less dough now than we had in the beginning? Is it the same amount?

3. *Science*
   a. Compare the textures of the different ingredients.
   b. Compare the distinct color differences and make use of prediction skills ("What color do you think it will be if we mix everything together?").
   c. Discuss how dry milk may be changed from a powder to a liquid by adding water.
4. *Motor development.* The stirring, mixing, and rolling of the dough facilitate motor development.

Crispy Baked Potatoes

MATERIALS: Cookie sheet, timer, sharp knife for cutting.

Medium baking potatoes
Butter or margarine

Cut potatoes in half, lengthwise, and place flat side down on a buttered cookie sheet, Bake at 400° F for 30 minutes.

ACTIVITIES: This classroom cooking activity is useful in teaching the following:

1. *Math.* The children can compare the concepts of "whole" and "half."
   a. How many halves equal whole?
   b. How does the shape of the potato change after being cut in half?
2. *Nutrition and safety*
   a. Teach the proper handling of sharp knives.
   b. Teach the precautions necessary for working with a hot oven.
   c. Stress the importance of cleaning the potatoes before baking. "Scrub the potato skins to get them clean—we can eat the skins because they have vitamins and minerals, too."
3. *Socioemotional development.* Because each potato is halved, two children will share one original potato. Stress the importance of sharing and encourage an atmosphere of cooperation.
4. *Science.* Potatoes are grown all over the world. Children can be taught that they grow under the ground and are called *tubers.*

SUMMARY

- By integrating food and nutrition concepts into various curriculum areas, the total early childhood curriculum can be used and enhanced.
- The menu can be considered the major raw material in planning and implementing learning activities in early childhood education.
- The major consideration in selecting a food for use in the curriculum should be the nutritional quality of the food.
- Curriculum objectives for preschool programs usually emphasize the following areas of development: personal and social, sensorimotor, language, and perceptual-cognitive.

- To write an effective nutrition curriculum, one must possess a knowledge of basic food and nutrition concepts.
- A systematic approach to instruction must be operational for a curriculum to be successful. The elements involved must be recognized as interrelated; steps in the system contribute to improved nutrient intake through nutrition education.
- Teaching preschoolers that words have value is very important for reading readiness. A recipe can be rewritten by simplifying, reorganizing, and including symbols or illustrations to facilitate the child's reading and understanding of it.
- An important component of nutrition education is safety during food preparation. Safety precautions should be emphasized, and supervision is imperative.

DISCUSSION QUESTIONS

1. Explain how mealtime experiences can function as settings for nutrition education.
2. Why is the menu considered the major raw material in planning and implementing learning activities in early childhood education?
3. Discuss the importance of selecting foods high in nutrient density for use in the curriculum.
4. Name and explain the four developmental areas used to integrate food and nutrition activities into the learning environment.
5. List and describe the steps involved in a systematic approach to instruction.
6. How are learning objectives crucial to the development of an effective curriculum?
7. Explain how you would convert a recipe from a standard cookbook into one that would stimulate learning in preschoolers.
8. List some precautions to be observed when cooking in the classroom.

REFERENCES

1. Clemens, B.: Presentation in elementary education 422 health and nutrition class, Edwardsville, 1976, Southern Illinois University.

2. Gerlach, V. S., and Ely, D. P.: Teaching and media: a systematic approach, Englewood Cliffs, NJ, 1971, Prentice-Hall, Inc.

SUGGESTED READINGS

Elkind, D.: Child development and education—a Piagetian perspective, New York, 1976, Oxford University Press, Inc.

Hendrick, J.: Total learning: developmental curriculum for the young child, 3rd ed., Columbus, OH, 1990, Merrill Publishing Co.

Hendrick, J.: The whole child, Columbus, OH, 1988, Merrill Publishing Co.

Marotz, L., Rush, J., and Cross, M.: Health, safety and nutrition for the young child, Albany, NY, 1985, Delmar Inc.

Rockwell, R. E., Sherwood, E. A., and Williams, R. A.: Hug a tree and other things to do outdoors with young children, Mt. Rainier, MD, 1983, Gryphon House, Inc.

Williams, R. A., Rockwell, R. E., and Sherwood, E. A.: Mudpies to magnets—a preschool science curriculum, Mt. Rainier, MD, 1987, Gryphon House, Inc.

APPENDIX 8-A Goals for an Effective Early Childhood Program

The State of Missouri Department of Elementary and Secondary Education suggests the following goals for establishing effective early childhood education programs in its *Focus on Early Childhood Education: Resource Guide for the Education of Children Ages Three to Six* (Jefferson City, MO, 1974). The child should be able to:

1. Develop and maintain a positive feeling about himself and about his own abilities to create and to learn.
2. Expand his awareness of the world around him through many sensory experiences—opportunities to see, hear, taste, feel, smell—that are prerequisites for developing concepts and solving problems.
3. Develop language through listening, speaking, and dramatic play activities, which form the basis for reading, writing, and other communication skills.
4. Develop maximum physical growth and health through motor activities and proper nutrition.
5. Understand his strengths and limitations, and cope with success, failure, and change.
6. Express verbal and nonverbal feelings, such as joy, happiness, fear, and anger, in acceptable ways.
7. See himself as a part of mankind who shows respect and concern for the rights and property of others.
8. Develop a reverence for life.
9. Become self-directing, with the ability to use freedom by providing him with opportunities to explore, create, and make choices.

Students will be able to

- Describe the value of parent involvement in early childhood nutrition programs
- List several methods of contacting parents regarding the nutrition education program
- Identify and describe ways in which parents' contributions of time and talent can be used for nutrition education programs
- Describe the need for evaluation of parent-involvement programs
- Identify and describe methods of recognizing parent contributions of time and talent

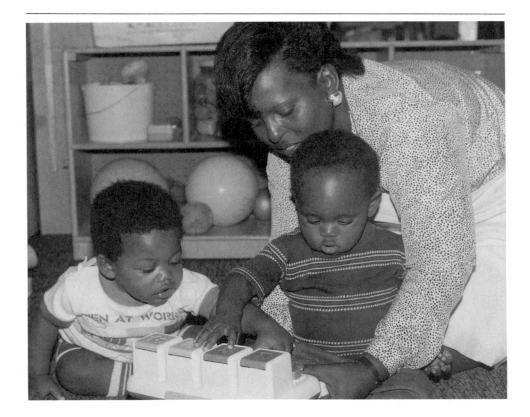

9

Parent Involvement in Nutrition Education

The child masters many skills during the first 6 years of life. Learning to eat is one of the most important. What the parent learns about nutrition, food, food preparation, and the importance of mealtime in the home all help to mold the child's food habits and attitudes.

Early childhood programs provide an excellent setting for nutrition education for the entire family. Therefore, it seems only practical that some ideas and approaches for working effectively with parents be discussed (Figure 9–1).

There has been an increasing interest, which has gained momentum over the past decade, in parent involvement at both the preschool and elementary school levels. Parent involvement has long been recognized as an essential part of a high-quality educational experience. Programs generated by the Great Cities Projects of the sixties, the Elementary and Secondary Education Act, and the War on Poverty have all placed heavy emphasis on some form of parent participation [1]. The major focus of this emphasis has been founded on the theory that if the school and parents work together as partners, the result will be success for the child at school.

WHY INVOLVE PARENTS?

Parents and early childhood programs need to be involved with each other because they have a common element—children. The home and preschool are important functional areas for the young child. To assist the child and to provide the most effective learning environment, both preschool and home must be in cooperation, pulling together to benefit the child. Lack of cooperation and

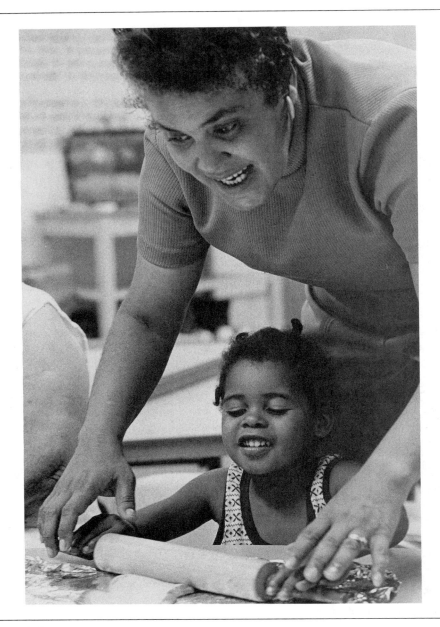

Figure 9–1
Nutrition education involves the entire family.

understanding between the two forces most instrumental in a young child's development can serve only to foster frustration and anxiety. Explicit conflict of purposes may result. When parents participate, the child knows the parents care enough to become involved. Lines of communication are open because there is an additional bond. The early childhood nutrition program can provide an avenue to unite parent and child in sound nutrition practices.

In a position statement on nutrition standards in day-care programs, the American Dietetic Association stresses, "Day care providers should develop and implement a nutrition education plan that will help children, parents, families, and personnel involved in the care of children make informal decisions affecting their health and well being [2]."

A by-product of parental involvement is that parents themselves benefit. The sense of being needed and useful is evident among those parents who have become involved in various center programs. There is a sense of giving of oneself. At the same time parents learn how they may best help their youngsters at home, how they can provide a nutritious meal and snacks, or exciting ways in which they can introduce new foods.

Finally, the children's care givers benefit from parental involvement. For example, parent contributions of time and talent often free teachers for instruction and perhaps allow more time for individualization. In addition, parents provide a basis for a more thorough understanding of a child and the child's nutritional habits, thereby assisting the teacher in providing a stimulus to help the child acquire better food habits. The answer to why early childhood programs should seek to involve parents is to enhance the overall development of the children.

First Steps in Getting Parents Involved

If it is agreed that parent involvement is beneficial to children, how can early childhood educators encourage such parent participation in the nutrition program? Where does a teacher begin? Which methods may be worth trying? The following sections give several methods of initiating parent involvement. One or several of the methods may be used to motivate participation in children's learning experiences about food. Modifications and adaptations for specific neighborhoods and their specific needs must be made, of course, but by taking advantage of these ideas some forward movement in parent-teacher cooperation should be evident.

Informal Contacts.   Most of the initial contacts with parents can be made on an informal basis. Some will be incidental, a matter of taking advantage of a given situation. Perhaps when a parent stops by to pick up a child for a doctor appointment, if time permits, a teacher should move toward the door with a smile and at least say a few words about the eating activities of the child. In casual conversations so often a parent says, "If there is anything I can do, please let me know." They do not really expect the teacher to say, "As a matter of fact, there is something you can do." But the gate is open, and a teacher or director can step in with a simple way in which that parent can assist the child or the program.

The same procedure of openness and friendly conversation can be used during a center open house, parent-teacher conference periods, and parent meetings. When parents feel at ease and get the idea that their child will benefit, they are more willing to contribute their time and talent.

Registration. Another opportunity for the center to encourage parent participation occurs at registration. If a parent is asked to fill out a registration form, a simple and general statement such as "I will volunteer to help the center in food and nutrition activities (yes _____ no _____)" might be included. Or an open-ended statement such as "I will volunteer to assist my child in the program by _____ " could be used. If a secretary or teacher fills out a registration form while interviewing the parents, willingness to help could be ascertained through casual conversation. However, the interviewer must be careful to broach the subject in a matter-of-fact way so that no pressure to participate is felt by the parent.

Resource Person. Once the children are in the classroom, the teacher should be alert to any comments they might make about what their parents do. For example, if a child casually mentions that his family has beehives in the backyard, the teacher should determine through reviews of the records or even a phone call to the parents whether the family would be willing to share their special interest. Perhaps the parents have some slides, a beehive, or just some frames with honey on them to show the children. They might enjoy bringing samples of honey for the children to taste or sitting and talking with the children about bees. Pictures or slides might be provided by the teacher so the learning situation would be a cooperative effort. Many parents have skills or hobbies in which children are interested, and they might be flattered to be asked to share them in the center. It may be necessary for the teacher to reassure them and to preplan together, but parents are often fine resources for specific areas of study and should never be overlooked.

A Special Letter. A direct way to find out whether parents are willing volunteers is to send a letter telling them that their help is needed. Specific tasks for which they could volunteer should be included in an interest inventory that accompanies the letter. The inventory should provide an open-ended section to enable the parent volunteer to suggest activities that may not have been listed. Frequently parents are most willing to volunteer their talents, but when asked to list them, they respond in a limited manner.

Orientation. Just a few days before the beginning of a program year, all parents may be invited to attend an informal "get-acquainted-with-our-room" program—an orientation. Each parent is invited to the center and meets with the teacher and all the other parents. The teacher presents the routine for activities as well as the food and nutrition program. During this time the teacher extends an invitation for parental assistance and has a prepared list of some kinds of activities for which help is needed. For example, if parent aides are to be used daily for eating activities, a sign-up sheet should be available. Those parents who would like to go on field trips or who could provide transportation could sign another sheet so labeled. The teacher might merely keep a list of those who say they would like to help and then determine later which specific contribution might be preferred by the parent. However, advanced planning helps parents commit their time.

Standardized Informational Techniques. Techniques for exchanging information between the parents and the care giver must be standardized and clear, particularly in infant programs. Nutritional information passed between the home and center always involves the accurate recording of daily and nightly occurrences such as times of feeding and types and amounts of food. In addition, naps, diaper changes, amount of sleep, unusual behavior, and home routines are recorded on standardized forms (see Appendixes 9-A, 9-B, 9-C, 9-D, 9-E). Sharing information helps to establish a sense of trust and a partnership between the home and the center as it contributes to an accurate 24-hour record of the child's health and well-being.

Newsletter. Another method of maintaining home-center contact is the newsletter. A monthly newsletter can include a copy of the menus and the activities that have been used to help children "get to know" the foods on the menu. The newsletter also provides an opportunity to list materials needed from home for classroom activities involving food, to present recipes used, and to solicit recipes parents have used with children. Nutrition information may also be included.

Home Visits. The most time-consuming method of contact with parents, but probably the most successful and beneficial to all, is the home visit. It takes a special type of teacher—one who is extroverted and personable—to call on parents in the home. The first visit should be brief and introductory and should provide a basis for future participation and involvement in *all* aspects of the program. During such visits, which preferably are arranged ahead of time, it is imperative that the teacher convey understanding and interest in the child and his family. During the visit it may become apparent that the family does not have the financial resources to supply the child with a wide variety of food experiences, as has been advocated in earlier chapters. However, use of the food stamp or commodity program can help the family continue the nutrition education objectives of the center.

Ways in Which to Use Parent Contributions

Once parent-center contacts have been made—and this may be a continuing process throughout the year—initiation of actual involvement must begin. Parent contributions will be more meaningful if parents are given an opportunity to plan with the care giver those areas that they mutually believe can be of benefit to the program. One goal for the care giver is to be organized but not so static that parents think their suggestions and ideas are not welcomed. In presenting options to the parent, the care giver may wish to organize activities into the following categories. It should be noted that contributions listed in one area may also be pertinent to another category of parent–care giver cooperation.

1. Ways in which parents may assist children during center hours
2. Ways in which parents may work with materials and equipment during center hours
3. Ways in which parents may contribute time and effort to the program after center hours
4. Ways in which parents may participate without leaving their homes

Assisting Children During Center Hours. The following listing offers some ideas for parental assistance with children in the child-care center. Some parents may want and need on-the-job training. Remember that some states may require a health examination for all persons helping with preparation of food. It is important to capitalize on parents' strengths, hobbies, and interests. For example, someone who has worked as a food service employee in a restaurant would have contributions to make concerning food preparation and occupational information about food. Parents may participate in the following ways:

1. Supervise and contribute to learning centers
   a. Talk with children to develop language skills, that is, discuss food concepts following procedure described in Chapter 7; supervise games; tell and read stories about foods to children; listen to children read aloud
   b. Demonstrate and supervise a garden plot
   c. Demonstrate and supervise a cooking center
   d. Lead and supervise science and mathematics as food-related activities
2. Share hobbies and demonstrate how they are done (as food related)
3. Share and demonstrate career information (as food related)
4. Prepare snacks and interact with children during eating times (Figure 9–2)
5. Prepare basic mixes with children (Chapter 6) or for food service personnel
6. Supervise bathrooms and handwashing, especially before mealtime and food preparation activities
7. Share cleanup of kitchen equipment, table, and chairs with the children, or assist food service personnel

Working with Materials and Equipment During Center Hours. Some ways in which parents may be involved in clerical tasks at the center during, before, or after class hours include:

1. Typing menus
2. Taking pictures of food and making food displays or scrapbooks
3. Assisting with meal service, purchasing, preparation, and cleanup
4. Laminating materials, such as food pictures, child-developed recipe books, and recipe cards
5. Collecting food containers
6. Making food boxes for center

Contributing Time and Effort at School After Center Hours. One of the most common forms of parent-teacher contact takes place at parent-teacher conferences. However, informal committees, discussion groups, and personal phone calls may provide for parent-teacher cooperation, too. Workshops are especially enjoyable and provide an inviting format for the care giver to offer information regarding basic nutrition, how nutrition objectives are met in the center program, and how the parents can work cooperatively with the staff to achieve objectives.

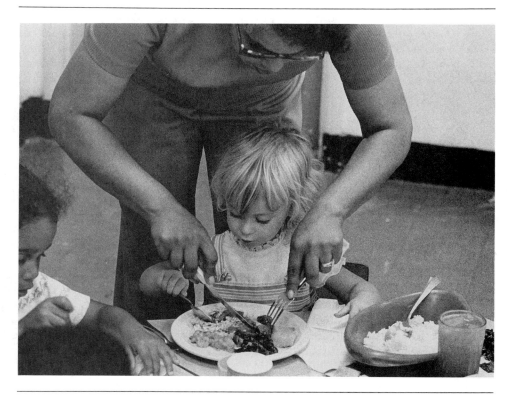

Figure 9-2
Parents can assist and interact with children.

Early in the year, possibly even before the program starts, a teacher should list a number of activities that parents might work on during workshops. The list should be long enough so that an element of choice is offered to the parents at each gathering. Some of the following ideas might be considered and specific tasks planned around them:

1. Inviting nutritionists and other health professionals from the local health department, hospitals, and other community agencies to discuss basic nutrition concepts, it is important that these discussions
   a. Be organized, with the presentation of basic nutrition concepts first as a home foundation to the use of food and nutrition.
   b. Directly involve parents with hands-on nutrition experiences (Appendix 9–F presents a guideline for preplanning, conducting, and evaluating a nutritionally oriented family workshop.)
2. Creating work jobs, games, and toys that can be used in nutrition education, for example, preparing pocket charts for categorizing and classifying food items, pictures and designs for a food bulletin board, or taste jars (for additional ideas, see Chapter 8)
3. Meeting with care givers and food service personnel to plan menus that can demonstrate the teaching of specific nutrition concepts
4. Inviting parents to share with professionals the importance of physical activities as related to food consumption
5. Sharing nutritious recipes, that is, recipes with high nutrient density
6. Sharing activities that parents have used to encourage their children to accept a wide variety of foods

Some programs may find parent advisory boards advantageous, although several words of caution should be noted. Parents should be free to suggest and recommend anything, but final authority and decision making probably should remain with the professionals, those trained educators who are responsible for all of the children at the center. This is particularly true of decisions about curriculum or specific individual behavior problems. In addition, parents should not be allowed to have access to an individual child's records or to discuss a specific child's problems, especially if names or the data being discussed would identify the child. Those responsibilities must be retained by the care givers and administrators.

Participating Without Leaving the Homes. One important way in which parents may participate at home is to help the child with developmental activities. The care giver may list activities or games that provide nutrition experiences and readiness for later learning. For example, a care giver may suggest some of the following for follow-up activities to strengthen nutrition principles learned in the centers.

1. While walking through a store together, talk to your child about the various products and their uses.

2. Look around the house for objects or foods whose first letters sound alike—cup, can, cap; pickle, pear, peach, pineapple.
3. Encourage your child to talk with you about food.
4. While preparing food, allow your child to help.
5. Let child share in cleanup activities.
6. Test new food activities at home. Provide feedback to teacher on strengths and weaknesses of activities.

Only imagination will limit the number of ways in which parents may help their children at home. The suggestions will vary from year to year and community to community, although some may be duplicated. Ideally, they would vary from child to child, so the suggestions would be geared to individual needs. Several short lists of ideas sent home at different times are more effective than one long list at the beginning of the year. Some of the same activities may be discussed during casual conversations or even at workshops, if parents express an interest. The purpose is to help parents realize they may take advantage of incidental learning opportunities as they arise.

Often parents are willing to help children in the center but cannot take time away from home. Perhaps they work full-time or have younger children at home. Perhaps a handicap prohibits them from coming to the center. Nonetheless, there are ways in which these parents may be encouraged to help provide a better learning environment for their children.

Teachers frequently request that parents provide snacks and treats for birthdays and holidays. High-calorie foods with few nutrients are most often sent. This problem can only be avoided by developing a policy that endorses the provision of nutritious foods for party times. Parents, teachers, and children can work together to develop the party snack list, which can be presented to parents in a letter or a parent handbook at the beginning of the school year. Appendix 9–G provides an example of a letter that can be sent to parents as well as a list of nutritious treats parents and children can prepare at home.

EVALUATION OF PARENT INVOLVEMENT

A simple method to help evaluate the effectiveness of parental participation is to keep attendance records from workshops, discussion groups, and programs. Of course, such statistics on attendance cannot indicate the quality of participation; they indicate only the number of participants. Although exposure of parents to program purposes and activities may be advantageous, evaluation should not be based exclusively on program turnout.

Evaluating the quality of participation is much more difficult than counting noses or calculating percentage of parent participation. Both long-range (perhaps yearly) and short-range (daily) objectives need to be considered. Observations and discussions between parents and care givers, possibly with checklists, are means of informal evaluation. Parent grievances to administrators and care givers may indicate areas toward which improvement efforts need to be directed. All these sources of evaluative information should be used.

Each area of parent-school involvement must be evaluated. For example, after a parent acts as a volunteer, the parent and the care giver should immediately review both positive and negative points of that particular day's activities. The aim is to improve the quality of interaction on succeeding days. Neither parent nor care giver should be afraid of criticism, which needs to be given and accepted in a positive way.

Evaluations of clerical tasks should be done in two ways, one aimed at the self-fulfillment of the participant and the other at the quality of work. Do the participants feel useful and needed? Excessive typographical errors cannot be tolerated, nor can equipment constantly in need of repair because of mishandling. If the clerical chores involve total class interruptions, then alternate methods of completing the tasks must be created. Wastefulness of materials might be noted, also. As with other areas of evaluation, any benefit must be a result of frank and open discussion between parent participant and care giver.

After workshops or programs, a short, informal checklist could be passed to each parent in attendance. They should be encouraged, but not required to fill it out. Questions might include: Was this gathering worth your time and effort? What did you like about it? What did you dislike about it? Was it too long? Too short? Just right? What would you like to do at a future meeting? How could our gatherings be improved? (If there were an outside resource person or persons, a question such as, "Would you invite him or her back? Why not?" might be included.) Parents need not sign their names. From these informal instruments some worthwhile suggestions for improvement of a parent-participation program may be forthcoming.

The teacher and care giver might use a checklist to help evaluate their own involvement with parents. Such a list might be scanned several times a year as a reminder of some important points to remember when cooperating with parent volunteers [3].

1. Am I a good listener?
2. Do I try to make parents feel needed?
3. Have I given personal recognition in the form of compliments and notes to all participants? Have I had the children send thank-you notes? Would a year-end recognition coffee session be useful?
4. Do I try to learn about each parent's interests, hobbies, or work so that each may contribute according to his or her strengths and training?
5. Do I accept all suggestions for activity and discuss programs and problems openly?
6. Do I preplan alone or with the parents?
7. Am I a dictator?
8. Do I keep all meetings and workshops informal and encourage interaction?
9. Do I keep parents informed through meetings, newsletters, notes, or phone calls?

10. Do I provide baby-sitting and transportation services if needed for greater participation?
11. Have I elicited cooperation and understanding of the center administration?
12. Am I careful not to discuss children in front of their parents? Am I sure all records are confidential and unavailable to any parents?
13. Am I aware that some parents may force their views on others?
14. Do I believe there are too many interruptions in the center when parents are involved?
15. Do I expect every parent to be involved? Do I exploit their generosity of time, talent, and effort?

At the end of the year, suggestions for improving the program should be solicited from all parent participants—clerical aides, parent resources, and home participants. A letter could be sent home and returned with each child. Some portions of the programs may be dropped, others added, and some modified according to the combined responses of parents, children, director, and care giver.

RECOGNITION

Every parent volunteer, regardless of the time devoted to the program, should receive frequent praise and encouragement for service. Much satisfaction can be gained when parents believe they have been accepted as colleagues by their coworkers. Another form of satisfaction results when parents believe they have contributed to the progress and growth of an individual child or group of children. Teachers must make a continual effort to express their acceptance of the volunteers and the skills they are contributing.

A special "thank you" is in order for the parents. This can be done at a meeting where the main order of business is the public recognition of parents for their services. Some form of tangible recognition is recommended: a certificate of appreciation, a letter of congratulations, a "good egg award," a happy-gram. It should be something the volunteer can take as a memento of the experience [4]. Newspaper and television coverage of the awards and recognition ceremonies can be helpful in drawing public attention to the program.

Recognition, no matter which form it takes, is essential. A single thank you as the parent volunteer leaves is a courtesy that will pay dividends. A parent volunteer who enjoys the work is thanked in many ways. The general reception and attitude that the staff expresses toward the volunteer is a form of recognition. In addition, the parent volunteer represents the people of the community. When we recognize the volunteer, we recognize the community.

Parents, care givers, and children may all benefit from effective participation based on clear-cut objectives and goals. It is natural that as the year progresses, more and more responsibility and freedom may be allowed parent participants, according to their responsiveness and abilities. Effective participation grows like a seed, a little each day. If properly nutured, it produces fine fruit by the end of a growing season.

SUMMARY

- Children and their well-being are major concerns for parents and early childhood educators. Parent involvement in early childhood nutrition programs provides unity for the parent and child in sound educational experiences about food.
- Benefits of parent participation are realized by parents, early childhood care givers, and the children involved.
- Effectiveness of parent recruitment is maximized when several methods are used. Contacts can be made through informal conversation during various parent-teacher meetings, letters, newsletters, home visits, and inclusion of appropriate questions on registration forms.
- To ensure maximum participation, parents should be given options for involvement. Suggested categories for contribution include (1) assisting children during center hours, (2) working with materials and equipment during center hours, (3) contributing time and effort to the program after center hours, and (4) participating without leaving the home.
- Ideas for parental assistance are vast; the strengths, hobbies, and interests of parents should be explored. Parents can also serve as valuable resource persons for early childhood nutrition education.
- Evaluating the effectiveness of a parent involvement program is necessary to maintain and improve the quality of interaction. Suggested evaluation techniques are attendance records at various meetings, questionnaires, parent/care giver feedback, and self-evaluation by teachers concerning involvement with parents.
- Recognition of parent participation is vital. Frequent praise or other tangible expressions of appreciation provide encouragement and satisfaction for parents.

DISCUSSION QUESTIONS

1. Discuss the value of parent involvement in early childhood nutrition programs.
2. Briefly outline the methods of initiating parent involvement in a nutrition education program.
3. What purpose do home visits serve in nutrition education?
4. Describe four ways parents can contribute to the early childhood nutrition program during center hours.
5. Discuss opportunities for parents to contribute to the school's nutrition program after center hours.

6. List three suggestions for parents to use at home to reinforce nutrition concepts learned at school.
7. Discuss the necessity of evaluating a parent involvement program. Which aspects of the program should be evaluated?
8. Describe methods of recognizing parents for their involvement in early childhood nutrition programs. Why is this important?

REFERENCES

1. Liddle, G., Rockwell, R. E., and Sacadat, E.: Education improvement for the disadvantaged, Springfield, IL, 1967, Charles C. Thomas, Publisher.
2. Position paper on nutrition standards in day care programs for children, J. Am. Diet Assoc. 87:502, 1987.
3. Rockwell, R. E., and Grafford, K. J.: Tips: teachers involve parent services, Edwardsville, 1977, Department of Elementary and Early Childhood Education, Southern Illinois University.
4. Rockwell, R. E., and Comer, J. M.: School volunteer program, a manual for coordinators, midwest teachers corp network, Athens, OH, 1978, College of Education, Ohio University.

SUGGESTED READINGS

Berger, E. H.: Parents as partners in education, Columbus, OH, 1987, Merrill Publishing Co.

Bigner, J. J.: Parent-child relations, New York, 1979, Macmillian Publishing Co.

Bromwich, R.: Working with parents and infants—an international approach, Baltimore, 1981, University Park Press.

Ferguson-Florissant School District: Parents as first teachers, Ferguson, MO, 1985, Ferguson-Florissant School District.

Gestwicki, C.: Home, school and community relations: a guide to working with parents, Albany, NY: 1987, Delmar Inc.

Margolin, E.: Teaching young children at school and home, New York, 1982, Macmillan Publishing Co.

Rutherford, R. B., Jr., and Edgard, E.: Teachers and parents—a guide to interaction and cooperation, Boston, 1979, Allyn & Bacon, Inc.

APPENDIX 9–A   Center Feeding Chart

CENTER FEEDING CHART

Date: March 23   Sample:

	Time: 9:15		
John	Solids Milk	1/2 j 8 oz.	1/4 j 6 oz.

Name	1st feeding Food prepared/eaten			2nd feeding Food prepared/eaten			3rd feeding Food prepared/eaten			4th feeding Food prepared/eaten		
Amy	Time: 9:40			Time: 1:10			Time:			Time:		
	formula	8 oz.	6 oz	milk	4 oz	all						
	cereal	3T	all	fruit meat	4T 2T	2T 1T						
Cathie	Time: 9:30			Time: 11:36			Time: 3:15			Time:		
	juice	4 oz	all	sandwich	1/2	1/4	milk	4 oz	1 oz			
	cracker	1		milk fruit	8 oz 1/2 jar	6 oz all	fruit	1/2 jar	all			
Emmy	Time: 10:07			Time:			Time:			Time:		
	milk	4 oz	2 oz									
	fruit	1 jar	all									
Frances	Time: 10:05			Time: 12:37			Time: 3:04			Time:		
	cereal	1 jar	3/4 j.	meat veg.	1/2 jar 1/2 jar	1/2 jar all	juice	8 oz	6 oz			
	fruit	1/2 jar	all	milk	6 oz	all						
Kerry	Time: 11:45			Time:			Time:			Time:		
	meat veg. fruit	1/2 jar 1/2 jar 1/2 jar	all	juice	4 oz	all						
Leigh	Time: 12:30			Time: 2:45			Time:			Time:		
	banana	1	3/3	juice	8 oz	all						
	milk	4 oz	3 oz	sandwich	1/2							
Leslie	Time: 10:09			Time: 1:15			Time:			Time:		
	milk	6 oz	3 oz	juice	8 oz	all						
	cereal	2T	ref.	sandwich	1/2							
Munro	Time: 1:13			Time:			Time:			Time:		
	sandwich cheese fruit milk	1 slice 1 jar 8 oz	1/2 all all all									
Oliver	Time: 9:30			Time: 12:30			Time: 3:10			Time:		
	juice	6 oz	all	meat + veg. fruit milk	1 jar 1/2 jar 4 oz	all all	milk	8 oz	all			

Source: Herbert-Jackson, E., O'Brien, M., Porterfield, J., and Risley, T. R.: The infant center, Baltimore, 1977, University Park Press.

APPENDIX 9–B Notes for Parents of 3- to 18-Month-Old Infants

Parent Report   Date _____

Name _____ Leaving _____

Last fed: _____ Last slept from: _____ To: _____

Parent's instructions for today:

Medicines:

Give phone number if different from the one we have on file: _____

Center Report

Your baby slept from: Diapering

_____ to _____   _____   _____

_____ to _____   _____   _____

_____ to _____   _____   _____

_____ to _____   _____   _____

                                     _____   _____

Your baby ate:

<u>When</u>   <u>What</u>

1st

2nd

3rd

4th

Some of the activities your   Disposition:
baby participated in were:

Center Comments:

Source: St. Louis Community College at Florissant Valley, Child Development Center, 1988.

APPENDIX 9–C Notes for Parents of 18- to 24-Month-Old Toddlers

Name: _____

Date: _____

Did your child sleep
well last night?

Yes _____   No _____

Is your child having a
hard morning?

Yes _____   No _____

Reason:

Give phone number if

different: _____

Special instructions for
today:

FOOD INTAKE

+   =   good

1   =   one serving

0   =   nothing

Breakfast _____

Lunch   _____

Snack   _____

SLEEPING

_____ to _____

_____ to _____ .

EXTRA COMMENTS:

DIAPERING (bowel movements)

L   =   Loose

H   =   Hard

N   =   Normal

_____

_____

_____

ACTIVITIES

Source: St. Louis Community College at Florissant Valley, Child Development Center, 1988.

APPENDIX 9-D   Parent Report Form

San Antonio College
Child Development Center
Two Year Old Class

Parent Report

Day _____ Departure time _____ Child's name _____

Did your child sleep well last night? _____ Has your child had breakfast? _____

Any special instructions for today?   Phone number if different for today: _____

Today's play activities

Individual

Art or science

Large group

Helping

Outdoor

Other

Meals

ⵜ = type of snack food served
+ = ate lots
1 = ate one serving
0 = ate little

	a.m. Snack	Lunch	p.m. Snack
Protein source			
Fruit/juice			
Vegetable			
Bread/cereal			
Milk product			

General disposition

Nap: Slept from _____ to _____

Potty: Number of accidents _____

Comments:

Permission to Give Medication

I authorize the Director or employed staff member to administer the following medication(s):

Medication or Prescription No.	Dosage	Hours of Day	Staff use only (Date, Time, Initials)

Parent's Signature _____

Date _____

Source: San Antonio College Child Development Center.

St. Louis Community College at Florissant Valley
Child Development Center

Sign-in/Sign-out

Classroom: _____ **Date:** _____

Child's Name	Parent's Signature	Arrival Time	Parent's Signature	Departure Time	Comments
1.					
2.					
3.					
4.					
5.					
6.					
7.					
8.					
9.					
10.					
11.					
12.					
13.					
14.					
15.					
16.					
17.					
18.					
19.					
20.					

Source: St. Louis Community College at Florissant Valley, Child Development Center, 1988.

WORKSHOP AGENDA

Workshop title:
Show, Tell, and Taste Snacks: a Fun Way to Eat for Nutrition

Theme:
Nutritious snacks

Purpose:

- To promote family togetherness
- To increase parents' awareness of what their children eat
- To teach children to choose, make, and enjoy nutritious food and snacks
- To help families choose nutritious snacks
- To suggest that children keep a record of the snacks they eat
- To know the difference between nutritious snacks and those that are not

Advance preparation:
Three weeks before:

1. Clear meeting with principal.
2. Secure authorization for room use.
3. Secure room for babysitting facility.
4. Make arrangements for several babysitters— one on "standby" status.
5. Form committee to make arrangements for possible transportation for parents.
6. Set up food committee with chairman. Pass out food sign-up sheet.

Two weeks before:

1. Make invitations.
2. Remind parents of food items they signed up for use as workshop materials or refreshments.
3. Organize games (include extra one if time permits).
4. Prepare on paper physical arrangement of the room.

One week before:

1. Prepare name tags.
2. Prepare mixer.
3. Prepare evaluation form and box.
4. Organize material for workshop.
5. Check with food committee to see what items are still lacking.
6. Prepare and organize materials for snack kit.
7. Send invitations.

One day before:

1. Remind parents of meeting.
2. Check progress of food committee.
3. Remind baby-sitters of the date and time.
4. Check with transportation committee to verify rides for parents needing them.

Day of the meeting:

1. Set up tables and activity centers.
2. Put posters, name tags, handouts in place.

Mixer

Materials:
1. Posters of meat group, milk group, grain group, and fruit/vegetable group
2. Paper plate depicting balanced meal
3. Eight envelopes of food pictures
   a. Two envelopes of meat pictures
   b. Two envelopes of milk pictures
   c. Two envelopes of grain pictures
   d. Two envelopes of fruit/vegetable pictures
4. Eight plates

Activity:
1. Each person receives a food envelope and a paper plate.

2. Each person must ask others for food items to place on his/her plate until a balanced meal is received.

NAME TAGS

Name tags are cut in the shape of a glass from orange construction paper (orange juice) or white construction paper (milk) with space for a name to be written in marker.

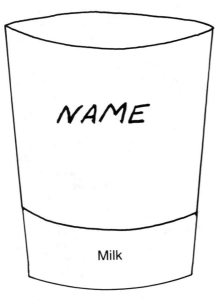

Milk

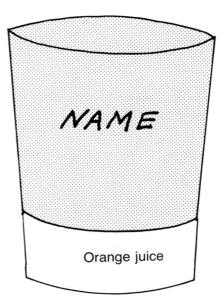

Orange juice

WORKSHOP SCHEDULE

Time	Activity	Technique	Resources	Person Responsible
12:45–12:55	Welcome	Name tags	Paper, markers, pins	Janet
		Mixer	Paper plates, tape, food pictures	Susan
12:55–1:05	Introduction of meeting Purpose: Choosing nutritious snacks	Good nutrition is important. We can make nutritious food more interesting and fun to eat, especially snacks. This can be a family or child project.	Basic food groups posters	Donna
	Parents go to the six activity centers (see next section)	Explain each activity center. Look at the number on your name tag. Begin at that station and continue wherever your interest takes you.	Name tags Activity centers	Amanda
1:05–1:30	Activity centers			
	1. Peanut butter play dough	Follow recipe #1 in parent handout.	Peanut butter, dry milk	Amanda
	2. Bugs on a log	Follow recipe #2 in parent handout.	Peanut butter, celery, raisins	Donna
	3. Peanut butter fruitwich	Follow recipe #3 in parent handout.	Crushed cereal, banana, peanut butter	Erma
	4. Fruit face and variations	Follow recipe #4 in parent handout.	Apple slices, raisins, pineapple chunks, shredded carrots, orange	Susan
	5. Decorated crackers	Follow recipe #5 in parent handout.	Crackers, cheese spread in a can	Katie
	6. Bread cut-outs	Follow recipe #6 in parent handout.	Whole wheat bread, cookie cutters, cream cheese	Janet
1:30–1:45	Refreshments	Serve yourself juice; eat snacks prepared.	Fruit punch, bowl cups	All
	Conclusion	Pass out evaluation sheet.	Pencils, parent handout	Katie

EVALUATION SHEET

We are interested in knowing whether you enjoyed our meeting this afternoon. Please put a check in the box below that best describes your feeling about the meeting. The space provided at the bottom of this page is for any suggestions you might have concerning our parent group meetings. We would be happy to hear from you, so feel free to comment!

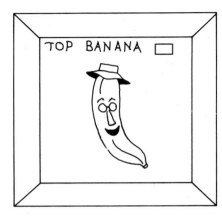 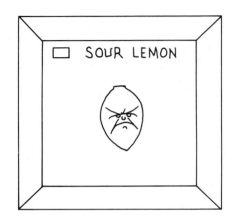

Comments:

_____

_____

_____

_____

_____

RECIPES FOR SNACKS
PREPARED AT ACTIVITY CENTERS

#1   Peanut butter play dough
(Meat and milk groups)

18 oz peanut butter
6 tbsp honey
Nonfat dry milk to right consistency
Cocoa (optional)

Mix together and form into shapes. Eat and enjoy!

#2   Bugs on a log
(meat and fruit/vegetable groups)

Celery washed and cut into 4″ lengths
Peanut butter
Raisins

Spread peanut butter in celery. Arrange 3 or 4 raisins on top of peanut butter.

#3   Peanut butter fruitwich
(fruit/vegetable and grain or meat groups)

Banana cut in half lengthwise
Peanut butter to spread on banana
Crushed cereal or nuts

Reassemble the bananas and roll in the crushed cereal or nuts.
Slice in round if desired.

#4   Fruit face
(fruit/vegetable group)

Apple, cut into quarters
Pineapple chunk
2 raisins
2 orange slices
½ C shredded carrots
Paper plate

Arrange ¼ apple below center of plate for mouth. Put two quarters on either side for ears. A pineapple chunk in the middle becomes the nose. Use two raisins for eyes and two orange slices for eyebrows. Shredded carrots at the top make hair. Substitute any fruit and vegetables you like.

#5   Decorated crackers
(grain and milk groups)

Whole wheat or whole-grain crackers
Cheese in a can

Create designs, faces, animals with the cheese on the crackers, or spread cream cheese on preshaped crackers.

#6   Bread cut-outs
(grain and milk groups)

Whole wheat bread
Cheese from a can or cream cheese
Cookie cutters

Cut shapes from a slice of whole wheat bread with cookie cutters. Decorate with cheese from a can. Or spread cream cheese on the bread with a knife.

ADDITIONAL RECIPES TO TRY AT HOME

#7   Pudding finger paint

1 package pudding mix, cooked type
2 C milk
Waxed paper, large sheet

Cook pudding according to package directions. Pour a small amount (¼ C) on the waxed paper. Make designs with fingers or spoon. Lick fingers as necessary. Eat remainder of "painting" with spoon.

#8   Meal face

Hot dog, poached egg, or bacon strip fried for
    mouth
Carrot or celery slices for eyes and nose
Tomato slices for ears
Shredded cheese, lettuce, or slaw for hair
Paper plate

Assemble foods to make face. Or use any favorite foods to arrange a face on the plate.

#9   Sandwich special

Cottage cheese and shredded carrots on whole
   wheat raisin bread
Peanut butter between apple rings
Honey butter (mix equal parts of honey and soft butter) between graham crackers (much better for
   a snack or dessert than cookies)
Chopped leftover meat (moisten with mayonnaise)
   and a lettuce slice
Peanut butter and alfalfa sprouts or tomato slices
   on whole wheat bread

#10   Banana pops

Banana on a stick
Yogurt
Nuts, coconut, or granola

Dip banana in yogurt, then roll in nuts, coconut, or
granola. Freeze.

#11   Crunchy bananas

Banana cut into 1″ thick slices
Popsicle stick
Orange juice
Coconut, wheat germ, or chopped peanuts

Spear banana slices with stick, dip in juice, and
roll in favorite topping.

#12   Homemade granola

Unsweetened cereal, any variety
Raisins
Coconut
Peanuts

Mix all together.

#13   Banana candle

Pineapple slice on a plate
Banana, peeled and cut in half
Maraschino cherry

Cut off ends of banana. Stand up the half banana
in the pineapple ring. Put a cherry on top for the
flame.

#14   Meat kabobs

Vienna sausage rounds
Cherry tomato
Toothpick
Italian dressing

Thread sausage on toothpick with tomato. Marinate
in Italian dressing if desired.

#15   Cheese kabobs

Cubed cheese
Toothpicks
Fruit chunks, any variety

Thread cubes of cheese on toothpicks, alternating
with fruit.

#16   Cheese balls

Cream cheese
Milk
Chopped peanuts

Soften cream cheese with a little milk; form into
balls. Roll in chopped peanuts.

#17   Cheese crunchies

Cheese cubes
Pretzel sticks
Wheat germ

Spear cheese cube with pretzel stick and roll in
wheat germ.

#18   Popcorn with cheese

Popcorn, popped
Cheese melted or dried to sprinkle on popcorn

#19   Popcorn-peanut nibbler

Popped corn
Roasted peanuts
Butter and salt

Mix and toast in oven approximately 10 minutes.

#20   Finger Jello (Knox Blox)

7 envelopes unflavored gelatin (or 4 envelopes unflavored gelatin and 3 envelopes flavored)
4 C boiling fruit juice (or 4 C boiling water)

Mix and pour into a 13″ × 9″ pan. Chill until firm and cut into approximately 100 squares.

#21   Toad-in-a-Hole

1 slice of bread
1 tbsp butter
1 egg

With a cookie cutter cut out a circle in the center of the bread. Melt butter in pan and brown bread on both sides. Break an egg in the hole. Cook covered until the egg doesn't jiggle.

#22   Bunny Salad

1 lettuce leaf
1 canned pear half
4 orange sections
1 maraschino cherry cut into 6 slices (or substitute pieces of apple or tomato for the cherry)

Put the lettuce leaf on the table. Put the pear half cut side down on the lettuce leaf. Add orange sections for ears. Use cherry or apple or tomato slices for eyes, nose, mouth and inside of ears.

#23   Mellow Yellow

2 slices of bread, buttered
1 slice of cheese between the bread slices
1 tbsp. butter melted in a pan

Brown bread on both sides. Cut into triangles and share with a friend.

SNACKS

The following list is a list of simple, economical, and nutritious snack ideas you may find practical.

Remember, to make snacks more tempting have them readily accessible and attractive for eye-catching appeal.

Milk group

Flavored milk drink—½ C milk with ½ C any fruit juice
Cheese cubes
Ice cream

Meat group

Sunflower seeds, pumpkin seeds
Toasted soybeans
Assorted nuts
Peanut butter
Peanut butter balls rolled in sesame seeds
Beef jerky
Eggs sliced with pickle
Walnut, pecan halves with soft cheese spread as filling

Fruits and Vegetables

Using any fresh fruit or vegetable, experiment with imaginative shapes (minted or dilled cucumbers, radish fans, celery branches, pepper strips, carrot curls, or cauliflower buds).
Make fruit juice by rolling unpeeled orange between hands until soft; insert straw.
Cut apples into small wedges and place on toothpick with raisins.
Freeze orange juice on sticks in ice cube trays to make sunshine pops.

Grains

Chow Mein noodles
Crackers—use cheese and whole-grain varieties
Unsugared, ready-to-eat cereal
Taco shells (broken into chips)

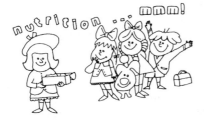

Dear Parents,

If you panic when someone tells you to bring a "nutritious" snack, relax. Here are some guidelines for choosing and making nutritious snacks.

Use plain simple foods which are low in sugar, salt, and fat and high in food value.

Why low in sugar? Because sugar promotes tooth decay, is a concentrated source of calories with no nutrients, and displaces more nutritious foods in our diet.

Why low in salt? Because we consume 2 to 10 times more salt than we need and excessive salt intake may trigger hypertension in susceptible people.

Why low in fat? Because fat contains twice the calories of carbohydrate or protein and while we do need some fat in our diets, we generally get much more than we need.

Why high in food value? Because preschool appetites are quite variable from day to day, even meal to meal, and most young children cannot consume all the nutrients they need in three meals a day. Snacks become an important part of the child's nutrient intake so these foods need to be carefully chosen to balance the child's diet.

Why worry at this age? Because preschool children are establishing eating habits that will last a lifetime—hopefully, a long healthy lifetime.

This doesn't mean you must throw out your 5 lb. bag of sugar or empty the salt shaker into the trash can and serve dry toast in the morning. Moderation is a better idea.

It may interest you to know that nutrition surveys have revealed that most preschoolers do not get enough iron, calcium and vitamin A in their diets.

Snack time is an important time of the preschool day, a time of learning as well as physical satisfaction. Involving your child in snack preparation at home for class can be a meaningful and educational experience.

Thanks,

The Teachers

Source: Barbara L. Goldenhersh, Director of Presbyterian Community Preschool, Belleville, IL, 1988.

NUTRITIOUS SNACK SUGGESTIONS
PRESBYTERIAN COMMUNITY PRESCHOOL

Fresh fruit kabobs

Cut bite-size pieces of melon, pineapple, grapes, strawberries, apples, etc. Place on a plastic straw. Dip in lemon juice to keep fresh.

Orange smiles

Cut each orange into eight wedges. Leave peel on.

"Gorp"

Mixture of raisins, dried fruits, sunflower seeds, and nuts in small cups or sandwich bags.

Banana bread, pumpkin bars, blueberry muffins

Home-made breads and muffins are always a special treat. These make excellent birthday snacks.

"Ants on a log"

Spread celery pieces with peanut butter or cheese. Add raisins on top for the "ants."

Raw veggies and dip

Celery, cucumber, green pepper, cherry tomatoes, carrot sticks, broccoli "trees," and cauliflower "flowers" are great with dip. Dill dip is quite popular with preschoolers.

Popcorn

For variety sprinkle with cinnamon or Parmesan cheese.

Sandwiches

Peanut butter and jelly or honey, tuna, egg or chicken salad, and bologna sandwiches are fine snacks. A quarter or half sandwich per child is appropriate.

Rice Krispie squares, triangles, or rectangles

Face cookies

Spread peanut butter on graham cracker. Make a face with raisins.

Jello or pudding

Make in small paper cups.

Celery and pineapple sticks

Mash two 8 oz packages of cream cheese. Add one large can of crushed pineapple drained. Mix and spread on celery pieces.

Dried fruit assortment

Mix an assortment of dried fruits: apricots, peaches, dates, apples, raisins, etc. Serve in small paper cups.

Happy faces

Spread bread circles with peanut butter. Add raisins for features and grated carrots or cheese for hair.

Applewiches

Core an apple, slice into circles and dip in lemon juice to prevent discoloration. Spread peanut butter on apple slices and close to make sandwiches.

Popsicles

Blend one 6 oz can softened frozen juice (grape is excellent), 1 can water and 1 pint vanilla ice cream. Pour into molds or small paper cups, insert sticks, and freeze.

Orange juice-icles

Mix one 6 oz can frozen orange juice, 3 cans cold water, 1 egg white and 2 tbsp honey in blender. Pour into molds or small paper cups, insert sticks, and freeze.

Source: Nutritious snack suggestions courtesy of Barbara L. Goldenhersh, Director of Presbyterian Community Preschool, Belleville, IL, 1988.

Appendixes

Appendix I Nutritive Values of the Edible Part of Foods[1]

Food, approximate measure, and weight (in grams)		Food energy	Protein	Fat (total lipid)	Fatty acids			Carbohydrate	Calcium	Iron	Vitamin A value	Thiamine	Riboflavin	Niacin	Ascorbic acid
					Saturated (total)	Unsaturated Oleic	Unsaturated Linoleic								
	gm.	(Calories)	(gm.)	(gm.)	(gm.)	(gm.)	(gm.)	(gm.)	(mg.)	(mg.)	(I.U.)	(mg.)	(mg.)	(mg.)	(mg.)

Milk, cream, cheese (related products)

Food, approximate measure, and weight (in grams)		Food energy	Protein	Fat (total lipid)	Saturated (total)	Oleic	Linoleic	Carbohydrate	Calcium	Iron	Vitamin A value	Thiamine	Riboflavin	Niacin	Ascorbic acid
Milk, cow's															
Fluid, whole (3.5% fat)	1 cup	244	160	9	9	5	3	Trace	12	288	0.1	350	0.08	0.42	0.1	2
Fluid, nonfat (skim)	1 cup	246	90	9	Trace	—	—	—	13	298	.1	10	.10	.44	.2	2
Buttermilk, cultured, from skim milk	1 cup	246	90	9	Trace	—	—	—	13	298	.1	10	.09	.44	.2	2
Evaporated, unsweetened, undiluted	1 cup	252	345	18	20	11	7	1	24	635	.3	820	.10	.84	.5	3
Condensed, sweetened, undiluted	1 cup	306	980	25	27	15	9	1	166	802	.3	1,090	.23	1.17	.5	3
Dry, whole	1 cup	103	515	27	28	16	9	1	39	936	.5	1,160	.30	1.50	.7	6
Dry, nonfat, instant	1 cup	70	250	25	Trace	—	—	—	36	905	.4	20	.24	1.25	.6	5
Milk, goat's															
Fluid, whole	1 cup	244	165	8	10	6	2	Trace	11	315	.2	390	.10	.27	.7	2
Cream															
Half-and-half (cream and milk)	1 cup	242	325	8	28	16	9	1	11	261	.1	1,160	.08	.38	.1	2
	1 tbsp.	15	20	Trace	2	1	1	Trace	1	16	Trace	70	Trace	.02	Trace	Trace
Light, coffee or table	1 cup	240	505	7	49	27	16	1	10	245	.1	2,030	.07	.36	.1	2
	1 tbsp.	15	30	Trace	3	2	1	Trace	1	15	Trace	130	Trace	.02	Trace	Trace
Whipping, unwhipped (volume about double when whipped)															
Light	1 cup	239	715	6	75	41	25	2	9	203	.1	3,070	.06	.30	.1	2
	1 tbsp.	15	45	Trace	5	3	2	Trace	1	13	Trace	190	Trace	.02	Trace	Trace
Heavy	1 cup	238	840	5	89	49	29	3	7	178	.1	3,670	.05	.26	.1	2
	1 tbsp.	15	55	Trace	6	3	2	Trace	Trace	11	Trace	230	Trace	.02	Trace	Trace

Food	Measure														
Cheese															
Blue or Roquefort type	1 oz.	28	105	6	9	5	3	Trace	1	89	.1	350	.01	.17	.1	0
Cheddar or American																
Ungrated	1 inch cube	17	70	4	5	3	2	Trace	Trace	128	.2	220	Trace	.08	Trace	0
Grated	1 cup	112	445	28	36	20	12	1	2	840	1.1	1,470	.03	.51	.1	0
	1 tbsp.	7	30	2	2	1	1	Trace	Trace	52	.1	90	Trace	.03	Trace	0
Cheddar, process	1 oz.	28	105	7	9	5	3	Trace	1	219	.3	350	Trace	.12	Trace	0
Cheese foods, Cheddar	1 oz.	28	90	6	7	4	2	Trace	2	162	.2	280	.01	.16	Trace	0
Cottage cheese, from skim milk																
Creamed	1 cup	225	240	31	9	5	3	Trace	7	212	.7	380	.07	.56	0.2	0
	1 oz.	28	30	4	1	1	Trace	Trace	1	27	.1	50	.01	.07	Trace	0
Uncreamed	1 cup	225	195	38	1	Trace	Trace	Trace	6	202	.9	20	.07	.63	.2	0
	1 oz.	28	25	5	Trace	—	—	—	1	26	.1	Trace	.01	.08	Trace	0
Cream cheese	1 oz.	28	105	2	11	6	4	Trace	1	18	.1	440	Trace	.07	Trace	0
	1 tbsp.	15	55	1	6	3	2	Trace	Trace	9	Trace	230	Trace	.04	Trace	0
Swiss (domestic)	1 oz.	28	105	8	8	4	3	Trace	1	262	.3	320	Trace	.11	Trace	0
Milk beverages																
Cocoa	1 cup	242	235	9	11	6	4	Trace	26	286	.9	390	.09	.45	.4	2
Chocolate-flavored milk drink (made with skim milk)	1 cup	250	190	8	6	3	2	Trace	27	270	.4	210	.09	.41	.2	2
Malted milk	1 cup	270	280	13	12	—	—	—	32	364	.8	670	.17	.56	.2	2
Milk desserts																
Cornstarch pudding, plain (blanc mange)	1 cup	248	275	9	10	5	3	Trace	39	290	.1	390	.07	.40	.1	2
Custard, baked	1 cup	248	285	13	14	6	5	1	28	278	1.0	870	.10	.47	.2	1
Ice cream, plain, factory packed																
Slice or cut brick, ⅛ of quart brick	1 slice or cut brick	71	145	3	9	5	3	Trace	15	87	.1	370	.03	.13	.1	1
Container	3½ fld. oz.	62	130	2	8	4	3	Trace	13	76	.1	320	.03	.12	.1	1
Container	8 fld. ozs.	142	295	6	18	10	6	1	29	175	.1	740	.06	.27	.1	1
Ice milk	1 cup	187	285	9	10	6	3	Trace	42	292	.2	390	.09	.41	.2	2
Yogurt, from partially skimmed milk	1 cup	246	120	8	4	2	1	Trace	13	295	.1	170	.09	.43	.2	2

Continued.

[1]Reprinted from Nutritive value of foods, U.S. Department of Agriculture, Home and Garden Bulletin No. 72.
Dashes show that no basis could be found for imputing a value although there was some reason to believe that a measurable amount of the constituent might be present.

Eggs

Food, approximate measure, and weight (in grams)	gm.	Food energy (Calories)	Protein (gm.)	Fat (total lipid) (gm.)	Fatty acids Saturated (total) (gm.)	Fatty acids Unsaturated Oleic (gm.)	Fatty acids Unsaturated Linoleic (gm.)	Carbohydrate (gm.)	Calcium (mg.)	Iron (mg.)	Vitamin A value (I.U.)	Thiamine (mg.)	Riboflavin (mg.)	Niacin (mg.)	Ascorbic acid (mg.)
Eggs, large, 24 ounces per dozen															
Raw															
Whole, without shell	1 egg	80	6	6	2	3	Trace	Trace	27	1.1	590	.05	.15	Trace	0
White of egg	1 white	15	4	Trace	—	—	—	Trace	3	Trace	0	Trace	.09	Trace	0
Yolk of egg	1 yolk	60	3	5	2	2	Trace	Trace	24	.9	580	.04	.07	Trace	0
Cooked															
Boiled, shell removed	2 eggs	160	13	12	4	5	1	1	54	2.3	1,180	.09	.28	.1	0
Scrambled, with milk and fat	1 egg	110	7	8	3	3	Trace	1	51	1.1	690	.05	.18	Trace	0
Meat, poultry, fish, shellfish (related products)															
Bacon, broiled or fried, crisp	2 slices	100	5	8	3	4	1	1	2	.5	0	.08	.05	.8	—
Beef, trimmed to retail basis[2], cooked															
Cuts braised, simmered, or pot-roasted															
Lean and fat	3 oz.	245	23	16	8	7	Trace	0	10	2.9	30	.04	.18	3.5	—
Lean only	2.5 oz.	140	22	5	2	2	Trace	0	10	2.7	10	.04	.16	3.3	—
Hamburger (ground beef), broiled															
Lean	3 oz.	185	23	10	5	4	Trace	0	10	3.0	20	.08	.20	5.1	—
Regular	3 oz.	245	21	17	8	8	Trace	0	9	2.7	30	.07	.18	4.6	—
Roast, oven-cooked, no liquid added															
Relatively fat, such as rib															
Lean and fat	3 oz.	375	17	34	16	15	1	0	8	2.2	70	.05	.13	3.1	—
Lean only	1.8 oz.	125	14	7	3	3	Trace	0	6	1.8	10	.04	.11	2.6	—
Relatively lean, such as heel of round															
Lean and fat	3 oz.	165	25	7	3	3	Trace	0	11	3.2	10	.06	.19	4.5	—
Lean only	2.7 oz.	125	24	3	1	1	Trace	0	10	3.0	Trace	.06	.18	4.3	—
Steak, broiled															
Relatively fat, such as sirloin															
Lean and fat	3 oz.	330	20	27	13	12	1	0	9	2.5	50	.05	.16	4.0	—
Lean only	2.0 oz.	115	18	4	2	2	Trace	0	7	2.2	10	.05	.14	3.6	—
Relatively lean, such as round															
Lean and fat	3 oz.	220	24	13	6	6	Trace	0	10	3.0	20	.07	.19	4.8	—
Lean only	2.4 oz.	130	21	4	2	2	Trace	0	9	2.5	10	.06	.16	4.1	—

Food, approximate measure	Weight (g)	Food energy (cal.)	Protein (g)	Fat (g)	Saturated fatty acids (g)	Unsaturated Oleic (g)	Unsaturated Linoleic (g)	Carbohydrate (g)	Calcium (mg)	Iron (mg)	Vitamin A (I.U.)	Thiamin (mg)	Riboflavin (mg)	Niacin (mg)	Ascorbic acid (mg)
Beef, canned															
Corned beef, 3 oz.	85	185	22	10	5	4	Trace	0	17	3.7	20	.01	.20	2.9	—
Corned beef hash, 3 oz.	85	155	7	10	5	4	Trace	9	11	1.7	—	.01	.08	1.8	—
Beef, dried or chipped, 2 oz.	57	115	19	4	2	2	Trace	0	11	2.9	—	.04	.18	2.2	—
Beef and vegetable stew, 1 cup	235	210	15	10	5	4	Trace	15	28	2.8	2,310	.13	.17	4.4	15
Beef potpie, baked: individual pie, 4¼-inch diameter, weight before baking about 8 oz., 1 pie	227	560	23	33	9	20	2	43	32	4.1	1,860	.25	.27	4.5	7
Chicken, cooked															
Flesh only, broiled, 3 oz.	85	115	20	3	1	1	1	0	8	1.4	80	0.05	0.16	7.4	—
Breast, fried, ½ breast															
With bone, 3.3 oz.	94	155	25	5	1	2	1	1	9	1.3	70	.04	.17	11.2	—
Flesh and skin only, 2.7 oz.	76	155	25	5	1	2	1	1	9	1.3	70	.04	.17	11.2	—
Drumstick, fried															
With bone, 2.1 oz.	59	90	12	4	1	2	1	Trace	6	.9	50	.03	.15	2.7	—
Flesh and skin only, 1.3 oz.	38	90	12	4	1	2	1	Trace	6	.9	50	.03	.15	2.7	—
Chicken, canned, boneless, 3 oz.	85	170	18	10	3	4	2	0	18	1.3	200	.03	.11	3.7	3
Chicken potpie—See Poultry potpie															
Chile con carne, canned															
With beans, 1 cup	250	335	19	15	7	7	Trace	30	80	4.2	150	.08	.18	3.2	—
Without beans, 1 cup	255	510	26	38	18	17	1	15	97	3.6	380	.05	.31	5.6	—
Heart, beef, lean, braised, 3 oz.	85	160	27	5	—	—	—	1	5	5.0	20	.21	1.04	6.5	1
Lamb, trimmed to retail basis,[2] cooked															
Chop, thick, with bone, broiled, 1 chop, 4.8 oz.	137	400	25	33	18	12	1	0	10	1.5	—	.14	.25	5.6	—
Lean and fat, 4.0 oz.	112	400	25	33	18	12	1	0	10	1.5	—	.14	.25	5.6	—
Lean only, 2.6 oz.	74	140	21	6	3	2	Trace	0	9	1.5	—	.11	.20	4.5	—
Leg, roasted															
Lean and fat, 3 oz.	85	235	22	16	9	6	Trace	0	9	1.4	—	.13	.23	4.7	—
Lean only, 2.5 oz.	71	130	20	5	3	2	Trace	0	9	1.4	—	.12	.21	4.4	—
Shoulder, roasted															
Lean and fat, 3 oz.	85	285	18	23	13	8	1	0	9	1.0	—	.11	.20	4.0	—
Lean only, 2.3 oz.	64	130	17	6	3	2	Trace	0	8	1.0	—	.10	.18	3.7	—
Liver, beef, fried, 2 oz.	57	130	15	6	—	—	—	3	6	5.0	30,280	.15	2.37	9.4	15

Continued.

[2]Outer layer of fat on the cut was removed to within approximately ½ inch of the lean. Deposits of fat within the cut were not removed.

Food, approximate measure, and weight (in grams)		(gm.)	Food energy (Calories)	Protein (gm.)	Fat (total lipid) (gm.)	Fatty acids Saturated (total) (gm.)	Unsaturated Oleic (gm.)	Unsaturated Linoleic (gm.)	Carbohydrate (gm.)	Calcium (mg.)	Iron (mg.)	Vitamin A value (I.U.)	Thiamine (mg.)	Riboflavin (mg.)	Niacin (mg.)	Ascorbic acid (mg.)
Pork, cured, cooked																
Ham, light cure, lean and fat, roasted	3 oz.	85	245	18	19	7	8	2	0	8	2.2	0	.40	.16	3.1	—
Luncheon meat																
Boiled ham, sliced	2 oz.	57	135	11	10	4	4	1	0	6	1.6	0	.25	.09	1.5	—
Canned, spiced or unspiced	2 oz.	57	165	8	14	5	6	1	1	5	1.2	0	.18	.12	1.6	—
Pork, fresh, trimmed to retail basis,[2] cooked																
Chop, thick, with bone	1 chop, 3.5 oz.	98	260	16	21	8	9	2	0	8	2.2	0	.63	.18	3.8	—
Lean and fat	2.3 oz.	66	260	16	21	8	9	2	0	8	2.2	0	.63	.18	3.8	—
Lean only	1.7 oz.	48	130	15	7	2	3	1	0	7	1.9	0	.54	.16	3.3	—
Roast, oven-cooked, no liquid added																
Lean and fat	3 oz.	85	310	21	24	9	10	2	0	9	2.7	0	.78	.22	4.7	—
Lean only	2.4 oz.	68	175	20	10	3	4	1	0	9	2.6	0	.73	.21	4.4	—
Cuts, simmered																
Lean and fat	3 oz.	85	320	20	26	9	11	2	0	8	2.5	0	.46	.21	4.1	—
Lean only	2.2 oz.	63	135	18	6	2	3	1	0	8	2.3	0	.42	.19	3.7	—
Poultry potpie (based on chicken potpie). Individual pie, 4 1/4-inch diameter, weigh before baking	1 pie	227	535	23	31	10	15	3	42	68	3.0	3,020	.25	.26	4.1	5
Sausage																
Bologna, slice, 4.1 by 0.1 inch	8 slices	227	690	27	62	—	—	—	2	16	4.1	—	.36	.49	6.0	—
Frankfurter, cooked	1	51	155	6	14	—	—	—	1	3	.8	—	.08	.10	1.3	—
Pork, links or patty, cooked	4 oz.	113	540	21	50	18	21	5	Trace	8	2.7	0	.89	.39	4.2	—
Tongue, beef, braised	3 oz.	85	210	18	14	—	—	—	Trace	6	1.9	—	.04	.25	3.0	—
Turkey potpie. See Poultry potpie																
Veal, cooked																
Cutlet, without bone, broiled	3 oz.	85	185	23	9	5	4	Trace	—	9	2.7	—	.06	.21	4.6	—
Roast, medium fat, medium done; lean and fat	3 oz.	85	230	23	14	7	6	Trace	0	10	2.9	—	.11	.26	6.6	—

Fish and shellfish																
Bluefish, baked or broiled	3 oz.	85	135	22	4	—	—	—	0	25	.6	40	.09	.08	1.6	—
Clams																
Raw, meat only	3 oz.	85	65	11	1	—	—	—	2	59	5.2	90	.08	.15	1.1	8
Canned, solids and liquid	3 oz.	85	45	7	1	—	—	—	2	47	3.5	—	.01	.09	.9	—
Crabmeat, canned	3 oz.	85	85	15	2	—	—	—	1	38	.7	—	.07	.07	1.6	—
Fish sticks, breaded, cooked, frozen; stick 3.8 by 1.0 by 0.5 inch	10 sticks or 8 oz. package	227	400	38	20	5	4	10	15	25	.9	—	.09	.16	3.6	—
Haddock, fried	3 oz.	85	140	17	5	1	3	—	5	34	1.0	—	0.03	0.06	2.7	2
Mackerel																
Broiled, Atlantic	3 oz.	85	200	19	13	—	—	—	0	5	1.0	450	.13	.23	6.5	—
Canned, Pacific, solids and liquid[3]	3 oz.	85	155	18	9	—	—	—	0	221	1.9	20	.02	.28	7.4	—
Ocean perch, breaded (egg and bread-crumbs), fried	3 oz.	85	195	16	11	—	—	—	6	28	1.1	—	.08	.09	1.5	—
Oysters, meat only. Raw, 13-19 medium selects	1 cup	240	160	20	4	—	—	—	8	226	13.2	740	.33	.43	6.0	—
Oyster stew, 1 part oysters to 3 parts milk by volume, 3-4 oysters	1 cup	230	200	11	12	—	—	—	11	269	3.3	640	.13	.41	1.6	—
Salmon, pink, canned	3 oz.	85	120	17	5	1	1	Trace	0	[4]167	.7	60	.03	.16	6.8	—
Sardines, Atlantic, canned in oil, drained solids	3 oz.	85	175	20	9	—	—	—	0	372	2.5	190	.02	.17	4.6	—
Shad, baked	3 oz.	85	170	20	10	—	—	—	0	20	.5	20	.11	.22	7.3	—
Shrimp, canned, meat only	3 oz.	85	100	21	1	—	—	—	1	98	2.6	50	.01	.03	1.5	—
Swordfish, broiled with butter or margarine	3 oz.	85	150	24	5	—	—	—	0	23	1.1	1,780	.03	.04	9.3	—
Tuna, canned in oil, drained solids	3 oz.	85	170	24	7	—	—	—	0	7	1.6	70	.04	.10	10.1	—
Mature dry beans and peas, nuts, peanuts (related products)																
Almonds, shelled	1 cup	142	850	26	77	6	52	15	28	332	6.7	0	.34	1.31	5.0	Trace

Continued.

[2]Outer layer of fat on the cut was removed to within approximately ½ inch of the lean. Deposits of fat within the cut were not removed.

[3]Vitamin values based on drained solids.

[4]Based on total contents of can. If bones are discarded, value will be greatly reduced.

Food, approximate measure, and weight (in grams)	gm.	Food energy (Calories)	Protein (gm.)	Fat (total lipid) (gm.)	Fatty acids Saturated (total) (gm.)	Unsaturated Oleic (gm.)	Unsaturated Linoleic (gm.)	Carbohydrate (gm.)	Calcium (mg.)	Iron (mg.)	Vitamin A value (I.U.)	Thiamine (mg.)	Riboflavin (mg.)	Niacin (mg.)	Ascorbic acid (mg.)
Beans, dry															
Common varieties, such as Great Northern, navy, and others, canned:															
Red 1 cup	256	230	15	1	—	—	—	42	74	4.6	Trace	.13	.10	1.5	—
White, with tomato sauce															
With pork 1 cup	261	320	16	7	3	3	1	50	141	4.7	340	.20	.08	1.5	5
Without pork 1 cup	261	310	16	1	—	—	—	60	177	5.2	160	.18	.09	1.5	5
Lima, cooked 1 cup	192	260	16	1	—	—	—	48	56	5.6	Trace	.26	.12	1.3	Trace
Brazil nuts 1 cup	140	915	20	94	19	45	24	15	260	4.8	Trace	1.34	.17	2.2	—
Cashew nuts, roasted 1 cup	135	760	23	62	10	43	4	40	51	5.1	140	.58	.33	2.4	—
Coconut															
Fresh, shredded 1 cup	97	335	3	34	29	2	Trace	9	13	1.6	0	.05	.02	.5	3
Dried, shredded, sweetened 1 cup	62	340	2	24	21	2	Trace	33	10	1.2	0	.02	.02	.2	0
Cowpeas or blackeye peas, dry, cooked 1 cup	248	190	13	1	—	—	—	34	42	3.2	20	.41	.11	1.1	Trace
Peanuts, roasted, salted															
Halves 1 cup	144	840	37	72	16	31	21	27	107	3.0	—	.46	.19	24.7	0
Chopped 1 tbsp.	9	55	2	4	1	2	1	2	7	.2	—	.03	.01	1.5	0
Peanut butter 1 tbsp.	16	95	4	8	2	4	2	3	9	.3	—	.02	.02	2.4	0
Peas, split, dry, cooked 1 cup	250	290	20	1	—	—	—	52	28	4.2	100	.37	.22	2.2	—
Pecans															
Halves 1 cup	108	740	10	77	5	48	15	16	79	2.6	140	.93	.14	1.0	2
Chopped 1 tbsp.	7.5	50	1	5	Trace	3	1	1	5	.2	10	.06	.01	.1	Trace
Walnuts, shelled															
Black or native, chopped 1 cup	126	790	26	75	4	26	36	19	Trace	7.6	380	.28	.14	.9	—
English or Persian															
Halves 1 cup	100	650	15	64	4	10	40	16	99	3.1	30	.33	.13	.9	3
Chopped 1 tbsp.	8	50	1	5	Trace	1	3	1	8	.2	Trace	.03	.01	.1	Trace
Vegetables and vegetable products															
Asparagus															
Cooked, cut spears 1 cup	175	35	4	Trace	—	—	—	6	37	1.0	1,580	.27	.32	2.4	46
Canned spears, medium															
Green 6 spears	96	20	2	Trace	—	—	—	3	18	1.8	770	.06	.10	.8	14
Bleached 6 spears	96	20	2	Trace	—	—	—	4	15	1.0	80	.05	.06	.7	14

Food	Measure															
Beans																
Lima, immature, cooked	1 cup	160	180	12	1	—	—	—	32	75	4.0	450	.29	.16	2.0	28
Snap, green																
Cooked																
In small amount of water, short time	1 cup	125	30	2	Trace	—	—	—	7	62	.8	680	.08	.11	.6	16
In large amount of water, long time	1 cup	125	30	2	Trace	—	—	—	7	62	0.8	680	0.07	0.10	0.4	13
Canned																
Solids and liquid	1 cup	239	45	2	Trace	—	—	—	10	81	2.9	690	.08	.10	.7	9
Strained or chopped (baby food)	1 oz.	28	5	Trace	Trace	—	—	—	1	9	.3	110	.01	.02	.1	Trace
Bean sprouts. See Sprouts.																
Beets, cooked, diced	1 cup	165	50	2	Trace	—	—	—	12	23	.8	40	.04	.07	.5	11
Broccoli spears, cooked	1 cup	150	40	5	Trace	—	—	—	7	132	1.2	3,750	.14	.29	1.2	135
Brussels sprouts, cooked	1 cup	130	45	5	1	—	—	—	8	42	1.4	680	.10	.18	1.1	113
Cabbage																
Raw																
Finely shredded	1 cup	100	25	1	Trace	—	—	—	5	49	.4	130	.05	.05	.3	47
Coleslaw	1 cup	120	120	1	9	2	2	5	9	52	.5	180	.06	.06	.3	35
Cooked																
In small amount of water, short time	1 cup	170	35	2	Trace	—	—	—	7	75	.5	220	.07	.07	.5	56
In large amount of water, long time	1 cup	170	30	2	Trace	—	—	—	7	71	.5	200	.04	.04	.2	40
Cabbage, celery or Chinese																
Raw, leaves and stalk, 1-inch pieces	1 cup	100	15	1	Trace	—	—	—	3	43	.6	150	.05	.04	.6	25
Cabbage, spoon (or pakchoy), cooked	1 cup	150	20	2	Trace	—	—	—	4	222	.9	4,650	.07	.12	1.1	23
Carrots																
Raw																
Whole, 5½ by 1 inch, (25 thin strips)	1	50	20	1	Trace	—	—	—	5	18	.4	5,500	.03	.03	.3	4
Grated	1 cup	110	45	1	Trace	—	—	—	11	41	.8	12,100	.06	.06	.7	9
Cooked, diced	1 cup	145	45	1	Trace	—	—	—	10	48	.9	15,220	.08	.07	.7	9
Canned, strained or chopped (baby food)	1 oz.	28	10	Trace	Trace	—	—	—	2	7	.1	3,690	.01	.01	.1	1
Cauliflower, cooked, flowerbuds	1 cup	120	25	3	Trace	—	—	—	5	25	.8	70	.11	.10	.7	66

Continued.

Food, approximate measure, and weight (in grams)			Food energy	Protein	Fat (total lipid)	Fatty acids Saturated (total)	Fatty acids Unsaturated Oleic	Fatty acids Unsaturated Linoleic	Carbohydrate	Calcium	Iron	Vitamin A value	Thiamine	Riboflavin	Niacin	Ascorbic acid
		gm.	(Calories)	(gm.)	(gm.)	(gm.)	(gm.)	(gm.)	(gm.)	(mg.)	(mg.)	(I.U.)	(mg.)	(mg.)	(mg.)	(mg.)
Celery, raw Stalk, large outer, 8 by about 1½ inches, at root end	1 stalk	40	5	Trace	Trace	—	—	—	2	16	.1	100	.01	.01	.1	4
Pieces, diced	1 cup	100	15	1	Trace	—	—	—	4	39	.3	240	.03	.03	.3	9
Collards, cooked	1 cup	190	55	5	1	—	—	—	9	289	1.1	10,260	.27	.37	2.4	87
Corn, sweet Cooked, ear 5 by 1¾ inches[5]	1 ear	140	70	3	1	—	—	—	16	2	.5	[6]310	.09	.08	1.0	7
Canned, solids and liquid	1 cup	256	170	5	2	—	—	—	40	10	1.0	[6]690	.07	.12	2.3	13
Cowpeas, cooked, immature seeds	1 cup	160	175	13	1	—	—	—	29	38	3.4	560	.49	.18	2.3	28
Cucumbers, 10 oz., 7½ by about 2 inches Raw, pared	1	207	30	1	Trace	—	—	—	7	35	.6	Trace	.07	.09	.4	23
Raw, pared, center slice ⅛-inch thick	6 slices	50	5	Trace	Trace	—	—	—	2	8	.2	Trace	.02	.02	.1	6
Dandelion greens, cooked	1 cup	180	60	4	1	—	—	—	12	252	3.2	21,060	.24	.29	—	32
Endive, curly (including escarole)	2 oz.	57	10	1	Trace	—	—	—	2	46	1.0	1,870	.04	.08	.3	6
Kale, leaves including stems, cooked	1 cup	110	30	4	1	—	—	—	4	147	1.3	8,140	—	—	—	68
Lettuce, raw Butterhead, as Boston types; head, 4-inch diameter	1 head	220	30	3	Trace	—	—	—	6	77	4.4	2,130	.14	.13	.6	18
Crisphead, as Iceberg; head, 4¾-inch diameter	1 head	454	60	4	Trace	—	—	—	13	91	2.3	1,500	.29	.27	1.3	29
Looseleaf, or bunching varieties, leaves	2 large	50	10	1	Trace	—	—	—	2	34	.7	950	.03	.04	.2	9
Mushrooms, canned, solids and liquid	1 cup	244	40	5	Trace	—	—	—	6	15	1.2	Trace	.04	.60	4.8	4
Mustard greens, cooked	1 cup	140	35	3	1	—	—	—	6	193	2.5	8,120	.11	.19	.9	68
Okra, cooked, pod 3 by ⅝ inch	8 pods	85	25	3	Trace	—	—	—	5	78	.4	420	.11	.15	.8	17

Onions																
Mature																
Raw, onion 2½-inch diameter	1	110	40	2	Trace	—	—	—	10	30	0.6	40	0.04	0.04	0.2	11
Cooked	1 cup	210	60	3	Trace	—	—	—	14	50	.8	80	.06	.06	.4	14
Young green, small, without tops	6	50	20	1	Trace	—	—	—	5	20	.3	Trace	.02	.02	.2	12
Parsley, raw, chopped	1 tbsp.	3.5	1	Trace	Trace	—	—	—	Trace	7	.2	300	Trace	.01	Trace	6
Parsnips, cooked	1 cup	155	100	2	1	—	—	—	23	70	.9	50	.11	.13	.2	16
Peas, green																
Cooked	1 cup	160	115	9	1	—	—	—	19	37	2.9	860	.44	.17	3.7	33
Canned, solids and liquid	1 cup	249	165	9	1	—	—	—	31	50	4.2	1,120	.23	.13	2.2	22
Canned, strained (baby food)	1 oz.	28	15	1	Trace	—	—	—	3	3	.4	140	.02	.02	.4	3
Peppers, hot, red, without seeds, dried (ground chili powder, added seasonings)	1 tbsp.	15	50	2	2	—	—	—	8	40	2.3	9,750	.03	.17	1.3	2
Peppers, sweet																
Raw, medium, about 6 per pound																
Green pod without stem and seeds	1 pod	62	15	1	Trace	—	—	—	3	6	.4	260	.05	.05	.3	79
Red pod without stem and seeds	1 pod	60	20	1	Trace	—	—	—	4	8	.4	2,670	.05	.05	.3	122
Canned, pimentos, medium	1 pod	38	10	Trace	Trace	—	—	—	2	3	.6	870	.01	.02	.1	36
Potatoes, medium (about 3 per pound raw)																
Baked, peeled after baking	1	99	90	3	Trace	—	—	—	21	9	.7	Trace	.10	.04	1.7	20
Boiled																
Peeled after boiling	1	136	105	3	Trace	—	—	—	23	10	.8	Trace	.13	.05	2.0	22
Peeled before boiling	1	122	80	2	Trace	—	—	—	18	7	.6	Trace	.11	.04	1.4	20
French-fried, piece 2 by ½ by ½ inch																
Cooked in deep fat	10 pieces	57	155	2	7	2	2	4	20	9	.7	Trace	.07	.04	1.8	12
Frozen, heated	10 pieces	57	125	2	5	1	1	2	19	5	1.0	Trace	.08	.01	1.5	12
Mashed																
Milk added	1 cup	195	125	4	1	—	—	—	25	47	.8	50	.16	.10	2.0	19
Milk and butter added	1 cup	195	185	4	8	4	3	Trace	24	47	.8	330	.16	.10	1.9	18

Continued.

[5] Measure and weight apply to entire vegetable or fruit including parts not usually eaten.

[6] Based on yellow varieties; white varieties contain only a trace of cryptoxanthin and carotenes, the pigments in corn that have biological activity.

Food, approximate measure, and weight (in grams)		gm.	Food energy (Calories)	Protein (gm.)	Fat (total lipid) (gm.)	Fatty acids Saturated (total) (gm.)	Unsaturated Oleic (gm.)	Unsaturated Linoleic (gm.)	Carbohydrate (gm.)	Calcium (mg.)	Iron (mg.)	Vitamin A value (I.U.)	Thiamine (mg.)	Riboflavin (mg.)	Niacin (mg.)	Ascorbic acid (mg.)
Potato chips, medium, 2-inch diameter	10 chips	20	115	1	8	3	2	4	10	8	.4	Trace	.04	.01	1.0	3
Pumpkin, canned	1 cup	228	75	2	1	—	—	—	18	57	.9	14,590	.07	.12	1.3	12
Radishes, raw, small, without tops	4	40	5	Trace	Trace	—	—	—	1	12	.4	Trace	.01	.01	.1	10
Sauerkraut, canned, solids and liquid	1 cup	235	45	2	Trace				9	85	1.2	120	.07	.09	.4	33
Spinach																
Cooked	1 cup	180	40	5	1	—	—	—	6	167	4.0	14,580	.13	.25	1.0	50
Canned, drained solids	1 cup	180	45	5	1	—	—	—	6	212	4.7	14,400	.03	.21	.6	24
Canned, strained or chopped (baby food)	1 oz.	28	10	1	Trace	—	—	—	2	18	.2	1,420	.01	.04	.1	2
Sprouts, raw																
Mung bean	1 cup	90	30	3	Trace	—	—	—	6	17	1.2	20	.12	.12	.7	17
Soybean	1 cup	107	40	6	2	—	—	—	4	46	.7	90	.17	.16	.8	4
Squash																
Cooked																
Summer, diced	1 cup	210	30	2	Trace	—	—	—	7	52	.8	820	.10	.16	1.6	21
Winter, baked, mashed	1 cup	205	130	4	1	—	—	—	32	57	1.6	8,610	.10	.27	1.4	27
Canned, winter, strained and chopped (baby food)	1 oz.	28	10	Trace	Trace	—	—	—	2	7	.1	510	.01	.01	.1	1
Sweetpotatoes																
Cooked, medium, 5 by 2 inches, weight raw about 6 oz.																
Baked, peeled after baking	1	110	155	2	1	—	—	—	36	44	1.0	8,910	.10	.07	.7	24
Boiled, peeled after boiling	1	147	170	2	1	—	—	—	39	47	1.0	11,610	.13	.09	.9	25
Candied, 3½ by 2¼ inches	1	175	295	2	6	2	3	1	60	65	1.6	11,030	.10	.08	.8	17
Canned, vacuum or solid pack	1 cup	218	235	4	Trace	—	—	—	54	54	1.7	17,000	.10	.10	1.4	30

Tomatoes		Grams	Food energy (Cal.)	Protein (g)	Fat (g)	Saturated (total) (g)	Unsaturated Oleic (g)	Unsaturated Linoleic (g)	Carbohydrate (g)	Calcium (mg)	Iron (mg)	Vitamin A (I.U.)	Thiamine (mg)	Riboflavin (mg)	Niacin (mg)	Ascorbic acid (mg)
Raw, medium, 2 by 2½ inches, about 3 per pound	1	150	35	2	Trace	—	—	—	7	20	.8	1,350	.10	.06	1.0	⁷34
Canned	1 cup	242	50	2	Trace	—	—	—	10	15	1.2	2,180	.13	.07	1.7	40
Tomato juice, canned	1 cup	242	45	2	Trace	—	—	—	10	17	2.2	1,940	.13	.07	1.8	39
Tomato catsup	1 tbsp.	17	15	Trace	Trace	—	—	—	4	4	.1	240	.02	.01	.3	3
Turnips, cooked, diced	1 cup	155	35	1	Trace	—	—	—	8	54	.6	Trace	.06	.08	.5	33
Turnip greens																
Cooked																
In small amount of water, short time	1 cup	145	30	3	Trace	—	—	—	5	267	1.6	9,140	.21	.36	.8	100
In large amount of water, long time	1 cup	145	25	3	Trace	—	—	—	5	252	1.4	8,260	.14	.33	.8	68
Canned, solids and liquid	1 cup	232	40	3	1	—	—	—	7	232	3.7	10,900	.04	.21	1.4	44
Fruits and fruit products																
Apples, raw, medium, 2½-inch diameter, about 3 per pound⁵	1	150	70	Trace	Trace	—	—	—	18	8	.4	50	.04	.02	.1	3
Apple brown betty	1 cup	230	345	4	8	4	3	Trace	68	41	1.4	230	.13	.10	.9	3
Apple juice, bottled or canned	1 cup	249	120	Trace	Trace	—	—	—	30	15	1.5	—	.01	.04	.2	2
Applesauce, canned																
Sweetened	1 cup	254	230	1	Trace	—	—	—	60	10	1.3	100	.05	.03	.1	3
Unsweetened or artificially sweetened	1 cup	239	100	Trace	Trace	—	—	—	26	10	1.2	100	.04	.02	.1	2
Applesauce and apricots, canned, strained or junior (baby food)	1 oz.	28	25	Trace	Trace	—	—	—	6	1	.1	170	Trace	Trace	Trace	1
Apricots																
Raw, about 12 per pound⁵	3 apricots	114	55	1	Trace	—	—	—	14	18	.5	2,890	.03	.04	.7	10
Canned in heavy syrup																
Halves and syrup	1 cup	259	220	2	Trace	—	—	—	57	28	.8	4,510	.05	.06	.9	10
Halves (medium) and syrup	4 halves; 2 tbsp. syrup	122	105	1	Trace	—	—	—	27	13	.4	2,120	.02	.03	.4	5

Continued.

⁵Measure and weight apply to entire vegetable or fruit including parts not usually eaten.
⁷Year-round average. Samples marketed from November through May average around 15 milligrams per 150-gram tomato; from June through October, around 39 milligrams.

Food, approximate measure, and weight (in grams)	gm.	Food energy (Calo-ries)	Pro-tein (gm.)	Fat (total lipid) (gm.)	Fatty acids Satu-rated (total) (gm.)	Fatty acids Unsaturated Oleic (gm.)	Fatty acids Linoleic (gm.)	Carbo-hydrate (gm.)	Cal-cium (mg.)	Iron (mg.)	Vita-min A value (I.U.)	Thia-mine (mg.)	Ribo-flavin (mg.)	Niacin (mg.)	Ascor-bic acid (mg.)
Apricots—cont'd															
Dried															
Uncooked, 40 halves, small — 1 cup	150	390	8	1	—	—	—	100	100	8.2	16,350	.02	.23	4.9	19
Cooked, unsweetened, fruit and liquid — 1 cup	285	240	5	1	—	—	—	62	63	5.1	8,550	.01	.13	2.8	8
Apricot nectar, canned — 1 cup	250	140	1	Trace	—	—	—	36	22	.5	2,380	.02	.02	.5	7
Avocados, raw															
California varieties, mainly Fuerte															
10-ounce avocado, about 3½ by 4¼ inches, peeled, pitted — ½	108	185	2	18	4	8	2	6	11	.6	310	.12	.21	1.7	15
½-inch cubes — 1 cup	152	260	3	26	5	12	3	9	15	.9	440	.16	.30	2.4	21
Florida varieties															
13 oz. avocado, about 4 by 3 inches, peeled, pitted — ½	123	160	2	14	3	6	2	11	12	.7	360	.13	.24	2.0	17
½-inch cubes — 1 cup	152	195	2	17	3	8	2	13	15	.9	440	.16	.30	2.4	21
Bananas, raw, 6 by 1½ inches, about 3 per pound[5] — 1	150	85	1	Trace	—	—	—	23	8	.7	190	.05	.06	.7	10
Blackberries, raw — 1 cup	144	85	2	1	—	—	—	19	46	1.3	290	.05	.06	.5	30
Blueberries, raw — 1 cup	140	85	1	1	—	—	—	21	21	1.4	140	.04	.08	.6	20
Cantaloups, raw; medium, 5-inch diameter, about 1⅔ pounds[5] — ½	385	60	1	Trace	—	—	—	14	27	.8	[8]6,540	.08	.06	1.2	63
Cherries															
Raw, sweet, with stems[5] — 1 cup	130	80	2	Trace	—	—	—	20	26	.5	130	.06	.07	.5	12
Canned, red, sour, pitted, heavy syrup — 1 cup	260	230	2	1	—	—	—	59	36	.8	1,680	.07	.06	.4	13
Cranberry juice cocktail, canned — 1 cup	250	160	Trace	Trace	—	—	—	41	12	.8	Trace	.02	.02	.1	(?)

Food	Measure	Grams	Food energy (Cal.)	Protein (g)	Fat (g)	Saturated (g)	Unsaturated, oleic (g)	Unsaturated, linoleic (g)	Carbohydrate (g)	Calcium (mg)	Iron (mg)	Vitamin A (I.U.)	Thiamine (mg)	Riboflavin (mg)	Niacin (mg)	Ascorbic acid (mg)
Cranberry sauce, sweetened, canned, strained	1 cup	277	405	Trace	1	—	—	—	104	17	.6	40	.03	0.3	.1	5
Dates, domestic, natural and dry, pitted, cut	1 cup	178	490	4	1	—	—	—	130	105	5.3	90	.16	.17	3.9	0
Figs																
Raw, small, 1½-inch diameter, about 12 per pound	3 figs	114	90	1	Trace	—	—	—	23	40	.7	90	.07	.06	.5	2
Dried, large, 2 by 1 inch	1 fig	21	60	1	Trace	—	—	—	15	26	.6	20	.02	.02	.1	0
Fruit cocktail, canned in heavy syrup, solids and liquid	1 cup	256	195	1	1	—	—	—	50	23	1.0	360	.04	.03	1.1	5
Grapefruit																
Raw, medium, 4¼-inch diameter, size 64																
White[5]	½	285	55	1	Trace	—	—	—	14	22	.6	10	.05	.02	.2	52
Pink or red[5]	½	285	60	1	Trace	—	—	—	15	23	.6	640	.05	.02	.3	52
Raw sections, white	1 cup	194	75	1	Trace	—	—	—	20	31	.8	20	.07	.03	.3	72
Canned, white																
Syrup pack, solids and liquid	1 cup	249	175	1	Trace	—	—	—	44	32	.7	20	.07	.04	.5	75
Water pack, solids and liquid	1 cup	240	70	1	Trace	—	—	—	18	31	.7	20	.07	.04	.5	72
Grapefruit juice																
Fresh	1 cup	246	95	1	Trace	—	—	—	23	22	.5	([10])	.09	.04	.4	92
Canned, white																
Unsweetened	1 cup	247	100	1	Trace	—	—	—	24	20	1.0	20	.07	.04	.4	84
Sweetened	1 cup	250	130	1	Trace	—	—	—	32	20	1.0	20	.07	.04	.4	78
Frozen, concentrate, unsweetened																
Undiluted, can, 6 fluid oz.	1 can	207	300	4	1	—	—	—	72	70	.8	60	.29	.12	1.4	286
Diluted with 3 parts water, by volume	1 cup	247	100	1	Trace	—	—	—	24	25	.2	20	.10	.04	.5	96
Frozen, concentrate, sweetened																
Undiluted, can, 6 fluid oz.	1 can	211	350	3	1	—	—	—	85	59	.6	50	.24	.11	1.2	245
Diluted with 3 parts water, by volume	1 cup	249	115	1	Trace	—	—	—	28	20	.2	20	.08	.03	.4	82

Continued.

[5] Measure and weight apply to entire vegetable or fruit including parts not usually eaten.

[8] Value based on varieties with orange-colored flesh; for green-fleshed varieties value is about 540 I.U. per ½ melon.

[9] About 5 milligrams per 8 fluid ounces is from cranberries. Ascorbic acid is usually added to approximately 100 milligrams per 8 fluid ounces.

[10] For white-fleshed varieties value is about 20 I.U. per cup; for red-fleshed varieties, 1,080 I.U. per cup.

Food, approximate measure, and weight (in grams)		gm.	Food energy (Calories)	Protein (gm.)	Fat (total lipid) (gm.)	Fatty acids Saturated (total) (gm.)	Fatty acids Unsaturated Oleic (gm.)	Fatty acids Unsaturated Linoleic (gm.)	Carbohydrate (gm.)	Calcium (mg.)	Iron (mg.)	Vitamin A value (I.U.)	Thiamine (mg.)	Riboflavin (mg.)	Niacin (mg.)	Ascorbic acid (mg.)
Grapefruit juice—cont'd Dehydrated																
Crystals, can, net weight 4 oz.	1 can	114	430	5	1	—	—	—	103	99	1.1	90	.41	.18	2.0	399
Prepared with water (1 pound yields about 1 gal.)	1 cup	247	100	1	Trace	—	—	—	24	22	.2	20	.10	.05	.5	92
Grapes, raw																
American type (slip skin), such as Concord, Delaware, Niagara, Catawba, and Scuppernong[5]	1 cup	153	65	1	1	—	—	—	15	15	.4	100	.05	.03	.2	3
European type (adherent skin), such as Malaga, Muscat, Thompson Seedless, Emperor, and Flame Tokay[5]	1 cup	160	95	1	Trace	—	—	—	25	17	.6	140	.07	.04	.4	6
Grape juice, bottled or canned	1 cup	254	165	1	Trace	—	—	—	42	28	.8	—	.10	.05	.6	Trace
Lemons, raw, medium, 2½-inch diameter, size 150[5]	1 lemon	106	20	1	Trace	—	—	—	6	18	.4	10	.03	.01	.1	38
Lemon juice																
Fresh	1 cup	246	60	1	Trace	—	—	—	20	17	.5	40	.08	.03	.2	113
	1 tbsp.	15	5	Trace	Trace	—	—	—	1	1	Trace	Trace	Trace	Trace	Trace	7
Canned, unsweetened	1 cup	245	55	1	Trace	—	—	—	19	17	.5	40	.07	.03	.2	102
Lemonade concentrate, frozen, sweetened																
Undiluted, can, 6 fluid oz.	1 can	220	430	Trace	Trace	—	—	—	112	9	.4	40	.05	.06	.7	66
Diluted with 4½ parts water, by volume	1 cup	248	110	Trace	Trace	—	—	—	28	2	.1	10	.01	.01	.2	17
Lime juice																
Fresh	1 cup	246	65	1	Trace	—	—	—	22	22	.5	30	.05	.03	.03	80
Canned	1 cup	246	65	1	Trace	—	—	—	22	22	.5	30	.05	.03	.3	52

Limeade concentrate, frozen, sweetened																
Undiluted, can, 6 fluid oz.	1 can	218	410	Trace	Trace	—	—	—	108	11	.2	Trace	.02	.02	.3	26
Diluted with 4⅓ parts water, by volume	1 cup	248	105	Trace	Trace	—	—	—	27	2	Trace	Trace	Trace	Trace	Trace	6
Oranges, raw																
California, Navel (winter), 2⅘-inch diameter, size 88[5]	1 orange	180	60	2	Trace	—	—	—	16	49	.5	240	.12	.05	.5	75
Florida, all varieties, 3-inch diameter[5]	1	210	75	1	Trace	—	—	—	19	67	.3	310	.16	.06	.6	70
Orange juice																
Fresh																
California, Valencia (summer)	1 cup	249	115	2	1	—	—	—	26	27	.7	500	.22	.06	.9	122
Florida varieties																
Early and mid-season	1 cup	247	100	1	Trace	—	—	—	23	25	.5	490	.22	.06	.9	127
Late season, Valencia	1 cup	248	110	1	Trace	—	—	—	26	25	.5	500	.22	.06	.9	92
Canned, unsweetened	1 cup	249	120	2	Trace	—	—	—	28	25	1.0	500	.17	.05	.6	100
Frozen concentrate																
Undiluted, can, 6 fluid oz.	1 can	210	330	5	Trace	—	—	—	80	69	.8	1,490	.63	.10	2.4	332
Diluted with 3 parts water, by volume	1 cup	248	110	2	Trace	—	—	—	27	22	.2	500	.21	.03	.8	112
Dehydrated																
Crystals, can, net weight 4 oz.	1 can	113	430	6	2	—	—	—	100	95	1.9	1,900	.76	.24	3.3	406
Prepared with water, 1 lb. yields about 1 gal.	1 cup	248	115	1	Trace	—	—	—	27	25	.5	500	.20	.06	.9	108
Orange and grapefruit juice																
Frozen concentrate																
Undiluted, can, 6 fluid oz.	1 can	209	325	4	1	—	—	—	78	61	.8	790	.47	.06	2.3	301
Diluted with 3 parts water, by volume	1 cup	248	110	1	Trace	—	—	—	26	20	.3	270	.16	.02	.8	102
Papayas, raw, ½-inch cubes	1 cup	182	70	1	Trace	—	—	—	18	36	.5	3,190	.07	.08	.5	102

Continued.

[5]Measure and weight apply to entire vegetable or fruit including parts not usually eaten.

Food, approximate measure, and weight (in grams)	gm.	Food energy (Calories)	Protein (gm.)	Fat (total lipid) (gm.)	Fatty acids Saturated (total) (gm.)	Fatty acids Unsaturated Oleic (gm.)	Fatty acids Unsaturated Linoleic (gm.)	Carbohydrate (gm.)	Calcium (mg.)	Iron (mg.)	Vitamin A value (I.U.)	Thiamine (mg.)	Riboflavin (mg.)	Niacin (mg.)	Ascorbic acid (mg.)
Peaches															
Raw															
Whole, medium, 2-inch diameter, about 4 per pound[5]	1 / 114	35	1	Trace	—	—	—	10	9	.5	[11]1,320	.02	.05	1.0	7
Sliced	1 cup / 168	65	1	Trace	—	—	—	16	15	.8	[11]2,230	.03	.08	1.6	12
Canned, yellow-fleshed, solids and liquid															
Syrup pack, heavy															
Halves or slices	1 cup / 257	200	1	Trace	—	—	—	52	10	.8	1,100	.02	.06	1.4	7
Halves (medium) and syrup	2 halves and 2 tbsp. syrup / 117	90	Trace	Trace	—	—	—	24	5	.4	500	.01	.03	.7	3
Water pack	1 cup / 245	75	1	Trace	—	—	—	20	10	.7	1,100	.02	.06	1.4	7
Strained or chopped (baby food)	1 oz. / 28	25	Trace	Trace	—	—	—	6	2	.1	140	Trace	.01	.2	1
Dried															
Uncooked	1 cup / 160	420	5	1	—	—	—	109	77	9.6	6,240	.02	.31	8.5	28
Cooked, unsweetened, 10-12 halves and 6 tbsp. liquid	1 cup / 270	220	3	1	—	—	—	58	41	5.1	3,290	.01	.15	4.2	6
Frozen															
Carton, 12 oz., not thawed	1 carton / 340	300	1	Trace	—	—	—	77	14	1.7	2,210	.03	.14	2.4	[12]135
Can, 16 oz., not thawed	1 can / 454	400	2	Trace	—	—	—	103	18	2.3	2,950	.05	.18	3.2	[12]181
Peach nectar, canned	1 cup / 250	120	Trace	Trace	—	—	—	31	10	.5	1,080	.02	.05	1.0	1
Pears															
Raw, 3 by 2½-inch diameter[5]	1 / 182	100	1	1	—	—	—	25	13	.5	30	.04	.07	.2	7
Canned, solids and liquid															
Syrup pack, heavy															
Halves or slices	1 cup / 255	195	1	1	—	—	—	50	13	.5	Trace	.03	.05	.3	4
Halves (medium) and syrup	2 halves and 2 tbsp. syrup / 117	90	Trace	Trace	—	—	—	23	6	.2	Trace	.01	.02	.2	2

Food, approximate measure, and weight (grams)		Food energy (calories)	Protein (grams)	Fat (grams)	Fatty acids Saturated (total)	Unsaturated Oleic	Unsaturated Linoleic	Carbohydrate (grams)	Calcium (milligrams)	Iron (milligrams)	Vitamin A value (I.U.)	Thiamine (milligrams)	Riboflavin (milligrams)	Niacin (milligrams)	Ascorbic acid (milligrams)
Water pack	1 cup / 243	80	Trace	Trace	—	—	—	20	12	.5	Trace	.02	.05	.3	4
Strained or chopped (baby food)	1 oz. / 28	20	Trace	Trace	—	—	—	5	2	.1	10	Trace	.01	.1	1
Pear nectar, canned	1 cup / 250	130	1	Trace	—	—	—	33	8	.2	Trace	.01	.05	Trace	1
Persimmons, Japanese or kaki, raw, seedless, 2½-inch diameter[5]	1 / 125	75	1	Trace	—	—	—	20	6	.4	2,740	.01	.02	.1	11
Pineapple															
Raw, diced	1 cup / 140	75	1	Trace	—	—	—	19	24	.7	100	.12	.04	.3	24
Canned, heavy syrup pack, solids and liquid															
Crushed	1 cup / 260	195	1	Trace	—	—	—	50	29	.8	120	.20	.06	.5	17
Sliced, slices and juice	2 small or 1 large and 2 tbsp. juice / 122	90	Trace	Trace	—	—	—	24	13	.4	50	.09	.03	.2	8
Pineapple juice, canned	1 cup / 249	135	1	Trace	—	—	—	34	37	.7	120	.12	.04	.5	22
Plums, all except prunes															
Raw, 2-inch diameter, about 2 ounces[5]	1 / 60	25	Trace	Trace	—	—	—	7	7	.3	140	.02	.02	.3	3
Canned, syrup pack (Italian prunes)															
Plums (with pits) and juice[5]	1 cup / 256	205	1	Trace	—	—	—	53	22	2.2	2,970	.05	.05	.9	4
Plums (without pits) and juice	3 plums and 2 tbsp. juice / 122	100	Trace	Trace	—	—	—	26	11	1.1	1,470	.03	.02	.5	2
Prunes, dried, "softenized," medium															
Uncooked[5]	4 / 32	70	1	Trace	—	—	—	18	14	1.1	440	.02	.04	.4	1
Cooked, unsweetened, 17-18 prunes and ⅓ cup liquid[5]	1 cup / 270	295	2	1	—	—	—	78	60	4.5	1,860	.08	.18	1.7	2
Prunes with tapioca, canned, strained or junior (baby food)	1 oz. / 28	25	Trace	Trace	—	—	—	6	2	.3	110	.01	.02	.1	1
Prune juice, canned	1 cup / 256	200	1	Trace	—	—	—	49	36	10.5	—	.02	.03	1.1	4
Raisin, dried	1 cup / 160	460	4	Trace	—	—	—	124	99	5.6	30	.18	.13	.9	2

Continued.

[5]Measure and weight apply to entire vegetable or fruit including parts not usually eaten.

[11]Based on yellow-fleshed varieties; for white-fleshed varieties value is about 50 I.U. per 114-gram peach and 80 I.U. per cup of sliced peaches.

[12]Average weighted in accordance with commercial freezing practices. For products without added ascorbic acid, value is about 37 milligrams per 12-ounce carton and 50 milligrams per 16-ounce can; for those with added ascorbic acid, 139 milligrams per 12 ounces and 186 milligrams per 16 ounces.

Food, approximate measure, and weight (in grams)		(gm.)	Food energy (Calories)	Protein (gm.)	Fat (total lipid) (gm.)	Saturated (total) (gm.)	Unsaturated Oleic (gm.)	Unsaturated Linoleic (gm.)	Carbohydrate (gm.)	Calcium (mg.)	Iron (mg.)	Vitamin A value (I.U.)	Thiamine (mg.)	Riboflavin (mg.)	Niacin (mg.)	Ascorbic acid (mg.)
Raspberries, red																
Raw	1 cup	123	70	1	1	—	—	—	17	27	1.1	160	.04	.11	1.1	31
Frozen, 10 oz. carton, not thawed	1 carton	284	275	2	1	—	—	—	70	37	1.7	200	.06	.17	1.7	59
Rhubarb, cooked, sugar added	1 cup	272	385	1	Trace	—	—	—	98	212	1.6	220	.06	.15	.7	17
Strawberries																
Raw, capped	1 cup	149	55	1	1	—	—	—	13	31	1.5	90	.04	.10	1.0	88
Frozen, 10-oz. carton, not thawed	1 carton	284	310	1	1	—	—	—	79	40	2.0	90	.06	.17	1.5	150
Frozen, 16-ounce can, not thawed	1 can	454	495	2	1	—	—	—	126	64	3.2	150	.09	.27	2.4	240
Tangerines, raw, medium, 2½-inch diameter, about 4 per pound[5]	1	114	40	1	Trace	—	—	—	10	34	.3	350	.05	.02	.1	26
Tangerine juice																
Tangerine juice																
Canned, unsweetened	1 cup	248	105	1	Trace	—	—	—	25	45	.5	1,040	.14	.04	.3	56
Frozen concentrate																
Undiluted, can, 6 fluid oz.	1 can	210	340	4	1	—	—	1	80	130	1.5	3,070	.43	.12	.9	202
Diluted with 3 parts water, by volume	1 cup	248	115	1	Trace	—	—	—	27	45	.5	1,020	.14	.04	.3	67
Watermelon, raw, wedge, 4 by 8 inches (1/16 of 10 by 16-inch melon, about 2 pounds with rind)[5]	1 wedge	925	115	2	1	—	—	—	27	30	2.1	2,510	.13	.13	.7	30
Barley, pearled, light, uncooked	1 cup	203	710	17	2	Trace	1	1	160	32	4.1	0	.25	.17	6.3	0
Biscuits, baking powder with enriched flour, 2½-inch diameter	1	38	140	3	6	2	3	1	17	46	.6	Trace	.08	.08	.7	Trace
Bran flakes (40 percent bran) added thiamine	1 oz.	28	85	3	1	—	—	—	23	20	1.2	0	.11	.05	1.7	0

Bread	Measure															
Boston brown bread, slice, 3 by ¾ inch	1 slice	48	100	3	1	—	—	—	22	43	.9	0	.05	.03	.6	0
Cracked-wheat bread																
Loaf, 1-pound, 20 slices	1 loaf	454	1,190	39	10	2	5	2	236	399	5.0	Trace	.53	.42	5.8	Trace
Slice	1	23	60	2	1	—	—	—	12	20	.3	Trace	.03	.02	.3	Trace
French or Vienna bread																
Enriched, 1-pound loaf	1 loaf	454	1,315	41	14	3	8	2	251	195	10.0	Trace	1.26	.98	11.3	Trace
Unenriched, 1-pound loaf	1 loaf	454	1,315	41	14	3	8	2	251	195	3.2	Trace	.39	.39	3.6	Trace
Italian bread																
Enriched, 1-pound loaf	1 loaf	454	1,250	41	4	Trace	1	2	256	77	10.0	0	1.31	.93	11.7	0
Unenriched, 1-pound loaf	1 loaf	454	1,250	41	4	Trace	1	2	256	77	3.2	0	.39	.27	3.6	0
Raisin bread																
Loaf, 1-pound, 20 slices	1 loaf	454	1,190	30	13	3	8	2	243	322	5.9	Trace	.24	.42	3.0	Trace
Slice	1	23	60	2	1	—	—	—	12	16	.3	Trace	.01	.02	.2	Trace
Rye bread																
American, light (⅓ rye, ⅔ wheat) Loaf, 1-pound, 20 slices	1 loaf	454	1,100	41	5	—	—	—	236	340	7.3	0	.81	.33	6.4	0
Slice	1	23	55	2	Trace	—	—	—	12	17	.4	0	.04	.02	.3	0
Pumpernickel, loaf, 1 pound	1 loaf	454	1,115	41	5	—	—	—	241	381	10.9	0	1.05	.63	5.4	0
White bread, enriched																
1 to 2 percent nonfat dry milk Loaf, 1-pound, 20 slices	1 loaf	454	1,225	39	15	3	8	2	229	318	10.9	Trace	1.13	.77	10.4	Trace
Slice	1 slice	23	60	2	1	Trace	Trace	Trace	12	16	.6	Trace	.06	.04	.5	Trace
3 to 4 percent nonfat dry milk[13]																
Loaf, 1-pound	1	454	1,225	39	15	3	8	2	229	381	11.3	Trace	1.13	.95	10.8	Trace
Slice, 20 per loaf	1	23	60	2	1	Trace	Trace	Trace	12	19	.6	Trace	.06	.05	.6	Trace
Slice, toasted	1	20	60	2	1	Trace	Trace	Trace	12	19	.6	Trace	.05	.05	.6	Trace
Slice, 26 per loaf	1	17	45	1	1	Trace	Trace	Trace	9	14	.4	Trace	.04	.04	.4	Trace

Continued.

[5] Measure and weight apply to entire vegetable or fruit including parts not usually eaten.

[13] When the amount of nonfat dry milk in commercial white bread is unknown, values for bread with 3 to 4% nonfat dry milk are suggested.

Food, approximate measure, and weight (in grams)		gm.	Food energy (Calories)	Protein (gm.)	Fat (total lipid) (gm.)	Fatty acids Saturated (total) (gm.)	Fatty acids Unsaturated Oleic (gm.)	Fatty acids Unsaturated Linoleic (gm.)	Carbohydrate (gm.)	Calcium (mg.)	Iron (mg.)	Vitamin A value (I.U.)	Thiamine (mg.)	Riboflavin (mg.)	Niacin (mg.)	Ascorbic acid (mg.)
Bread—cont'd																
White bread, enriched—cont'd																
5 to 6 percent nonfat dry milk																
Loaf, 1-pound, 20 slices	1 loaf	454	1,245	41	17	4	10	2	228	435	11.3	Trace	1.22	.91	11.0	Trace
Slice	1	23	65	2	1	Trace	Trace	Trace	12	22	.6	Trace	.06	.05	.6	Trace
White bread, unenriched																
1 to 2 percent nonfat dry milk																
Loaf, 1-pound, 20 slices	1 loaf	454	1,225	39	15	3	8	2	229	318	3.2	Trace	.40	.36	5.6	Trace
Slice	1	23	60	2	1	Trace	Trace	Trace	12	16	.2	Trace	.02	.02	.3	Trace
3 to 4 percent nonfat dry milk[13]																
Loaf, 1-pound	1 loaf	454	1,225	39	15	3	8	—	229	381	3.2	Trace	.31	.39	5.0	Trace
Slice, 20 per loaf	1 slice	23	60	2	1	Trace	Trace	Trace	12	19	.2	Trace	.02	.02	.3	Trace
Slice, toasted	1	20	60	2	1	Trace	Trace	Trace	12	19	.2	Trace	.01	.02	.3	Trace
Slice, 26 per loaf	1 slice	17	45	1	1	Trace	Trace	Trace	9	14	.1	Trace	.01	.01	.2	Trace
5 to 6 percent nonfat dry milk																
Loaf, 1-pound, 20 slices	1 loaf	454	1,245	41	17	4	10	2	228	435	3.2	Trace	.32	.39	4.1	Trace
Slice	1	23	65	2	1	Trace	Trace	Trace	12	22	.2	Trace	.02	.03	.2	Trace
Whole-wheat bread, made with 2 percent nonfat dry milk																
Loaf, 1-pound, 20 slices	1 loaf	454	1,105	48	14	3	6	3	216	449	10.4	Trace	1.17	.56	12.9	Trace
Slice	1	23	55	2	1	Trace	Trace	Trace	11	23	.5	Trace	.06	.03	.7	Trace
Slice, toasted	1	19	55	2	1	Trace	Trace	Trace	11	22	.5	Trace	.05	.03	.6	Trace
Breadcrumbs, dry, grated	1 cup	88	345	11	4	1	2	1	65	107	3.2	Trace	.19	.26	3.1	Trace
Cakes[14]																
Angelfood cake; sector, 2-inch (1/12 of 8-inch-diameter cake)	1 sector	40	110	3	Trace	—	—	—	24	4	.1	0	Trace	.06	.1	0
Chocolate cake, chocolate icing; sector, 2-inch (1/16 of 10-inch-diameter layer cake)	1 sector	120	445	5	20	8	10	1	67	84	1.2	15190	.03	.12	.3	Trace

Fruitcake, dark (made with enriched flour); piece, 2 by 2 by ½ inch	1 piece	30	115	1	5	1	3	1	18	22	.8	[15]40	.04	.04	.2	Trace
Gingerbread (made with enriched flour); piece, 2 by 2 by 2 inches	1 piece	55	175	2	6	1	4	Trace	29	37	1.3	50	.06	.06	.5	0
Plain cake and cupcakes, without icing																
Piece, 3 by 2 by 1½ inches	1	55	200	2	8	2	5	1	31	35	.2	[15]90	.01	.05	.1	Trace
Cupcake, 2¾-inch diameter	1	40	145	2	6	1	3	Trace	22	26	.2	[15]70	.01	.03	.1	Trace
Plain cake and cupcakes, with chocolate icing																
Sector, 2-inch (1/16 of 10-inch-layer cake)	1	100	370	4	14	5	7	1	59	63	.6	[15]180	.02	.09	.2	Trace
Cupcake, 2¾-inch diameter	1	50	185	2	7	2	4	Trace	30	32	.3	[15]90	.01	.04	.1	Trace
Poundcake, old-fashioned (equal weights flour, sugar, fat, eggs); slice, 2¾ by 3 by ⅝ inch	1 slice	30	140	2	9	2	5	1	14	6	.2	[15]80	.01	.03	.1	0
Sponge cake; sector, 2-inch (1/12 of 8-inch-diameter cake)	1	40	120	3	2	1	1	Trace	22	12	.5	180	.02	.06	.1	Trace
Cookies																
Plain and assorted, 3-inch diameter	1 cooky	25	120	1	5	—	—	—	18	9	.2	20	.01	.01	.1	Trace
Fig bars, small	1	16	55	1	1	—	—	—	12	12	.2	20	.01	.01	.1	Trace
Corn, rice and wheat flakes, mixed, added nutrients	1 oz.	28	110	2	Trace	—	—	—	24	11	.5	0	.11	—	.9	0
Corn flakes, added nutrients																
Plain	1 oz.	28	110	2	Trace	—	—	—	24	5	.4	0	.12	.02	.6	0
Sugar-covered	1 oz.	28	110	1	Trace	—	—	—	26	3	.3	0	.12	.01	.5	0

Continued.

[13] When the amount of nonfat dry milk in commercial white bread is unknown, values for bread with 3 to 4% nonfat dry milk are suggested.

[14] Unenriched cake flour and vegetable cooking fat used unless otherwise specified.

[15] If the fat used in the recipe is butter or fortified margarine, the vitamin A value for chocolate cake with chocolate icing will be 490 I.U. per 2-inch sector; 100 I.U. for fruitcake; for plain cake without icing, 300 I.U. per piece; 220 I.U. per cupcake; for plain cake with icing, 440 I.U. per 2-inch sector; 220 I.U. per cupcake; and 300 I.U. for poundcake.

Food, approximate measure, and weight (in grams)	Weight (gm.)	Food energy (Calories)	Protein (gm.)	Fat (total lipid) (gm.)	Fatty acids — Saturated (total) (gm.)	Fatty acids — Unsaturated Oleic (gm.)	Fatty acids — Unsaturated Linoleic (gm.)	Carbohydrate (gm.)	Calcium (mg.)	Iron (mg.)	Vitamin A value (I.U.)	Thiamine (mg.)	Riboflavin (mg.)	Niacin (mg.)	Ascorbic acid (mg.)
Corn grits, degermed, cooked															
Enriched 1 cup	242	120	3	Trace	—	—	—	27	2	[16].7	[17]150	[16].10	[16].07	[16]1.0	0
Unenriched 1 cup	242	120	3	Trace	—	—	—	27	2	.2	[17]150	.05	.02	.5	0
Cornmeal, white or yellow, dry															
Whole ground, unbolted 1 cup	118	420	11	5	1	2	2	87	24	2.8	[17]600	.45	.13	2.4	0
Degermed, enriched 1 cup	145	525	11	2	Trace	1	1	114	9	[16]4.2	[17]640	[16].64	[16].38	[16]5.1	0
Corn muffins, made with enriched degermed cornmeal and enriched flour; muffin, 2¾-inch diameter 1 muffin	48	150	3	5	2	2	Trace	23	50	.8	[18]80	.09	.11	.8	Trace
Corn, puffed, pre-sweetened, added nutrients 1 oz.	28	110	1	Trace	—	—	—	26	3	.5	0	.12	.05	.6	0
Corn, shredded, added nutrients 1 oz.	28	110	2	Trace	—	—	—	25	1	.7	0	.12	.05	.6	0
Crackers															
Graham, plain 4 small or 2 medium	14	55	1	1	—	—	—	10	6	.2	0	.01	.03	.2	0
Saltines, 2 inches squares 2 crackers	8	35	1	1	—	—	—	6	2	.1	0	Trace	Trace	.1	0
Soda															
Cracker, 2½ inches square 2 crackers	11	50	1	1	Trace	1	Trace	8	2	.2	0	Trace	Trace	.1	0
Oyster crackers 10 crackers	10	45	1	1	Trace	1	Trace	7	2	.2	0	Trace	Trace	.1	0
Cracker meal 1 tbsp.	10	45	1	1	Trace	1	Trace	7	2	.1	0	.01	Trace	.1	0
Doughnuts, cake type 1 doughnut	32	125	1	6	1	4	Trace	16	13	[19].4	30	[19].05	[19].05	[19].4	0
Farina, regular, enriched, cooked 1 cup	238	100	3	Trace	—	—	—	21	10	[16].7	0	[16].11	[16].07	[16]1.0	Trace
Macaroni, cooked															
Enriched															
Cooked, firm stage (8 to 10 minutes; undergoes additional cooking in a food mixture) 1 cup	130	190	6	1	—	—	—	39	14	[16]1.4	0	[16].23	[16].14	[16]1.9	0

Food	Measure														
Cooked until tender Unenriched	1 cup	140	155	5	1	—	—	—	32	11	[16]1.3	0	[16].19	[16].11	[16]1.5	0
Cooked, firm stage (8 to 10 minutes; undergoes additional cooking in a food mixture)	1 cup	130	190	6	1	—	—	—	39	14	.6	0	.02	.02	.5	0
Cooked until tender	1 cup	140	155	5	1	—	—	—	32	11	.6	0	.02	.02	.4	0
Macaroni (enriched) and cheese, baked	1 cup	220	470	18	24	11	10	1	44	398	2.0	950	.22	.44	2.0	Trace
Muffins, with enriched white flour; muffin, 2¾-inch diameter	1	48	140	4	5	1	3	Trace	20	50	.8	50	.08	.11	.7	Trace
Noodles (egg noodles), cooked Enriched	1 cup	160	200	7	2	1	1	Trace	37	16	[16]1.4	110	[16].23	[16].14	[16]1.8	0
Unenriched	1 cup	160	200	7	2	1	1	Trace	37	16	1.0	110	.04	.03	.7	0
Oats (with or without corn) puffed, added nutrients	1 oz.	28	115	3	2	Trace	1	1	21	50	1.3	0	.28	.05	.5	0
Oatmeal or rolled oats, regular or quick-cooking, cooked	1 cup	236	130	5	2	Trace	1	1	23	21	1.4	0	.19	.05	.3	0
Pancakes (griddlecakes), 4-inch diameter Wheat, enriched flour (home recipe)	1 cake	27	60	2	2	Trace	1	Trace	9	27	.4	30	.05	.06	.3	Trace
Buckwheat (buckwheat pancake mix, made with egg and milk)	1 cake	27	55	2	2	1	1	Trace	6	59	.4	60	.03	.04	.2	Trace
Piecrust, plain, baked Enriched flour Lower crust, 9-inch shell	1	135	675	8	45	10	29	3	59	19	2.3	0	.27	.19	2.4	0
Double crust, 9-inch pie	1	270	1,350	16	90	21	58	7	118	38	4.6	0	.55	.39	4.9	0

[16] Iron, thiamine, riboflavin, and niacin are based on the minimum levels of enrichment specified in standards of identity promulgated under the Federal Food, Drug, and Cosmetic Act.

[17] Vitamin A value based on yellow product. White product contains only a trace.

[18] Based on recipe using white cornmeal; if yellow cornmeal is used, the vitamin A value is 140 I.U. per muffin.

[19] Based on product made with enriched flour. With unenriched flour, approximate values per doughnut are: Iron, 0.2 milligram; thiamine, 0.01 milligram; riboflavin, 0.03 milligram; niacin, 0.2 milligram.

Continued.

Food, approximate measure, and weight (in grams)	gm.	Food energy (Calories)	Protein (gm.)	Fat (total lipid) (gm.)	Fatty acids Saturated (total) (gm.)	Fatty acids Unsaturated Oleic (gm.)	Fatty acids Unsaturated Linoleic (gm.)	Carbohydrate (gm.)	Calcium (mg.)	Iron (mg.)	Vitamin A value (I.U.)	Thiamine (mg.)	Riboflavin (mg.)	Niacin (mg.)	Ascorbic acid (mg.)
Piecrust, plain, baked—cont'd															
Unenriched flour															
Lower crust, 9-inch shell — 1	135	675	8	45	10	29	3	59	19	.7	0	.04	.04	.6	0
Double crust, 9-inch pie — 1	270	1,350	16	90	21	58	7	118	38	1.4	0	.08	.07	1.3	0
Pies (piecrust made with unenriched flour); sector, 4-inch, 1/7 of 9-inch-diameter pie															
Apple — 1 sector	135	345	3	15	4	9	1	51	11	.4	40	.03	.02	.5	1
Cherry — 1 sector	135	355	4	15	4	10	1	52	19	.4	590	.03	.03	.6	1
Custard — 1 sector	130	280	8	14	5	8	1	30	125	.8	300	.07	.21	.4	0
Lemon meringue — 1 sector	120	305	4	12	4	7	1	45	17	.6	200	.04	.10	.2	4
Mince — 1 sector	135	365	3	16	4	10	1	56	38	1.4	Trace	.09	.05	.5	1
Pumpkin — 1 sector	130	275	5	15	5	7	1	32	66	.6	3,210	.04	.13	.6	Trace
Pizza (cheese); 5½-inch sector; ⅛ of 14-inch-diameter pie — 1 sector	75	185	7	6	2	3	Trace	27	107	.7	290	.04	.12	.7	4
Popcorn, popped, with added oil and salt — 1 cup	14	65	1	3	2	Trace	Trace	8	1	.3	—	—	.01	.2	0
Pretzels, small stick — 5 sticks	5	20	Trace	Trace	—	—	—	4	1	0	0	Trace	Trace	Trace	0
Rice, white (fully milled or polished), enriched, cooked															
Common commercial varieties, all types — 1 cup	168	185	3	Trace	—	—	—	41	17	[20] 1.5	0	[20] .19	[20] .01	[20] 1.6	0
Long grain, parboiled — 1 cup	176	185	4	Trace	—	—	—	41	33	[20] 1.4	0	[20] .19	[20] .02	[20] 2.0	0
Rice, puffed, added nutrients (without salt) — 1 cup	14	55	1	Trace	—	—	—	13	3	.3	0	.06	.01	.6	0
Rice flakes, added nutrients — 1 cup	30	115	2	Trace	—	—	—	26	9	.5	0	.10	.02	1.6	0
Rolls															
Plain, pan; 12 per 16 ounces															
Enriched — 1 roll	38	115	3	2	Trace	1	Trace	20	28	.7	Trace	.11	.07	.8	Trace
Unenriched — 1 roll	38	115	3	2	Trace	1	Trace	20	28	.3	Trace	.02	.03	.3	Trace
Hard, round; 12 per 22 oz. — 1 roll	52	160	5	2	Trace	1	Trace	31	24	.4	Trace	.03	.05	.4	Trace
Sweet, pan; 12 per 18 oz. — 1 roll	43	135	4	4	1	2	Trace	21	37	.3	30	.03	.06	.4	Trace

Food	Measure															
Rye wafers, whole-grain, 1⅞ by 3½ inches	2 wafers	13	45	2	Trace	—	—	—	10	7	.5	0	.04	.03	.2	0
Spaghetti																
Cooked, tender stage (14 to 20 minutes)																
Enriched	1 cup	140	155	5	1	—	—	—	32	11	[16]1.3	0	[16].19	[16].11	[16]1.5	0
Unenriched	1 cup	140	155	5	1	—	—	—	32	11	.6	0	.02	.02	.4	0
Spaghetti with meat balls in tomato sauce (home recipe)	1 cup	250	335	19	12	4	6	1	39	125	3.8	1,600	.26	.30	4.0	22
Spaghetti in tomato sauce with cheese (home recipe)	1 cup	250	260	9	9	2	5	1	37	80	2.2	1,080	.24	.18	2.4	14
Waffles, with enriched flour, ½ by 4½ by 5½ inches	1	75	210	7	7	2	4	1	28	85	1.3	250	.13	.19	1.0	Trace
Wheat, puffed																
With added nutrients (without salt)	1 oz.	28	105	4	Trace	—	—	—	22	8	1.2	0	.15	.07	2.2	0
With added nutrients, with sugar and honey	1 oz.	28	105	2	1	—	—	—	25	7	.9	0	.14	.05	1.8	0
Wheat, rolled; cooked	1 cup	236	175	5	1	—	—	—	40	19	1.7	0	.17	.06	2.1	0
Wheat, shredded, plain (long, round, or bite-size)	1 oz.	28	100	3	1	—	—	—	23	12	1.0	0	.06	.03	1.2	0
Wheat and malted barley flakes, with added nutrients	1 oz.	28	110	2	Trace	—	—	—	24	14	.7	0	.13	.03	1.1	0
Wheat flakes, with added nutrients	1 oz.	28	100	3	Trace	—	—	—	23	12	1.2	0	.18	.04	1.4	0
Wheat flours																
Whole-wheat, from hard wheats, stirred	1 cup	120	400	16	2	Trace	1	1	85	49	4.0	0	.66	.14	5.2	0
All-purpose or family flour																
Enriched, sifted	1 cup	110	400	12	1	Trace	Trace	Trace	84	18	[16]3.2	0	[16].48	[16].29	[16]3.8	0
Unenriched, sifted	1 cup	110	400	12	1	Trace	Trace	Trace	84	18	.9	0	.07	.05	1.0	0
Self-rising, enriched	1 cup	110	385	10	1	Trace	Trace	Trace	82	292	[16]3.2	0	[16].49	[16].29	[16]3.9	0
Cake or pastry flour, sifted	1 cup	100	365	8	1	Trace	Trace	Trace	79	17	.5	0	.03	.03	.7	0
Wheat germ, crude, commercially milled	1 cup	68	245	18	7	1	2	4	32	49	6.4	0	1.36	.46	2.9	0

[16]Iron, thiamine, riboflavin, and niacin are based on the minimum levels of enrichment specified in standards of identity promulgated under the Federal Food, Drug, and Cosmetic Act. *Continued.*

[20]Iron, thiamine, and niacin are based on the minimum levels of enrichment specified in standards of identity promulgated under the Federal Food, Drug, and Cosmetic Act. Riboflavin is based on unenriched rice. When the minimum level of enrichment for riboflavin specified in the standards of identity becomes effective the value will be 0.12 milligram per cup of parboiled rice and of white rice.

Fats, oils

Food, approximate measure, and weight (in grams)			Food energy	Protein	Fat (total lipid)	Fatty acids			Carbohydrate	Calcium	Iron	Vitamin A value	Thiamine	Riboflavin	Niacin	Ascorbic acid
						Saturated (total)	Unsaturated Oleic	Unsaturated Linoleic								
		(gm.)	(Calories)	(gm.)	(gm.)	(gm.)	(gm.)	(gm.)	(gm.)	(mg.)	(mg.)	(I.U.)	(mg.)	(mg.)	(mg.)	(mg.)
Butter, 4 sticks per pound																
Sticks, 2	1 cup	227	1,625	1	184	101	61	6	1	45	0	21 7,500	—	—	—	0
Stick, ⅛	1 tbsp.	14	100	Trace	11	6	4	Trace	Trace	3	0	21 460	—	—	—	0
Pat or square (64 per pound)	1	7	50	Trace	6	3	2	Trace	Trace	1	0	21 230	—	—	—	0
Fats, cooking																
Lard	1 cup	220	1,985	0	220	84	101	22	0	0	0	0	0	0	0	0
Lard	1 tbsp.	14	125	0	14	5	6	1	0	0	0	0	0	0	0	0
Vegetable fats	1 cup	200	1,770	0	200	46	130	14	0	0	0	—	0	0	0	0
Vegetable fats	1 tbsp.	12.5	110	0	12	3	8	1	0	0	0	—	0	0	0	0
Margarine, 4 sticks per pound																
Sticks, 2	1 cup	227	1,635	1	184	37	105	33	1	45	0	22 7,500	—	—	—	0
Stick, ⅛	1 tbsp.	14	100	Trace	11	2	6	2	Trace	3	0	22 460	—	—	—	0
Pat or square (64 per pound)	1 pat	7	50	Trace	6	1	3	1	Trace	1	0	22 230	—	—	—	0
Oils, salad or cooking																
Corn	1 tbsp.	14	125	0	14	1	4	7	0	0	0	—	0	0	0	0
Cottonseed	1 tbsp.	14	125	0	14	4	3	7	0	0	0	—	0	0	0	0
Olive	1 tbsp.	14	125	0	14	2	11	1	0	0	0	—	0	0	0	0
Soybean	1 tbsp.	14	125	0	14	2	3	7	0	0	0	—	0	0	0	0
Salad dressings																
Blue cheese	1 tbsp.	16	80	1	8	2	2	4	1	13	Trace	30	Trace	.02	Trace	Trace
Commercial, mayonnaise type	1 tbsp.	15	65	Trace	6	1	1	3	2	2	Trace	30	Trace	Trace	Trace	—
French	1 tbsp.	15	60	Trace	6	1	1	3	3	2	.1	—	—	—	—	—
Home cooked, boiled	1 tbsp.	17	30	1	2	1	1	Trace	3	15	.1	80	.01	.03	Trace	Trace
Mayonnaise	1 tbsp.	15	110	Trace	12	2	3	6	Trace	3	.1	40	Trace	.01	Trace	—
Thousand island	1 tbsp.	15	75	Trace	8	1	2	4	2	2	.1	50	Trace	Trace	Trace	Trace
Sugars, sweets																
Candy																
Caramels	1 oz.	28	115	1	3	2	1	Trace	22	42	.4	Trace	.01	.05	Trace	Trace
Chocolate, milk, plain	1 oz.	28	150	2	9	5	3	Trace	16	65	.3	80	.02	.09	.1	Trace
Fudge, plain	1 oz.	28	115	1	3	2	1	Trace	21	22	.3	Trace	.01	.03	.1	Trace

Food	Measure	Weight (g)	Food energy	Protein	Fat	Saturated fatty acids	Oleic	Linoleic	Carbohydrate	Calcium	Iron	Vitamin A	Thiamine	Riboflavin	Niacin	Ascorbic acid
Hard candy	1 oz.	28	110	0	Trace	—	—	—	28	6	.5	0	0	0	0	0
Marshmallows	1 oz.	28	90	1	Trace	—	—	—	23	5	.5	0	0	Trace	Trace	0
Chocolate sirup, thin type	1 tbsp.	20	50	Trace	Trace	Trace	Trace	Trace	13	3	.3	—	Trace	.01	.1	0
Honey, strained or extracted	1 tbsp.	21	65	Trace	0	—	Trace	—	17	1	.1	0	Trace	.01	.1	Trace
Jams and preserves	1 tbsp.	20	55	Trace	Trace	—	—	—	14	4	.2	Trace	Trace	.01	Trace	Trace
Jellies	1 tbsp.	20	55	Trace	Trace	—	—	—	14	4	.3	Trace	Trace	.01	Trace	1
Molasses, cane: Light (first extraction)	1 tbsp.	20	50	—	—	—	—	—	13	33	.9	—	.01	.01	Trace	—
Blackstrap (third extraction)	1 tbsp.	20	45	—	—	—	—	—	11	137	3.2	—	.02	.04	.4	—
Sirup, table blends (chiefly corn, light and dark)	1 tbsp.	20	60	0	0	—	—	—	15	9	.8	0	0	0	0	0
Sugars (cane or beet): Granulated	1 cup	200	770	0	0	—	—	—	199	0	.2	0	0	0	0	0
	1 tbsp.	12	45	0	0	—	—	—	12	0	Trace	0	0	0	0	0
Lump, 1⅛ by ¾ by ⅜	1 lump	6	25	0	0	—	—	—	6	0	Trace	0	0	0	0	0
Powdered, stirred before measuring	1 cup	128	495	0	0	—	—	—	127	0	.1	0	0	0	0	0
	1 tbsp.	8	30	0	0	—	—	—	8	0	Trace	0	0	0	0	0
Brown, firm-packed	1 cup	220	820	0	0	—	—	—	212	187	7.5	0	.02	.07	.4	0
	1 tbsp.	14	50	0	0	—	—	—	13	12	.5	0	Trace	Trace	Trace	0
Miscellaneous items																
Beer (average 3.6 percent alcohol by weight)	1 cup	240	100	1	0	—	—	—	9	12	Trace	—	.01	.07	1.6	—
Beverages, carbonated: Cola type	1 cup	240	95	0	0	—	—	—	24	—	—	0	0	0	0	0
Ginger ale	1 cup	230	70	0	0	—	—	—	18	—	—	0	0	0	0	0
Bouillon cube, ⅝ inch	1 cube	4	5	1	Trace	—	—	—	Trace	—	—	—	—	—	—	—
Chili powder. See Vegetables, peppers																
Chili sauce (mainly tomatoes)	1 tbsp.	17	20	Trace	Trace	—	—	—	4	3	.1	240	.02	.01	.3	3
Chocolate: Bitter or baking	1 oz.	28	145	3	15	8	6	Trace	8	22	1.9	20	.01	.07	.4	0
Sweet	1 oz.	28	150	1	10	6	4	Trace	16	27	.4	Trace	.01	.04	.1	Trace
Cider. See Fruits, apple juice																

21 Year-round average.
22 Based on the average vitamin A content of fortified margarine. Federal specifications for fortified margarine require a minimum of 15,000 I.U. of vitamin A per pound.

Continued.

Food, approximate measure, and weight (in grams)		Food energy	Protein	Fat (total lipid)	Fatty acids			Carbohydrate	Calcium	Iron	Vitamin A value	Thiamine	Riboflavin	Niacin	Ascorbic acid
					Saturated (total)	Unsaturated Oleic	Linoleic								
	gm.	(Calories)	(gm.)	(gm.)	(gm.)	(gm.)	(gm.)	(gm.)	(mg.)	(mg.)	(I.U.)	(mg.)	(mg.)	(mg.)	(mg.)
Gelatin, dry															
Plain	1 tbsp.	10	35	9	Trace	—	—	—	—	—	—	—	—	—	—	—
Dessert powder, 3-oz. package	½ cup	85	315	8	0	—	—	—	75	—	—	—	—	—	—	—
Gelatin dessert, ready-to-eat															
Plain	1 cup	239	140	4	0	—	—	—	34	—	—	—	—	—	—	—
With fruit	1 cup	241	160	3	Trace	—	—	—	40	—	—	—	—	—	—	—
Olives, pickled															
Green	4 medium or 3 extra large or 2 giant	16	15	Trace	2	Trace	2	Trace	Trace	8	.2	40	—	—	—	—
Ripe: Mission	3 small or 2 large	10	15	Trace	2	Trace	2	Trace	Trace	9	.1	10	Trace	Trace	—	—
Pickles, cucumber															
Dill, large, 4 by 1¾ inches	1	135	15	1	Trace	—	—	—	3	35	1.4	140	Trace	.03	Trace	8
Sweet, 2¾ by ¾ inches	1	20	30	Trace	Trace	—	—	—	7	2	.2	20	Trace	Trace	Trace	1
Popcorn. See Grain products															
Sherbet, orange	1 cup	193	260	2	2	—	—	—	59	31	Trace	110	.02	.06	Trace	4
Soups, canned; ready-to-serve (prepared with equal volume of water)															
Bean with pork	1 cup	250	170	8	6	1	2	2	22	62	2.2	650	.14	.07	1.0	2
Beef noodle	1 cup	250	70	4	3	1	1	1	7	8	1.0	50	.05	.06	1.1	Trace

	Measure	Weight (g)														
Beef bouillon, broth, consomme	1 cup	240	30	5	0	0	0	0	3	Trace	.5	Trace	Trace	.02	1.2	—
Chicken noodle	1 cup	250	65	4	2	Trace	1	1	8	10	.5	50	.02	.02	.8	Trace
Clam chowder	1 cup	255	85	2	3	—	—	—	13	36	1.0	920	.03	.03	1.0	—
Cream soup (mushroom)	1 cup	240	135	2	10	1	3	5	10	41	.5	70	.02	.12	.7	Trace
Minestrone	1 cup	245	105	5	3	—	—	—	14	37	1.0	2,350	.07	.05	1.0	—
Pea, green	1 cup	245	130	6	2	—	1	Trace	23	44	1.0	340	.05	.05	1.0	7
Tomato	1 cup	245	90	2	2	Trace	1	1	16	15	.7	1,000	.06	.05	1.1	12
Vegetable with beef broth	1 cup	250	80	3	2	—	—	—	14	20	.8	3,250	.05	.02	1.2	—
Starch (cornstarch)	1 cup	128	465	Trace	Trace	—	—	—	112	0	0	0	0	0	0	0
	1 tbsp.	8	30	Trace	Trace	—	—	—	7	0	0	0	0	0	0	0
Tapioca, quick-cooking granulated, dry, stirred before measuring	1 cup	152	535	1	Trace	—	—	—	131	15	.6	0	0	0	0	0
	1 tbsp.	10	35	Trace	Trace	—	—	—	9	1	Trace	0	0	0	0	0
Vinegar	1 tbsp.	15	2	0	—	—	—	—	1	1	.1	—	—	—	—	—
White sauce, medium	1 cup	265	430	10	33	18	11	1	23	305	.5	1,220	.12	.44	.6	Trace
Yeast																
Baker's Compressed	1 oz.	28	25	3	Trace	—	—	—	3	4	1.4	Trace	.20	.47	3.2	Trace
Dry active	1 oz.	28	80	10	Trace	—	—	—	11	12	4.6	Trace	.66	1.53	10.4	Trace
Brewer's, dry, debittered	1 tbsp.	8	25	3	Trace	—	—	—	3	17	1.4	Trace	1.25	.34	3.0	Trace

Yogurt. See Milk, cream, cheese; related products

Appendix II Recommended Dietary Allowances (RDA), Revised 1980

Designed for the maintenance of good nutrition of practically all healthy people in the United States

	Age (years)	Weight kg	Weight lb	Height cm	Height in	Protein (g)	Fat-Soluble Vitamins Vita-min A (µg RE†)	Vita-min D (µg)‡	Vitamin E (mg α-TE§)	Vita-min C (mg)
Infants	0.0-0.5	6	13	60	24	kg × 2.2	420	10	3	35
	0.5-1.0	9	20	71	28	kg × 2.0	400	10	4	35
Children	1-3	13	29	90	35	23	400	10	5	45
	4-6	20	44	112	44	30	500	10	6	45
	7-10	28	62	132	52	34	700	10	7	45
Males	11-14	45	99	157	62	45	1000	10	8	50
	15-18	66	145	176	69	56	1000	10	10	60
	19-22	70	154	177	70	56	1000	7.5	10	60
	23-50	70	154	178	70	56	1000	5	10	60
	51 +	70	154	178	70	56	1000	5	10	60
Females	11-14	46	101	157	62	46	800	10	8	50
	15-18	55	120	163	64	46	800	10	8	60
	19-22	55	120	163	64	44	800	7.5	8	60
	23-50	55	120	163	64	44	800	5	8	60
	51 +	55	120	163	64	44	800	5	8	60
Pregnant						+ 30	+ 200	+ 5	+ 2	+ 20
Lactating						+ 20	+ 400	+ 5	+ 3	+ 40

*The allowances are intended to provide for individual variations among most normal persons as they live in the United States under usual environmental stresses. Diets should be based on a variety of common foods in order to provide other nutrients for which human requirements have been less well defined.

†Retinol equivalents. 1 retinol equivalent = 1 µg retinol or 6 µg carotene.

‡As cholecalciferol. Ten µg cholecalciferol = 400 IU vitamin D.

§α-Tocopherol equivalents. 1 mg D-α-tocopherol = 1 αTE.

Water-Soluble Vitamins						Minerals					
Thiamin (mg)	Ribo-flavin (mg)	Niacin (mg NE‖)	Vita-min B_6 (mg)	Folacin (µg)¶	Vita-min B_{12} (µg)	Calcium (mg)	Phos-phorus (mg)	Mag-nesium (mg)	Iron (mg)	Zinc (mg)	Iodine (µg)
0.3	0.4	6	0.3	30	0.5#	360	240	50	10	3	40
0.5	0.6	8	0.6	45	1.5	540	360	70	15	5	50
0.7	0.8	9	0.9	100	2.0	800	800	150	15	10	70
0.9	1.0	11	1.3	200	2.5	800	800	200	10	10	90
1.2	1.4	16	1.6	300	3.0	800	800	250	10	10	120
1.4	1.6	18	1.8	400	3.0	1200	1200	350	18	15	150
1.4	1.7	18	2.0	400	3.0	1200	1200	400	18	15	150
1.5	1.7	19	2.2	400	3.0	800	800	350	10	15	150
1.4	1.6	18	2.2	400	3.0	800	800	350	10	15	150
1.2	1.4	16	2.2	400	3.0	800	800	350	10	15	150
1.1	1.3	15	1.8	400	3.0	1200	1200	300	18	15	150
1.1	1.3	14	2.0	400	3.0	1200	1200	300	18	15	150
1.1	1.3	14	2.0	400	3.0	800	800	300	18	15	150
1.0	1.2	13	2.0	400	3.0	800	800	300	18	15	150
1.0	1.2	13	2.0	400	3.0	800	800	300	10	15	150
+0.4	+0.3	+2	+0.6	+400	+1.0	+400	+400	+150	**	+5	+25
+0.5	+0.5	+5	+0.5	+100	+1.0	+400	+400	+150	**	+10	+50

‖One NE (niacin equivalent) is equal to 1 mg niacin or 60 mg dietary tryptophan.

¶The folacin allowances refer to dietary sources as determined by *Lactobacillus casei* assay after treatment with enzymes ("conjugases") to make polyglutanyl forms of the vitamin available to the test organism.

#The RDA for vitamin B_{12} in infants is based on average concentration of the vitamin in human milk. The allowances after weaning are based on energy intake (as recommended by the American Academy of Pediatrics) and consideration of other factors such as intestinal absorption.

**The increased requirement during pregnancy cannot be met by the iron content of habitual American diets or by the existing iron stores of many women; therefore the use of 30 to 60 mg of supplemental iron is recommended. Iron needs during lactation are not substantially different from those of nonpregnant women, but continued supplementation of the mother for 2 to 3 months after parturition is advisable in order to replenish stores depleted by pregnancy.

Mean heights and weights and recommended energy intake

Category	Age (years)	Weight kg	Weight lb	Height cm	Height in	Energy Needs (with range) kcal		Energy Needs (with range) MJ
Infants	0.0-0.5	6	13	60	24	kg × 115		kg × .48
	0.5-1.0	9	20	71	28	kg × 105		kg × .44
Children	1-3	13	29	90	35	1300	(900-1800)	5.5
	4-6	20	44	112	44	1700	(1300-2300)	7.1
	7-10	28	62	132	52	2400	(1650-3300)	10.1
Males	11-14	45	99	157	62	2700	(2000-3700)	11.3
	15-18	66	145	176	69	2800	(2100-3900)	11.8
	19-22	70	154	177	70	2900	(2500-3300)	12.2
	23-50	70	154	178	70	2700	(2300-3100)	11.3
	51-75	70	154	178	70	2400	(2000-2800)	10.1
	76+	70	154	178	70	2050	(1650-2450)	8.6
Females	11-14	46	101	157	62	2200	(1500-3000)	9.2
	15-18	55	120	163	64	2100	(1200-3000)	8.8
	19-22	55	120	163	64	2100	(1700-2500)	8.8
	23-50	55	120	163	64	2000	(1600-2400)	8.4
	51-75	55	120	163	64	1800	(1400-2200)	7.6
	76+	55	120	163	64	1600	(1200-2000)	6.7
Pregnancy						+300		
Lactation						+500		

From Recommended Dietary Allowances, revised 1980, Food and Nutrition Board, National Academy of Sciences-National Research Council, Washington, D.C.

The data in this table have been assembled from the observed median heights and weights of children shown in Table 1, together with desirable weights for adults given in Table 2 for the mean heights of men (70 inches) and women (64 inches) between the ages of 18 and 34 years as surveyed in the US population (HEW/NCHS data).

The energy allowances for the young adults are for men and women doing light work. The allowances for the two older age groups represent mean energy needs over these age spans, allowing for a 2% decrease in basal (resting) metabolic rate per decade and a reduction in activity of 200 kcal/day for men and women between 51 and 75 years, 500 kcal for men over 75 years and 400 kcal for women over 75. . . . The customary range of daily energy output is shown for adults in parentheses and is based on a variation in energy needs of ±400 kcal at any one age . . . emphasizing the wide range of energy intakes appropriate for any group of people.

Energy allowances for children through age 18 are based on median energy intakes of children these ages followed in longitudinal growth studies. The values in parentheses are 10th and 90th percentiles of energy intake, to indicate the range of energy consumption among children of these ages.

Appendix III U.S. Recommended Daily Allowance (U.S. RDA) for Children and Infants

	Infants Under 13 Months	Children Under 1 to 4 Years
Protein	25 g*	28 g*
Vitamin A	1500 IU	2500 IU
Vitamin C	35 mg	40 mg
Thiamin	0.5 mg	0.7 mg
Riboflavin	0.6 mg	0.8 mg
Niacin	8.0 mg	9.0 mg
Calcium	0.6 g	0.8 g
Iron	15 mg	10 mg
Vitamin D	400 IU	400 IU
Vitamin E	5 IU	10 IU
Vitamin B_6	0.4 mg	0.7 mg
Folacin	0.1 mg	0.2 mg
Vitamin B_{12}	2 μg	3 μg
Phosphorus	0.5 g	0.8 g
Iodine	45 μg	70 μg
Magnesium	70 mg	200 mg
Zinc	5 mg	8 mg
Copper	0.6 mg	1 mg
Biotin	0.15 mg	0.15 mg
Pantothenic acid	3 mg	5 mg

*If the protein efficiency ratio of protein is equal to or better than that of casein, the U.S. RDA is 20 g for children under 4 years of age.

Appendix IV   Dietary Screening Aids

24-HOUR RECALL

Name _____

Date and time of interview _____

Length of interview _____

Date of recall _____

Day of the week of recall (1—M, 2—T, 3—W, 4—Th, 5—F, 6—Sat, 7—Sun) ___

"I would like you to tell me everything you (your child) ate and drank from the time you (he) got up in the morning until you (he) went to bed at night and what you (he) ate during the night. Be sure to mention everything you (he) ate or drank at home, at work (school), and away from home. Include snacks and drinks of all kinds and everything else you (he) put in your (his) mouth and swallowed. I also need to know where you (he) ate the food, and now let us begin."

What time did you (he) get up yesterday? _____

Was it the usual time? _____
What was the first time you (he) ate or had anything to drink yesterday morning?
  (list on the form that follows)
Where did you (he) eat? (list on form that follows)
Now tell me what you (he) had to eat and how much?
(Occasionally the interviewer will need to ask:)
  When did you (he) eat again? Or, is there anything else?
  Did you (he) have anything to eat or drink during the night?

Was intake unusual in any way? Yes _____ No _____

(If answer is yes) Why? _____

            In what way? _____

What time did you (he) go to bed last night? _____
Do(es) you (he) take vitamin or mineral supplements?

            Yes _____ No _____

(If answer is yes) How many per day? _____

            Per week? _____
What kind? (Insert brand name if known)

Multivitamins _____

Ascorbic acid _____

From Screening children for nutritional status: suggestions for child health programs, Washington, D.C., 1971, U.S. Government Printing Office.

24-HOUR RECALL—cont'd

Vitamins A and D _____

Iron _____

Other _____

Suggested Form For Recording Food Intake

Time	Where Eaten*	Food	Type and/or Preparation	Amount	Food Code†	Amount Code†

*Code

   H—Home

   R—Restaurant, drugstore, or lunch
      counter

  CL—Carried lunch from home

  CC—Child-care center

   OH—Other home (friend, relative, baby-sitter,
      etc.)

    S—School, office, plant, or work

  FD—Food dispenser

   SS—Social center (e.g., Senior Citizen, etc.)

†Do not write in these spaces.

DIETARY QUESTIONNAIRE FOR CHILDREN

Name _____

Date _____

1. Does the child eat at regular times each day? _____
2. How many days a week does he eat?

    A morning meal? _____

    A lunch or midday meal? _____

    An evening meal? _____

    During the night?* _____

3. How many days a week does he have snacks?

    In midmorning? _____

    In midafternoon? _____

    In the evening? _____

    During the night? _____

From Screening children for nutritional status: suggestions for child health programs, Washington, D.C., 1971, U.S. Government Printing Office.

*Include formula feeding for young children.

Continued.

4. Which meals does he usually eat with your family?

    None _____ Breakfast _____ Noon meal _____ Evening meal _____

5. How many times per week does he eat at school, child-care center, or day camp?

    Breakfast _____ Lunch _____ Between meals _____

6. Would you describe his appetite as Good? _____ Fair? _____ Poor? _____

7. At what time of day is he most hungry?

    Morning _____ Noon _____ Evening _____

8. What foods does he dislike? _____
   _____

9. Is he on a special diet now? Yes _____ No _____
   If yes, why is he on a diet? (Check)

    _____ For weight reduction (own prescription)

    _____ For weight reduction (doctor's prescription)

    _____ For gaining weight

    _____ For allergy, specify _____

    _____ For other reason, specify _____

    If no, has he been on a special diet within the past year? Yes _____ No _____

    If yes, for what reason? _____

10. Does he eat anything that is not usually considered food? Yes _____ No _____

    If yes, with his fingers? _____ With a spoon? _____

11. Can he feed himself? Yes _____ No _____

    If yes, with his fingers? _____ with a spoon? _____

12. Can he use a cup or glass by himself? Yes _____ No _____

13. Does he drink from a bottle with a nipple? Yes _____ No _____

    If yes, how often? _____ At what time of day or night? _____

14. How many times per week does he eat the following foods (at any meal or between meals)? Circle the appropriate number:

Food		
Bacon _____	0 1 2 3 4 5 6 7	>7, specify _____
Tongue _____	0 1 2 3 4 5 6 7	>7, specify _____
Sausage _____	0 1 2 3 4 5 6 7	>7, specify _____
Luncheon meat	0 1 2 3 4 5 6 7	>7, specify _____
Hot dogs _____	0 1 2 3 4 5 6 7	>7, specify _____
Liver—chicken _____	0 1 2 3 4 5 6 7	>7, specify _____
Liver—other _____	0 1 2 3 4 5 6 7	>7, specify _____
Poultry _____	0 1 2 3 4 5 6 7	>7, specify _____
Salt pork _____	0 1 2 3 4 5 6 7	>7, specify _____
Pork or ham _____	0 1 2 3 4 5 6 7	>7, specify _____
Bones (neck or other) _____	0 1 2 3 4 5 6 7	>7, specify _____
Meat in mixtures (stew, tamales, casseroles, etc.) _____	0 1 2 3 4 5 6 7	>7, specify _____
Beef or veal _____	0 1 2 3 4 5 6 7	>7, specify _____
Other meat _____	0 1 2 3 4 5 6 7	>7, specify _____
Fish _____	0 1 2 3 4 5 6 7	>7, specify _____

DIETARY QUESTIONNAIRE FOR CHILDREN—cont'd

15. How many times per week does he eat the following foods (at any meal or between meals)? Circle the appropriate number:

Fruit juice _____ 0 1 2 3 4 5 6 7 >7, specify _____
Fruit _____ 0 1 2 3 4 5 6 7 >7, specify _____
Cereal—dry _____ 0 1 2 3 4 5 6 7 >7, specify _____
Cereal—cooked or instant _____ 0 1 2 3 4 5 6 7 >7, specify _____
Cereal—infant _____ 0 1 2 3 4 5 6 7 >7, specify _____
Eggs _____ 0 1 2 3 4 5 6 7 >7, specify _____
Pancakes or waffles _____ 0 1 2 3 4 5 6 7 >7, specify _____
Cheese _____ 0 1 2 3 4 5 6 7 >7, specify _____
Potato _____ 0 1 2 3 4 5 6 7 >7, specify _____
Other cooked vegetables _____ 0 1 2 3 4 5 6 7 >7, specify _____
Raw vegetables _____ 0 1 2 3 4 5 6 7 >7, specify _____
Dried beans or peas _____ 0 1 2 3 4 5 6 7 >7, specify _____
Macaroni, spaghetti, rice, or noodles 0 1 2 3 4 5 6 7 >7, specify _____
Ice cream, milk pudding, custard, or 0 1 2 3 4 5 6 7 >7, specify _____
    cream soup _____
Peanut butter or nuts _____ 0 1 2 3 4 5 6 7 >7, specify _____
Sweet rolls or doughnuts _____ 0 1 2 3 4 5 6 7 >7, specify _____
Crackers or pretzels _____ 0 1 2 3 4 5 6 7 >7, specify _____
Cookies _____ 0 1 2 3 4 5 6 7 >7, specify _____
Pie, cake, or brownies _____ 0 1 2 3 4 5 6 7 >7, specify _____
Potato chips or corn chips _____ 0 1 2 3 4 5 6 7 >7, specify _____
Candy _____ 0 1 2 3 4 5 6 7 >7, specify _____
Soft drinks, Popsicles, or Kool-Aid __ 0 1 2 3 4 5 6 7 >7, specify _____
Instant Breakfast _____ 0 1 2 3 4 5 6 7 >7, specify _____

16. How many servings per day does he eat of the following foods? Circle the appropriate number:

Bread (including sandwich), toast, rolls, muffins
    (1 slice or 1 piece is 1 serving) ___ 0 1 2 3 4 5 6 7 >7, specify _____
Milk (including on cereal or other foods)
    (8 ounces is 1 serving) _____ 0 1 2 3 4 5 6 7 >7, specify _____
Sugar, jam, jelly, syrup (1 tsp is 1 0 1 2 3 4 5 6 7 >7, specify _____
    serving)

17. What specific kinds of the following foods does he eat most often?

Fruit juices _____
Fruit _____
Vegetables _____
Cheese _____
Cooked or instant cereal _____
Dry cereal _____
Milk _____

Appendix V Sterilization Techniques for Formula Preparation

FIRST STEPS

1. Always wash your hands before preparing formula.
2. Wash all bottles, nipples, and equipment in hot, soapy water.
3. Squeeze water through nipple holes during washing and rinsing.
4. Rinse all bottles, nipples, and equipment with hot, clear water to remove soap film.
5. Before opening formula can, wash can top with hot, clear water; rinse well.
6. Shake can very well before opening.

TERMINAL HEATING METHOD*

Follow First Steps, then . . .

1. Measure prescribed amount of water into measuring cup or bowl according to doctor's instructions.
2. Add prescribed amount of concentrated formula to water. (The usual mixture is 1 part concentrated formula to 1 part water.) Stir.
3. Pour prepared formula into clean nursing bottles. If using disc seals, invert nipples.   Otherwise, put nipples upright on bottles, and cover with nipple covers. *Leave nipple collars loose on bottles.*
4. Set bottles on rack or on cloth on bottom of sterilizer or deep kettle. Add about 3 inches of water.
5. Cover sterilizer or kettle, bring water to a boil, and boil for 20 minutes. Remove kettle or sterilizer from heat, and let cool to touch (approximately 1 hour) before removing lid.
6. Remove bottles from sterilizer or kettle. Tighten collars and store in refrigerator. Use within 48 hours.

BOILING (ASEPTIC) METHOD

Follow First Steps, then . . .

1. Place clean bottles, nipples, and equipment in sterilizer or deep kettle. Add enough water to sterilizer or kettle to cover these items.
2. Cover sterilizer or kettle. Bring water to boil and boil for 5 minutes. Remove sterilizer from heat, and let cool to touch (approximately 1 hour) before

Source: Sterilization techniques for formula preparation provided courtesy Mead Johnson Nutritionals.

*Terminal Heating method is *not* recommended for preparing formula from powder.

removing lid. Remove equipment with tongs, and place on clean towel.

3. Boil water for formula in covered saucepan for 5 minutes. Remove saucepan from heat, and let cool to room temperature.
4. Measure prescribed amount of the boiled water and concentrated formula or powder into measuring cup or bowl according to doctor's instructions. (The usual mixture is 1 part concentrated formula to 1 part water or, if using powder, one level scoop powder to every 2 fl oz water.) Stir. If powder is used, mix formula with sterilized eggbeater.
5. Pour prepared formula into bottles. If using disc seals, invert nipples. Otherwise, put nipples upright on bottles, and cover with nipple covers.
6. Store bottled formula in refrigerator. Use formula prepared from concentrated formula within 48 hours. Use formula prepared from powder within 24 hours.

SINGLE-BOTTLE METHOD

Follow First Steps, then . . .

1. Sterilize bottles, nipple units and tongs according to the boiling (aseptic) method.
2. Store bottles and nipple units in a convenient place at room temperature until ready to use.
3. At feeding time, boil water for formula in saucepan for 5 minutes, then remove from heat and let cool to room temperature.
4. Pour prescribed amount of the boiled water into bottle according to doctor's instructions.
5. Add prescribed amount of concentrated liquid or powder to water in bottle. (The usual mixture is 1 part concentrated liquid to 1 part water; or, if using powder, 1 scoop to every 2 fl oz of water.)
6. Shake well before feeding.

MICROWAVES

Do *not* use a microwave oven for warming infant formulas. This practice is dangerous because it can result in serious burns to you or your baby. Microwaving easily can cause the formula to overheat or can form hot spots in the formula. Also, bottles or bags can explode or burst during heating or even after the bottle is removed from the oven. If you would like to warm your baby's formula before feeding, we would recommend placing the bottle in a pan of warm water.

Microwave ovens are also not effective for sterilizing formula, bottles, or nipples. Use either the terminal heating method or the boiling (aseptic) method for sterilizing.

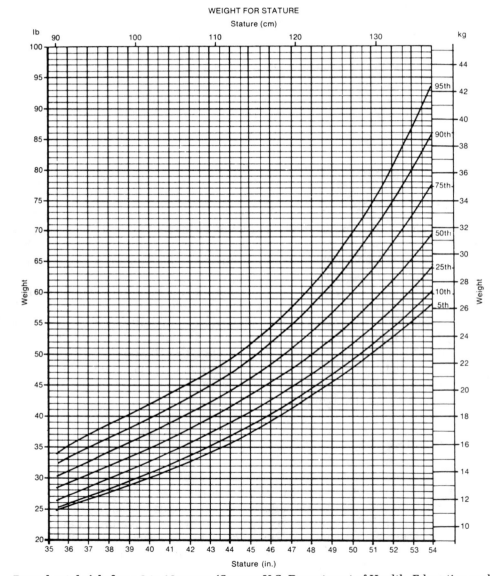

WEIGHT FOR STATURE

Prepubertal girls from 2 to 10 years. (*Source:* U.S. Department of Health, Education and Welfare, National Center for Health Statistics, 1979.)

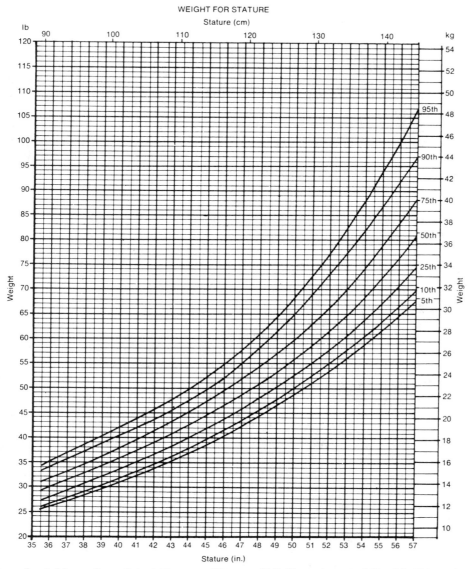

Prepubertal boys from 2 to 11½ years. (*Source:* U.S. Department of Health, Education and Welfare, National Center for Health Statistics, 1979.)

SOURCES OF FUNDING FOR FOOD SERVICE—CHILD CARE FOOD PROGRAM

The Child Care Food Program was begun in 1968 by the U.S. Department of Agriculture and was known as the Special Food Service Program for Children. Designed originally to serve especially needy children, the program provided assistance to nonresidential child-care centers serving children from low-income areas or from areas with significant numbers of working mothers.

In October 1975 new child nutrition legislation, Public Law 94–105, expanded and refocused the program. The law extended eligibility to all nonprofit day-care centers—those serving nonneedy as well as needy areas. It also opened participation to family and group day-care homes, allowing them to join under the sponsorship of a qualifying institution or organization.

Many centers would qualify but are unaware of the services. The following facts are presented to clarify the program:

The Child Care Food Program (CCFP) provides nutritious meals to children enrolled in child-care centers or day-care homes throughout the country. It also introduces young children to many different types of foods and helps teach them good eating habits.

Who Can Participate

The Program is limited to public and private nonprofit organizations providing licensed or approved nonresidential day-care services. Such organizations include, but are not limited to, day-care centers, outside-school-hours care centers, day-care homes, and institutions providing day-care services for handicapped children. Also, private for-profit centers may qualify if they receive compensation under Title XX of the Social Security Act for at least 25% of the children who are receiving nonresidential day care.

Child-care centers and outside-school-hours care centers can operate in the program either independently or under the auspices of a sponsoring organization, which accepts final administrative and financial responsibility for the program. Family day-care homes must participate under a sponsoring organization; they cannot enter the CCFP directly.

Children 12 and younger are eligible to participate in the program (except that for children of migrant workers, the age limit is 15 years). Physially or mentally handicapped people can participate regardless of age, if they receive care at a center or home where the majority of the enrollees are 18 or under.

Eligibility Requirements

All private institutions (except for-profit Title XX organizations) must have tax-exempt status under the Internal Revenue Code of 1954, or must have applied to the Internal Revenue Service (IRS) for it at the time they apply for the Child Care Food Program. If an institution takes part in other Federal programs for which it needs nonprofit status, it already meets this requirement. Family day-care homes are not required to be tax exempt, but their sponsoring organizations must have tax-exempt status if they are private. Local IRS offices can provide information on how to obtain tax-exempt status.

All institutions, except sponsoring organizations, must have child care *licensing or approval*. The administering agency can provide information on how to obtain a license or approval.

Meal Service

All participating institutions must serve meals that meet U.S. Department of Agriculture nutritional standards. Institutions may receive reimbursement for up to three meals per child per day. However, one of these meals must be a snack.

Available Assistance

The CCFP provides financial assistance to child-care centers and sponsoring organizations of day-care homes so that they can provide nutritious meals to the children enrolled for care.

Generally, program payments to child-care centers and outside-school-hours care centers are limited to the number of meals served to enrolled children multiplied by the appropriate rates for reimbursement. The rate of payment varies according to the family size and income of children participating in the program. Increased reimbursement is provided for needy children. Some state administering agencies may base reimbursement on the maximum rates or actual costs, whichever is less.

Meals served by day-care homes under the CCFP are reimbursed at different rates for each type of meal served that meets program requirements. The sponsoring organization must pass the full food service payment to the home, unless the sponsoring organization provides part of the home's food service. Day-care home providers receive reimbursement for meals served to their own children only when (1) their children meet the family size and income standards for free and reduced-price meals, and are participating in the CCFP, and (2) other nonresident enrolled children are present and participating in the program. Separate administrative funds are provided to sponsoring organizations based on the number of homes they administer.

Civil Rights

The CCFP is available to all eligible children regardless of race, color, national origin, sex, age, or handicap. If you believe that you have been treated unfairly in receiving food services for any of these reasons, write immediately to the Secretary of Agriculture, Washington, D.C. 20250. More information may be obtained from the Office of Equal Opportunity, U.S. Department of Agriculture, Washington, D.C. 20250.

Administering Agency

In most states, the program is administered by the State Department of Education. Where states do not administer the program, Food and Nutrition Service Regional Offices operate it directly.*

*From Facts about the Child Care Food Program, Food and Nutrition Service, INS-242, Aug. 1983.

Glossary

absorption   The process by which digestive products are transferred from the gastrointestinal tract into the blood or lymphatic system.

acid   A "sour" compound capable of reacting with an alkali.

acid-base balance   The equilibrium or relationship between acidic and alkaline compounds in the body.

additives (food)   Accidental or intentional substances incorporated in processed foods.

adipose tissue   Storehouse of fat in the body; chemically active tissue containing protein and other substances as well as fat.

alkaline substance   Any substance that can neutralize acids; basic in reaction.

amino acid   Organic molecule containing carbon, hydrogen, oxygen, and nitrogen; the structural unit of protein; contains an amino group ($-NH_2$) and a carboxyl or acidic group ($-COOH$).

anemia   Term literally meaning without blood; condition in which red blood cell and/or hemoglobin level is below normal.

anorexia   Disease state characterized by self-starvation; sometimes seen in achievement-oriented adolescents, particularly girls.

antacids   Substances that neutralize acidity, especially in the digestive tract. Common antacids include calcium carbonate, aluminum hydroxide, and sodium bicarbonate (baking soda).

antibodies   Proteins capable of combining with foreign substances (antigens) such as viruses, rendering them inactive or harmless.

antioxidant   Substances such as vitamin E that help prevent oxidative (oxygen-caused) destruction of body tissues and food substances.

appetite   Desire or craving for food that often occurs in the absence of hunger.

arteriosclerosis   Disease characterized by hardening and thickening of the walls of the arteries.

aspartame   A low-calorie, nutritive sweetener used as an additive in cold breakfast cereals, chewing gum, and other food products.

assessment   An evaluation of a child's knowledge, skills, behavior, and/or progress.

B vitamins   Group of water-soluble vitamins originally considered to be a single essential factor and now known to consist of eight separate vitamins.

base   An alkaline substance that can react with acids to neutralize the acid.

behavioral objective   Identifies exactly what the teacher will do, provide, or restrict, describes the learner's observable behavior, and defines how well the learner must perform.

bulimia   Condition characterized by binge eating or the compulsive ingestion of large amounts of food (as many as 5000 to 20,000 kcal) over a short period, and often followed by self-inducing vomiting.

Calorie   The heat required to raise the temperature of 1 kg water (at 1 atmosphere of pressure) 1 centigrade degree; also called a kilocalorie.

carbohydrates   Organic compounds composed of carbon, hydrogen, and oxygen. The hydrogen/oxygen ratio is that of water.

carbon   Chemical element present in all substances designated as organic, including proteins, carbohydrates, and fats. When a compound containing carbon combines with oxygen in the body, energy is liberated, and carbon dioxide is formed. Compounds that do not contain carbon are classified as inorganic.

carbon dioxide   Compound that is formed when carbon combines with oxygen. It leaves the body chiefly when air is exhaled from the lungs.

carotene   Yellow pigments that act as provitamin A; that is, they are converted into vitamin A in the body.

cell   Smallest structural unit of living material.

cellulose   A polysaccharide that provides roughage but is not digested by humans.

Child Care Food Program (CCFP)   Provides nutritious meals to children enrolled in child-care centers or day-care homes throughout the country (*Federal Register*, Vol. 47, No. 162, Aug. 20, 1982).

cholesterol   A steroid alcohol.

coenzyme   A component of an enzyme system (usually containing a vitamin) that is required for the activity of the enzyme.

cognition   All forms of knowing, including perceiving, imagining, reasoning, and judging.

cognitive development   The progression of an individual through a sequence of stages where thoughts, knowledge, interpretations, understandings, and ideas are developed.

comprehensive care   Care for children that encourages their social, emotional, physical, and intellectual growth.

coronary heart disease (CHD)   Arteriosclerosis in the arteries feeding the heart muscle.

curriculum   All of the specific features of a master teaching plan that have been chosen by a particular teacher for his or her classroom. Curricula may vary widely from school to school, but each curriculum reflects the skills, tasks, and behaviors that a school has decided are important for children to acquire.

daily food guide   Diet plan devised by the U.S. Department of Agriculture. It is based on the premise that persons selecting a specified number of servings each day from four food groups will meet their nutrient needs.

dental caries   Tooth decay.

dextrose   See **glucose**.

dietary guidelines   Set of general dietary recommendations formulated by the U.S. Department of Agriculture and the Department of Health and Human Services. It advocates dietary measures to prevent disease in terms that the average consumer can understand.

dietitian   Person who by taking college courses in nutrition, food science, food management, and related physical, biological, and social sciences and through formal work experience in an approved (usually clinical) setting has qualified to become a member of the American Dietetic Association.

digestion   Process of breaking down food into molecules that can be absorbed in the bloodstream.

disaccharide   Carbohydrate that breaks down to two monosaccharide molecules during digestion. Examples are sucrose, maltose, and lactose.

electrolyte   Any substance that dissociates into ions when dissolved.

element   Any one of the fundamental atoms of which all matter is composed.

energy   Capacity to do work against resistance.

enrichment   Addition of nutrients to food products.

enzyme   Proteins that catalyze reactions in the body. The names of enzymes frequently end with the suffix -ase, such as sucrase, the enzyme that effects the breakdown of sucrose.

essential amino acid   An amino acid needed for growth and maintenance of the body. It must be supplied in the diet.

essential fatty acid   Linoleic acid and possibly linolenic acid; a fatty acid that is a dietary essential.

evaluation   The process of analyzing and determining whether the desired objectives were achieved.

expressive language   Language used in communicating with other individuals.

fat-soluble vitamins   Vitamins A, D, E and K; vitamins that dissolve in fat but not in water.

fatty acid   An organic acid that can combine with glycerol.

feedback   Any kind of information being returned from a source that is useful in regulating behavior.

fiber (crude)   Insoluble organic material remaining from plants after prolonged acid and base hydrolysis.

fiber (dietary)   Generic term that includes those plant constituents, mostly carbohydrates, that are not digestible by humans.

fine motor skills   Activities with the fingers and hands.

Food and Drug Administration   Agency associated with the U.S. Department of Health and Human Services that has jurisdiction over the safety of food shipped interstate.

Food and Nutrition Board   Group of scientists in food and nutrition or related fields who act in an advisory capacity to the National Research Council of the National Academy of Sciences.

fortification   Addition of one or more nutrients to a food item that is not normally a good source of the nutrient, such as the addition of iodine to salt or vitamin D to milk.

fructose   A monosaccharide found in fruits and corn.

galactose   A monosaccharide or simple sugar with a chemical formula identical to that of glucose but with a different structure; component of lactose (milk sugar) and seldom found in nature uncombined.

genetics   The study of heredity and its variations.

glucose   A monosaccharide; the sugar of the blood.

goals   General statements that tell what teaching is expected to accomplish, for example, "to improve Mary's fine motor skills."

gross motor skills   Activities using large muscles such as running, climbing, throwing, and jumping.

hemoglobin   The oxygen-carrying pigment of red blood cells. Normal hemoglobin (Hb) values for adults are about 14 to 16 g/100 ml. Values for children will vary depending on the age of the child. In general after 6 months of age a hemoglobin value of 10 g/100 ml or greater is desirable.

hormone   A compound secreted by an endocrine gland that influences the functioning of an organ in another part of the body.

hunger   Complex of unpleasant sensations felt after prolonged food deprivation that will impel an animal or human to seek, work for, or fight for immediate relief by ingestion of food.

hydrogenation   The controlled addition of hydrogen to an unsaturated fatty acid. This process changes the melting point, thus producing solid fats from oils, depending on the extent of hydrogenation.

hydrolysis   The breaking apart of chemical bonds during digestion with the addition of water.

hyperactivity   A set of behavioral symptoms such as restlessness, excitability, short attention span, and a need for instant gratification.

hypertension   Abnormally high blood pressure.

inorganic   Pertaining to chemical compounds that do not contain carbon.

integration   Nutrition activities taking place in a variety of curricular areas, such as mathematics, science, music, motor skills, art, and social studies.

interest inventory   Identifies specific tasks for which parents can volunteer.

intrinsic factor   Substance produced in the stomach and needed for the absorption of vitamin B_{12} from the small intestine.

ketogenesis   Formation of ketones from fatty acids and some amino acids.

kilocalorie   The amount of heat required to raise 1 kg of water (at 1 atmosphere of pressure) 1 centigrade degree; same as a Calorie.

kinesthetic tactile   A combination of muscles, tendons, joints, and touch receptors yielding information about objects as well as the position of the body in space.

lactase   Enzyme that breaks down lactose in milk to glucose and galactose.

lactovegetarian   Person who consumes plant foods and dairy products but no meat or eggs.

lactoovovegetarian   Person who consumes dairy products and eggs in addition to plant foods but no meat.

lactose   Milk sugar; a disaccharide that is a combination of glucose and galactose.

low birth weight   A birth weight of less than 2500 g or about 5½ pounds.

linoleic acid   Polyunsaturated fatty acid that is an essential nutrient.

lipids   Organic compounds composed of carbon, hydrogen, and oxygen and generally immiscible with water; fats or fatlike substances.

lipoprotein   Compound composed of a lipid and a protein.

lipoprotein (high density)   Blood lipoproteins that help protect against coronary heart disease, probably by helping prevent cholesterol deposition in the tissues and blood vessels.

lipoprotein (low density)   Blood lipoprotein that carries large amounts of cholesterol to the tissues, where it is deposited.

macrominerals   Minerals present in the body in relatively large amounts.

megadose   Usually an intake of a vitamin or a mineral that exceeds recommended levels by about 10 times.

membrane   Thin, soft, pliable layers of animal or vegetable tissue, usually composed of layers of protein and lipid.

metabolism   All the chemical changes that occur from the time nutrients are absorbed until they are built into body substances or eliminated from the body.

microminerals   Minerals present in the body in relatively small amounts; also called trace elements.

monosaccharide   Carbohydrate in its simplest form. Examples are fructose, glucose, and galactose.

monounsaturated fatty acid   Fatty acid containing one double bond.

National Research Council (NCR)   Group of leading scientists appointed by the National Academy of Sciences to coordinate the efforts of major scientific and technical societies of the United States advising the government.

natural foods   Used loosely for foods made from ingredients of plant or animal origin that are altered as little as possible and do not contain artificial ingredients or additives.

nutrition labeling   Mandatory nutrition information carried on packages of all foods shipped interstate for which a nutritional claim is made, as well as on other foods at the discretion of the manufacturer. Mandatory information includes serving size, kilocalories, protein, carbohydrate, and fat content per serving and percentage of the U.S. RDA provided by the eight leading nutrients.

nutritional assessment   Determination of a person's or a group's nutritional status by means of (1) dietary analysis, (2) anthropometric measures (height, weight, skinfold thickness), (3) physical examination, and (4) determination of nutrient or metabolite levels in blood and urine.

obesity   Condition of being 20% or more above desirable or standard weight.

osteomalacia   Vitamin D deficiency disease of adults characterized by bone demineralization.

osteoporosis   Prolonged chronic reduction in bone mass in which reduced bone formation and or accelerated reabsorption may occur.

overweight   Body weight 10% above desirable or standard weight.

oxalate   Substance present in some plant foods such as spinach that binds calcium and various other minerals in the digestive tract and prevents their absorption.

oxidation   The loss of electrons; also combining with oxygen or removal of hydrogen.

pantothenic acid   One of the B vitamins.

pH   Negative logarithm of the effective hydrogen ion concentration; a means of expressing relative acidity or alkalinity, with pH 7 representing neutrality. Numbers lower than 7 indicate acidic; numbers greater than 7 indicate alkaline.

perception   The process of interpreting what is received by the five senses.

perceptual-motor interaction   The interaction of various channels of perception with motor activity, for example, the act of kicking is a perceptual-motor interaction between sight and gross motor responses.

performance objective   See **behavioral objective.**

peristalsis   Motions of the alimentary tract to move the food through the tract.

phospholipid   A fat containing phosphate and a nitrogenous substance in place of one of the fatty acids.

physiological   Refers to the science of physiology, which deals with functions of living organisms or their parts.

phytates   Substances often found with fiber in plant foods that bind zinc, calcium, and other minerals.

picture recipe   A recipe designed especially for nonreaders using illustrations rather than words.

plaque   Sticky film that forms on teeth; the lipid-containing substance that deposits on the inner walls of blood vessels.

plasma   Colorless fluid portion of the blood from which the cells have been removed.

polysaccharide   Complex carbohydrate molecule often consisting of 10,000 or more monosaccharides.

polyunsaturated fatty acid (PUFA)   Fatty acid with two or more double bonds in its carbon chain; present in large amounts in plant oils and liquid at room temperature.

protein   Class of nutrients made up of amino acids.

Public Law 94–142   The Education for All Handicapped Children Act (*Federal Register*, Vol. 42, No. 163, Aug. 23, 1977).

Recommended Dietary Allowances (RDA)   Quantities of specified vitamins, minerals, and protein needed daily that have been judged adequate for maintenance of good nutrition in the U.S. population, developed by the Food and Nutrition Board of the National Academy of Sciences National Research Council.

satiety   Cessation of desire for further nourishment.

saturated fatty acid   Fatty acid in which the carbons in its interior chain each have two hydrogens attached to them; present in large amounts in animal fats and usually solid at room temperature.

sensorimotor   Relating to a combination of input of sense organs and output of motor activity.

serum (blood serum)   Fluid portion of the blood that separates from the blood cells after clotting.

single-parent family   A family composed of children living with only one parent.

staff/child ratio   The number of child-care staff required in proportion to the number of children present. This ratio is necessary to ensure the safety and proper care of the children at all times.

starch   Polysaccharide consisting of many glucose molecules bonded together in both branched and straight chains; found in plant foods such as potatoes and corn.

sucrose   A disaccharide made up of glucose and frutose; table sugar.

supplements (dietary)   Substance or mixture of substances found in food but isolated in pure form or present in proportions untypical of a natural food product.

synthesis   Process by which a new substance is formed from its individual parts.

toxicity   Quality of a substance that makes it poisonous or toxic. It sometimes refers to the degree of severity of the poison or the possibility of being poisonous.

unsaturated fatty acid   Fatty acid with one or more sets of adjacent carbons held together with double bonds.

U.S. Recommended Daily Allowance (U.S. RDA)   A standard set of daily quantities of specified vitamins, minerals, and protein judged to be essential in human nutrition by the Food and Drug Administration. Values are taken from the Recommended Dietary Allowances developed by the Food and Nutrition Board of the National Academy of Sciences, National Research Council; used as a standard for nutrient labeling.

vegan   Person who does not consume animal products.

vitamin B$_6$ Water-soluble B vitamin.

vitamins   Organic nutrients that act as regulators of metabolic processes and are needed in the diet in small amounts.

volunteers   Unpaid personnel who usually work on a part-time basis performing important tasks that supplement, but do not replace, the work of employed staff.

whole-grain cereal   Cereal that contains all parts of the kernel of the grain from which it was made.

Index

WE VALUE YOUR OPINION—PLEASE SHARE IT WITH US

Merrill Publishing and our authors are most interested in your reactions to this textbook. Did it serve you well in the course? If it did, what aspects of the text were most helpful? If not, what didn't you like about it? Your comments will help us to write and develop better textbooks. We value your opinions and thank you for your help.

Text Title _____ Edition _____

Author(s) _____

Your Name (optional) _____

Address _____

City _____ State _____ Zip _____

School _____

Course Title _____

Instructor's Name _____

Your Major _____

Your Class Rank _____ Freshman _____ Sophomore _____ Junior _____ Senior

_____ Graduate Student

Were you required to take this course? _____ Required _____ Elective

Length of Course? _____ Quarter _____ Semester

1. Overall, how does this text compare to other texts you've used?

   _____ Superior _____ Better Than Most _____ Average _____ Poor

2. Please rate the text in the following areas:

	Superior	Better Than Most	Average	Poor
Author's Writing Style	_____	_____	_____	_____
Readability	_____	_____	_____	_____
Organization	_____	_____	_____	_____
Accuracy	_____	_____	_____	_____
Layout and Design	_____	_____	_____	_____
Illustrations/Photos/Tables	_____	_____	_____	_____
Examples	_____	_____	_____	_____
Problems/Exercises	_____	_____	_____	_____
Topic Selection	_____	_____	_____	_____
Currentness of Coverage	_____	_____	_____	_____
Explanation of Difficult Concepts	_____	_____	_____	_____
Match-up with Course Coverage	_____	_____	_____	_____
Applications to Real Life	_____	_____	_____	_____

3. Circle those chapters you especially liked:

    1 2 3 4 5 6 7 8 9

    What was your favorite chapter? _____

    Comments:

4. Circle those chapters you liked least:

    1 2 3 4 5 6 7 8 9

    What was your least favorite chapter? _____

    Comments:

5. List any chapters your instructor did not assign. _____

6. What topics did your instructor discuss that were not covered in the text?_____

    _____

7. Were you required to buy this book? _____ Yes _____ No

    Did you buy this book new or used? _____ New _____ Used

    If used, how much did you pay? _____

    Do you plan to keep or sell this book? _____ Keep _____ Sell

    If you plan to sell the book, how much do you expect to receive? _____

    Should the instructor continue to assign this book? _____ Yes _____ No

8. Please list any other learning materials you purchased to help you in this course (e.g., study guide, lab manual).

    _____

9. What did you like most about this text? _____

    _____

10. What did you like least about this text? _____

    _____

11. General comments:

    May we quote you in our advertising? _____ Yes _____ No

    Please mail to: Boyd Lane
                     College Division Research Department
                     P. O. Box 508
                     Columbus, Ohio 43216-0508